WHAT *are* YOU *eating?*

WHAT *are* YOU *eating?*

THE FOOD FACT FILE

Isabel Skypala

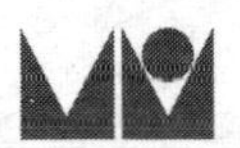

Michael O'Mara Books Limited

First published in Great Britain in 1998 by
Michael O'Mara Books Limited
9 Lion Yard, Tremadoc Road
London SW4 7NQ

A CIP catalogue record for this book is available
from the British Library

ISBN 1-85479-273-3 (hardback)
ISBN 1-85479-290-3 (paperback)

1 3 5 7 9 10 8 6 4 2

Designed and typeset by Martin Bristow

Printed and bound by Clays Ltd, Bungay, Suffolk

Contents

Introduction

Deciding what to eat has never been more difficult. Advanced technology enables us to eat most fruits and vegetables out of season. It has brought us a huge array of ready-prepared chilled, frozen, dried and canned foods. Our knowledge has increased and we face a daily barrage of information advising on healthy and unhealthy foods.

In the Middle Ages most people had little choice about the food they ate. Cereals such as bread and porridge, root vegetables, apples and pears, and small quantities of meat and fish were the staple diet of most people. By today's standards, this diet is very healthy, unlike that of the nobility who could afford to indulge and did so with seven-course meals featuring such delicacies as swan. It was the nineteenth-century Industrial Revolution and the consequent migration of country people to the towns that changed the British diet for ever. Previously most people had eaten food grown in their immediate vicinity, but once the majority of the population moved from the country, methods had to be developed to transport food to the towns and cities. Refrigeration, rail and other transport developments led to greater choice but also increased the uniformity of the diet. Industrialisation and the spread of the British Empire resulted in increasing prosperity, the creation of the middle classes and more money to buy food. However, cooking facilities in the cities were not always good or even available, and buying food ready-prepared was quite common. As any Dickens novel reveals, the take-away is not a twentieth-century phenomenon!

Our diet has probably changed more rapidly in the twentieth century than ever before. This is due not only to improvements in food technology, but also to food shortages after the Second World War which led to the development of intensive farming methods. Since the 1960s we have become more cosmopolitan, holidaying abroad and trying the food in the many Indian, Chinese and Italian restaurants which have become an established part of our lives. Advertising has changed our patterns of food consumption, and we have more money to spend on food as well as better ways of storing and preserving it.

Surveys reveal dramatic dietary changes in the last twenty-five years. In 1969 the average calorie intake was 2644kcals a day; figures from the 1994 national survey show that we now consume only

1880kcals per day. The types of food we eat have also changed, and although we are eating less overall, the consumption of some foods has increased. Cooked breakfasts, traditional meat and two veg meals and stodgy puds have been losing popularity for years. People are eating more convenience foods such as pizza, ice cream and ready-prepared salads. Most significant of all is the fact that in the last twenty years the amount of money we spend on eating out has almost doubled.

In 1991 the Government published *The Health of the Nation*, a document outlining a health strategy up to and beyond the year 2000. This has had a great impact on the health services, due to the targets it sets out for the NHS to achieve. Some targets aim to reduce deaths from major killer diseases such as heart disease and cancer; others are designed to stop the dramatic rise in the number of overweight and obese people in the UK. Since many of these diseases have a dietary link, the report had the effect of highlighting the need for a healthier diet for the nation. Another report published by the Department of Health in 1991 set out recommendations for the amount of energy, fat, protein, vitamins and minerals needed by men, women and children.

Despite these government guidelines, the confusion about the relationship between food and health has probably increased. Greater interest in food has led to the proliferation of food journalism, and the consequent rise of the food scare story. Research into food-related disease, often contradictory, also means that nutrition is such a rapidly changing field that even health professionals can give outdated nutritional advice, unless they are specialists such as dietitians. This makes the battle to eat a healthy diet one that is easily lost. Just when you thought that poly-unsaturated fat was the best thing on sliced bread, along comes olive oil. You successfully cut down on the booze and the experts decide we can all drink more alcohol. And if you thought that bread and potatoes were bad news because your old diet sheet told you so, think again!

But don't despair: look behind the health fads and media hype and you will find that the message about food for good health is the same as it has always been . . .

- Eat regular meals and don't eat more than you need
- Eat plenty of fruit and vegetables
- Avoid too many fried or fatty foods
- Keep snack foods and sweets to a minimum

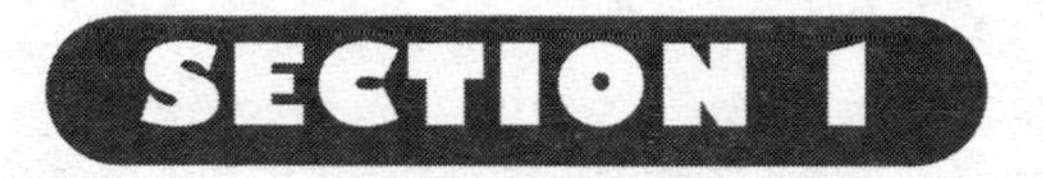

What Should We Eat?

Current recommended food intakes

In 1991 some new government guidelines on nutrient intake, *Dietary Reference Values for Food Energy and Nutrients for the United Kingdom** were published. Unlike previous guidelines, these included recommendations on fat, carbohydrate, fibre and some minerals such as zinc and selenium. All nutrients in our diet now have a recommended intake or a safe intake.

The tables at the beginning of this section will give you a general idea of what you should be consuming compared to the average UK intake. Then each nutrient will be discussed in detail, giving its function, good sources in the diet and additional data for the complete age range of recommended intakes. All figures for current average UK intakes are taken from the *National Food Survey 1994,* undertaken by the Ministry of Agriculture Fisheries and Food, and published by HMSO. For all recommended intakes, ages are given in years unless months are stated. Toddlers are generally aged one to three years. Not all nutrient requirements increase during pregnancy or whilst breast-feeding, but many do; figures for pregnant and breast-feeding women are the recommended daily intake of that nutrient for women aged nineteen to fifty, plus the extra amount they need.

*Department of Health, Report on Health and Social Subjects no 41, HMSO (1991)

Recommended daily intakes (RDI) for girls and women

Age in years	11–14	15–18	19–50	50+	Average UK intake (includes men and women)
Nutrients					
Energy (kcals)	1845	2110	1940	1900	1880
Protein (g)	41.2	45	45	46.5	63
Total fat (g)	—	—	71	70	82
Saturated fat (g)	—	—	21.5	21.1	31.9
Mono-unsat. fat (g)	—	—	12.9	12.6	30.5
Poly-unsat. fat (g)	—	—	25.8	25.3	14.1
Total carbohydrate (g)	—	—	243	238*	233
Sugar (g)	—	—	51.7	50.6	68
Fibre (g)	—	—	18	18	11.8
Sodium (mg)	1600	1600	1600	1600	2530
Potassium (mg)	3100	3500	3500	3500	2550
Calcium (mg)	800	800	700	700	830
Magnesium (mg)	280	300	270	270	229
Phosphorus (mg)	625	625	550	550	—
Iron (mg)	14.8	14.8	14.8	8.7	9.9
Copper (mg)	0.8	1.0	1.2	1.2	—
Zinc (mg)	9.0	7.0	7.0	7.0	7.8
Selenium (μg)	45	60	60	60	—
Vitamin A (μg)	600	600	600	600	1030
Vitamin D (μg)	—	—	—	10†	2.64
Vitamin E (mg)‡	—	—	5.0	5.0	6.0
Vitamin B_1 (mg)	0.7	0.8	0.8	0.8	1.29
Vitamin B_2 (mg)	1.1	1.1	1.1	1.1	1.61
Niacin (mg)	12	14	13	12	25.3
Vitamin B_6 (mg)	1.0	1.2	1.2	1.2	1.9
Vitamin B_{12} (μg)	1.2	1.5	1.5	1.5	4.8
Folate (μg)	200	200	200	200	241
Pantothenate (mg)‡	1.7	1.7	3-7	3-7	—
Biotin (μg)‡	10-200	10-200	10-200	10-200	—
Vitamin C (mg)	35	40	40	40	60

Key to symbols

* = average figure; † = over the age of 60 years; ‡ = no RDI, figure given is a safe amount

Recommended daily intakes (RDI) for boys and men

Age in years	11–14	15–18	19–50	50+	Average UK intake (both men and women)
Nutrients					
Energy (kcals)	2220	2755	2550	2270*	1880
Protein (g)	42.1	55.2	55.5	53.3	63
Total fat (g)	—	—	93.5	83.2	82
Saturated fat (g)	—	—	28.3	25.2	31.9
Mono-unsat. fat (g)	—	—	17	15.1	30.5
Poly-unsat. fat (g)	—	—	34	30.2	14.1
Total carbohydrate (g)	—	—	319	284*	233
Sugar (g)			68	60.5	68
Fibre (g)	—	—	18	18	11.8
Sodium (mg)	1600	1600	1600	1600	2530
Potassium (mg)	3100	3500	3500	3500	2550
Calcium (mg)	1000	1000	700	700	830
Magnesium (mg)	280	300	300	300	229
Phosphorus (mg)	775	775	550	550	—
Iron (mg)	11.3	11.3	8.7	8.7	9.9
Copper (mg)	0.8	1.0	1.2	1.2	—
Zinc (mg)	9.0	9.5	9.5	9.5	7.8
Selenium (µg)	45	70	75	75	—
Vitamin A (µg)	600	700	700	700	1030
Vitamin D (µg)	—	—	—	10†	2.64
Vitamin E (mg)‡	—	—	7.0	7.0	6.0
Vitamin B_1 (mg)	0.9	1.1	1.0	0.9	1.29
Vitamin B_2 (mg)	1.2	1.3	1.3	1.3	1.61
Niacin (mg)	15	18	17	16	25.3
Vitamin B_6 (mg)	1.2	1.5	1.4	1.4	1.9
Vitamin B_{12} (µg)	1.2	1.5	1.5	1.5	4.8
Folate (µg)	200	200	200	200	241
Pantothenate (mg)‡	1.7	1.7	3-7	3-7	—
Biotin (µg)‡	10-200	10-200	10-200	10-200	—
Vitamin C (mg)	35	40	40	40	60

Key to symbols
* = average figure; † = over the age of 60 years; ‡ = no RDI, figure given is a safe amount

Nutrients – what they are and why we need them

Protein

Protein is a vital part of all body cells and necessary for their growth and repair. When we eat protein it is broken down into substances called amino acids. Food contains twenty different amino acids. Of those twenty, eight cannot be made by the body and are known as essential amino acids. Meat, fish, eggs and milk contain all the amino acids including the essential ones. Plant foods do not contain all eight essential amino acids individually. Different plants contain different amino acids, and to make sure of all eight essential amino acids, plant foods need to be combined together if no animal protein is included in the diet. Combinations such as eating pulses with cereal foods or nuts with cereal foods ensure you are getting all eight. This is particularly important for vegans (see p. 49).

Most people in the UK eat far more protein than the recommended intake. We need to be more careful about what type of protein we are eating. It is best to eat protein from low-fat sources such as lean meat, poultry, game, fish, low-fat cheese, skimmed milk, beans and lentils. Many people still believe that a high-protein diet is essential for sportsmen and women, to improve muscle size, strength and overall performance. Actually, carbohydrate is far more important, and a high-carbohydrate low-fat diet is usually recommended. Athletes can only increase muscle size through intensive training. They might need slightly more protein than most people but, since our average intake is higher than that recommended, this amounts to eating a normal diet.

Foods high in protein include meat, liver, offal, chicken, poultry, game, fish, milk, eggs, beans, lentils, peas and nuts. There are also moderate amounts in rice, breakfast cereals, bread and pasta.

Recommended intakes of protein (grams per day – see also RDI tables on pp. 10–11)

0–6 months	7–12 months	1–3 years	4–6 years	7–10 years	Pregnant women	Breast-feeding from 0–4 months	Breast-feeding from 4+ months
12.5	13–15	14.5	19.7	28	51.0	56.0	53.0

Fat

Fat is a mixture of glycerol and fatty acids which can be either saturated or unsaturated. Unsaturated fatty acids can be further divided into mono-unsaturated and poly-unsaturated fatty acids. Poly-unsaturated fatty acids are also known as essential fatty acids because the body cannot make them. Fats are an important source of energy containing twice as many calories as carbohydrate (one gram of fat contains 9kcal). Some vitamins such as Vitamins A and D are fat-soluble and are only found in fatty foods. Fat also makes us feel full and satisfied – a property known as satiety. A meal high in fat will make you feel fuller for longer. The reverse is true for low-fat meals, which is why slimmers often find a plate of salad leaves them feeling hungry.

The amount of fat we eat has decreased over the years and we now eat about 82 grams a day, which represents about 39 per cent of our total energy intake. The decrease in fat intake is due to the increase in the number of us who drink semi-skimmed or skimmed milk, use low-fat spreads or eat less cheese. Even our meat now contains far less fat then it used to. Unfortunately our fat intake is still higher than it should be. More than a quarter of the fat we eat comes from the fat we cook with or spread on our bread. Perhaps we need to concentrate less on changing the sort of milk we drink, and more on how we cook our food.

It is not just the total amount of fat which is significant; it is also important to consume the right balance of fatty acids. 10 per cent of our food energy should come from saturated fat, 6 per cent from poly-unsaturated fat and 12 per cent from mono-unsaturated fat. Saturated fats have come in for a lot of bad press in the last ten years for being one of the main causes of a high cholesterol level. Our intake of saturated fats has now fallen; we are eating more poly-unsaturated fat in the form of margarine, and less butter.

One of the major changes in our fat intake in recent years is the increase in the amount of fat we eat in foods consumed away from home. These include crisps and snack foods, but most of this extra fat comes from meat products. Some high-fat foods are obvious but others less so. For example cheese contains more fat than chocolate, and two digestive biscuits contain as much fat as a bag of crisps or a piece of treacle tart.

Foods high in saturated fat include red meat, butter, milk, cream, cheese, suet, dripping, lard and hydrogenated margarine (any margarine which does not claim to be high in poly- or mono-unsaturated fat).

Foods high in mono-unsaturated fat include olive oil, olive oil margarines, peanuts.

Foods high in poly-unsaturated fat include corn oil, soya oil, safflower oil, sunflower oil, fatty fish such as mackerel, tuna, sardines, pilchards, herring and salmon.

Recommended intakes of fat (see RDI tables on pp. 10–11)

These figures are derived by taking the recommended percentage of total fat (35 per cent) and using the recommended energy figure to obtain an actual amount of fat. If your energy intake differs from the recommended level, your allowance of fat will be correspondingly higher or lower.

Carbohydrate

The main purpose of carbohydrates is to provide energy. One gram of carbohydrate contains 4kcal. There are three types of carbohydrate: sugars, starches and non-starch polysaccharides. Sugars come in two groups: monosaccharides (simple sugars) such as glucose or fructose (fruit sugar), and disaccharides such as sucrose (cane and beet sugar) and lactose (milk sugar). Disaccharides are two monosaccharides joined together. All these sugars are naturally sweet and dissolve in water. Starch is not sweet or soluble despite being made from large numbers of glucose units linked together. It is stored as granules and is found in all plants including cereals, vegetables and fruit. Animals, including man, store starch in the form of glycogen in the liver and muscles.

Another form of carbohydrate, non-starch polysaccharide, is better known as fibre. The old definition of fibre was that it could not be digested or absorbed by the body. We now know that this only applies to cellulose-containing foods. Cellulose is a type of insoluble carbohydrate which forms the cell walls of plants. It is found in the husk of cereal grains and the stem and skin of fruits and vegetables. However, there are also soluble fibres, such as pectin in apples, which dissolve in water to form a sticky solution or gel. The most important soluble fibres are found in peas, beans, lentils and oats.

Over the decades our intake of carbohydrate has fallen and we are eating less bread and potatoes, and although pasta and rice are becoming more popular, people do not eat the quantity of starch that they need. Few people in the UK now have bread with their meals, and bread and potatoes were considered taboo in the swinging sixties. The rest of our carbohydrate intake comes from simple sugars. This should only be a relatively small amount, but it is very easy to eat more than is healthy. For years health professionals have urged us to cut down on sugar, and, as a nation, we are putting less sugar in beverages, but unfortunately eating more sugary foods, such as sweets, chocolates and desserts. Foods often contain more sugar than you think. A fruit yoghurt and a slice of fruit cake both contain the equivalent of 5 teaspoons of sugar, and a glass of orange juice contains more sugar than a glass of orange squash.

Only 10 per cent of our total energy intake should be from natural or added sugar, so if you are eating 2000kcals daily, then only

200kcal should come from sugary foods. It is also recommended that our non-starch polysaccharide or fibre intake should be about 18 grams a day, which is the equivalent of one large tin of baked beans and a slice of wholemeal bread. There are no recommended amounts of carbohydrate and fibre for children, but it is important to remember that children are not small adults and have very different needs. Their overriding need is for energy, and too much fibre fills them up and affects their ability to absorb the nutrients from food, which can subsequently affect their growth.

Foods high in non-starch polysaccharide include beans (baked, kidney, broad, butter and others), lentils, peas, spinach, leeks, sweetcorn and berry fruits.

Foods high in starchy carbohydrate include bread, rolls, breakfast cereals, potatoes, rice and pasta.

Foods high in sugar include sweets, chocolates, fizzy drinks, tinned fruit in syrup, cakes, puddings, jam and marmalade.

Recommended intakes of carbohydrate (see RDI tables on pp. 10–11)

The recommended amount of carbohydrate is 47 per cent of our total energy intake. The major part of this should be provided by starchy foods; only one fifth should come from sugars (added or natural). The figures given in the tables are for intakes based on the recommended energy values for the different ages and sexes. If your energy intake is greater or less than the recommended level, you will need to adjust your carbohydrate intake accordingly.

Minerals

Minerals can be sub-divided into three groups: electrolytes, bone minerals and trace elements.

ELECTROLYTES

Sodium

Sodium is involved in the basic functioning of all body cells. It also regulates the body's internal fluid levels. We need about 1600mg a day but consume a great deal more. This is surprising since most foods contain only small amounts of sodium. However, much is added to food, both by manufacturers and ourselves, in the form of sodium chloride or salt. Eighty-five per cent of our entire sodium intake could come from the salt added to our food. We eat anything up to 9 grams of salt a day (⅓rd ounce) either in or on our food. Nine grams of salt contain 3600mg sodium, nearly twice the amount we need. Our bodies can cope with this excess by getting rid of it in the urine but, unfortunately this is not the end of the story. High blood pressure is much more common in countries whose population has a high salt intake. The Japanese, who eat about 25 grams of salt a day, have major problems with high blood pressure and strokes.

The current advice is to cut our salt intake to 6 grams a day. The difficulty is avoiding all of the sodium in the food we eat. Most of the salt in our diet comes from bread, breakfast cereals, butter and margarine, tinned food, processed meat and cheese. This does not mean you should stop eating bread or breakfast cereals, but eating fewer processed foods and more fresh foods will make a difference. Adding less salt during cooking and at the table is also important, but this is not easy if you like a lot of salt. Try using a salt mill or grinder, instead of an ordinary salt cellar. It will take time for your taste buds to adjust, but you can make food more interesting by using more herbs and spices.

Foods high in salt include bacon, ham, corned beef, smoked fish, canned anchovies, cheese, baked beans, tinned vegetables, bottled sauces, soups, salted snacks and olives in brine.

Recommended intakes of sodium (mg per day – see also RDI tables on pp. 10–11)

0–3 months	4–6 months	7–9 months	10–12 months	1–3 years	4–6 years	7–10 years
210	280	320	350	500	700	1200

Potassium

Potassium is part of the body's cells and helps with the functioning of nerves and muscles. The amount we need depends on how much muscle we have. It is important to eat enough potassium to help the kidneys excrete excess sodium from the body. For this reason the recommended amount of 3500mg is more than twice as much as that recommended for sodium, but the average intake is only 2550mg. Potassium is found in many animal and vegetable foods, but fruit and vegetables are often good sources. Potassium also has a role in the control of blood pressure. Eating more potassium-rich foods could be as helpful in reducing high blood pressure as cutting your salt intake. It is unusual for people to have too much potassium in their blood, but drugs and diseases can affect the potassium balance, making it too high or too low. A high or low potassium level can affect muscles causing weakness especially in the heart muscle, which in extreme cases can lead to heart failure.

Foods high in potassium include potatoes, spinach, chickpeas and other pulses, fatty fish, wheat, milk and red meat.

Recommended intakes of potassium (mg per day – see also RDI tables on pp. 10–11)

0–3 months	4–6 months	7–12 months	1–3 years	4–6 years	7–10 years
800	850	700	800	1100	200

BONE MINERALS

Calcium

Calcium is vital to the development and maintenance of the skeleton. To build good dense bones and protect against bone loss in later life, children need calcium and also, most importantly, plenty of exercise. This should start at an early age and continue until adulthood, but is particularly important for teenagers. Women are vulnerable to bone loss or osteoporosis after the menopause. Unfortunately, large doses of calcium do not guarantee protection against osteoporosis, so take the recommended amount and get plenty of exercise. More than half our calcium intake comes from milk; the rest coming from cereals, vegetables and meat. We take in about 830mg calcium a day which is only just above the recommended level. A pint of milk contains 700mg, but other foods are also good sources; a portion of spinach plus a medium-sized cheese and tomato pizza and a yoghurt would provide a similar amount.

Foods high in calcium include milk, cheese, yoghurt, canned fish, spinach, tofu, bread, green vegetables, figs, rhubarb, chocolate and hard water. Many brands of mineral water also contain high levels.

Recommended intakes of calcium (mg per day – see also RDI tables on pp. 10–11)

Babies	1–3 years	4–6 years	7–10 years	Breast-feeding women
525	350	450	550	1250

Magnesium

All human tissues contain magnesium, but most is found in the bones in combination with phosphorus. Because it is an essential part of the green pigment in plants (chlorophyll), vegetables are rich in magnesium. We eat about 230mg magnesium daily, which is slightly less than the amount recommended. However, our kidneys are very good at conserving magnesium, so even people with low intakes do not normally suffer any symptoms of deficiency. Only severe medical conditions can cause deficiency, the symptoms of which include depression, muscular weakness, vertigo and convulsions.

Foods high in magnesium include nuts, pulses, green vegetables, chocolate and wholegrain cereals.

Recommended intakes of magnesium (mg per day – see also RDI tables on pp. 10–11)

0–3 months	4–6 months	7–9 months	10–12 months	1–3 years	4–6 years	7–10 years	Breast-feeding women
55	60	75	80	85	120	200	320

Phosphorus

Phosphorus is found in all foods. Of the 1500mg we eat daily, about 150mg will come from phosphorus which has been added artificially to food. Most of the phosphorus in our body is present in our bones. We need to have a certain amount to balance our calcium levels but we are more than achieving the recommended level of 550mg a day.

Foods high in phosphorus include any which are rich in calcium (see p. 19)

Recommended intakes of phosphorus (mg per day – see also RDI tables on pp. 10–11)

Babies	1–3	4–6	7–10	Breast-feeding women
400	270	350	450	990

TRACE ELEMENTS

Iron

Iron is needed to carry oxygen in the blood to all body tissues. It is lost from the body whenever there is bleeding, and extra is also needed during pregnancy. For these reasons women need a lot more iron than men. The amount of iron absorbed depends on the type of food from which it comes. In animal foods, iron is present in a form called haem iron. This is absorbed much more easily than the iron found in vegetable foods. Haem iron absorption increases if there is a deficiency and decreases if the body has too much iron, so women can get the extra iron they need by absorbing twice as much iron from their food. Other factors can affect iron absorption. It is greatly helped by Vitamin C, and to a much lesser extent by alcohol. The tannin in tea decreases iron absorption, as does a substance called phytate. Although wholegrain cereals are rich in iron, its absorption is inhibited by the presence of phytate.

Iron-deficiency anaemia is the commonest nutritional disease in the world. It takes a long time to develop and is often hard to diagnose, but tiredness and lethargy are classic symptoms. Our average intake of iron is 9.9mg a day, which is above the recommended intake for men, but well below that for women. A typical way of getting that 9.9mg might be by eating two slices of wholemeal bread, a bowl of cereal, a steak and a portion of peas. Some groups of people are at particular risk of developing anaemia, including vegetarian and vegan women, pregnant women, children who are faddy eaters or on a restricted diet, and elderly people who live alone. People in these groups might benefit from taking iron supplements, but it is also worth remembering to have more Vitamin C, especially with vegetable sources of iron.

Foods high in iron include liver, red meat, kidney, black pudding, eggs, cockles, mussels, whelks, eggs, fatty fish, green vegetables, parsley, watercress, peas and beans, wholegrain cereals, treacle, chocolate, curry powder, nuts and liquorice.

Recommended intakes of iron (mg per day – see also RDI tables on pp. 10–11)

0–3 months	4–6 months	7–12 months	1–3 years	4–6 years	7–10 years
1.7	4.3	7.8	6.9	6.1	8.7

Copper

Copper is part of many different substances in the body, and a lack of copper causes a very rare type of anaemia. Normal adult diets provide 1–3mg a day which should be plenty for most people. Deficiency is only seen in children who cannot absorb copper as a result of a very rare disease called Menkes' syndrome. In contrast, sufferers from Wilson's disease have too much copper stored by the body. Apart from these two conditions, copper is not a nutrient most people need to worry about.

Foods high in copper include green vegetables, fish, oysters and liver.

Recommended intakes of copper (mg per day – see also RDI tables on pp. 10–11)

0–3 months	4–12 months	1–3 years	4–6 years	7–10 years	breast-feeding women
0.2	0.3	0.4	0.6	0.7	1.5

Zinc

Zinc is part of more than fifty different enzymes. There is zinc in the eye tissue and prostate, but most zinc is in the bones. The average diet can provide up to 17mg a day, but the average intake is 7.8mg, which is below that recommended for men. However, losses from the body are small and zinc deficiency is very rare. Zinc is important for good healing of wounds, is often used in the treatment of leg ulcers and is found in many nappy rash creams. It has also been linked to impotence, but nothing is proven. Interestingly, the oyster, which some believe to be an aphrodisiac, contains an incredible 18mg of zinc per oyster! Premature babies can become zinc-deficient as most zinc is laid down in the last three months of pregnancy.

Foods high in zinc include oysters, liver, meat and pulses.

Recommended intakes of zinc (mg per day – see also RDI tables on pp. 10–11)

0–6 months	7–12 months	1–3 years	4–6 years	7–10 years	Breast-feeding women
4.0	5.0	5.0	6.5	7.0	13.0

Selenium

Selenium is part of the body cell, protecting it from damage. It is found in soil, some soils are very rich in selenium and others very poor, and this will affect the amount found in cereals. The average intake in the UK of 65µg a day, is slightly less than that recommended for men, but covers women and children. Cereals provide about half of our selenium intake; the rest comes from meat and fish. It has been suggested that a high intake might prevent cancer, but there is no evidence for this.

Foods high in selenium include fish, meat and cereals.

Recommended intakes of selenium (µg per day – see also RDI tables on pp. 10–11)

0–3 months	4–6 months	7–12 months	1–3 years	4–6 years	7–10 years
10	13	10	15	20	30

Vitamins

Vitamins can be divided into two groups: fat-soluble and water-soluble. Fat-soluble vitamins include Vitamins A, D, E and K. Water-soluble vitamins include the Vitamin B complex and Vitamin C. The main difference between them is that fat-soluble vitamins are stored by the body, whereas water-soluble vitamins are not. For this reason, if you wish to take more than the recommended amount of a vitamin supplement you should check with your doctor first. Large doses of fat-soluble vitamins can be dangerous because your body cannot rid itself of any harmful excess and this can affect your liver.

FAT-SOLUBLE VITAMINS

Vitamin A or retinol

There are two forms of Vitamin A found in animal and vegetable foods. The type found in animal foods such as milk, cheese, eggs, some fatty fish and liver is called retinol: this is the most powerful form of Vitamin A. Fish liver oils are the richest source of retinol. However there is another very important source, the carotenes, which are found in red, yellow and green fruits and vegetables such as spinach, carrots, peaches and apricots. Carotenes are converted to retinol by the body but it takes 6 grams of carotene to make one gram of retinol. The most important carotene is beta carotene, which is associated with the green pigment found in vegetables called chlorophyll.

The average intake of Vitamin A in the UK is 1,030µg per person, and most of us already have enough stored in our liver to last for months if not years. Vitamin A is essential for the growth and normal development of the retina in the eye and the first sign of a deficiency is night blindness. This means that the old wives' tale about carrots helping you to see in the dark is true! If the night blindness is not treated, the child will go on to develop xerophthalmia which can lead to permanent blindness. Sadly xerophthalmia is widespread in South-east Asia, China and Africa, and is one of the seven most important preventable causes of blindness in the world. Closer to home, more people are at risk of having too much rather than too little Vitamin A. Taking large doses of the vitamin, or eating large quantities of carrots or liver, have featured in several special dietary regimes for cancer. It is very unwise to consume large doses of a vitamin which is stored by the body, or to follow extreme diets so unbalanced that they invariably do more harm than good.

Foods high in Vitamin A include liver, pâté, eggs, cheddar-type cheese, carrots, spinach, cantaloupe melon, nectarines, apricots, spring greens, yellow, red, orange and green peppers, butter, margarine, salmon, mackerel and full-cream milk.

Recommended intakes of Vitamin A (µg per day – see also RDI tables on pp. 10–11)

Babies	Toddlers	Children	Pregnant women
350	400	500	700

Vitamin D or cholecalciferol

Vitamin D is essential for the development of healthy bones, and controls the amount and use of calcium in the body. Unlike all other nutrients in the diet, food is not the main source of the vitamin. Our Vitamin D needs are met by the action of ultraviolet light on our skin. Contained in the skin's natural oils is a substance called 7-dehydrocholesterol, which produces cholecalciferol (natural Vitamin D) in the presence of sunlight. The average dietary intake is only 2.64µg a day, but most adults in the UK get all the Vitamin D they need from sunshine. Like Vitamin A, excess Vitamin D is stored by the body, so that we all have enough to see us through the winter months. However, adults who are housebound or who have very little exposure to sunlight may, like children, need extra Vitamin D from food. Very few foods naturally contain Vitamin D, the richest source being cod liver oil. Fatty fish and eggs also contain Vitamin D, and margarine and baby milks are fortified with the vitamin.

Rickets and osteomalacia, both caused by a lack of Vitamin D, result in bone deformities and joint problems for children and adults respectively. In Victorian times, a very poor diet and the thick pall of smoke which hung over most cities meant that three-quarters of all poor children were affected with the characteristic bow-legged appearance of rickets. After 1900 the incidence of rickets declined due to improvements in social conditions and the use of cod liver oil; by 1945 the disease had been eradicated in the UK. Unfortunately, because Vitamin D is stored by the body, some of the measures taken to rid the country of rickets resulted in children occasionally getting too much of the vitamin. It is still added to baby milks today but the amount is smaller, and there is no routine prescription of cod liver oil. This means that some children still risk developing rickets, especially those who do not spend much time outside. Osteomalacia, the adult version of rickets, is more likely to develop in women, especially pregnant women and elderly housebound women. The best way to increase Vitamin D levels is to get outside: even if it is not sunny, the ultraviolet rays will still be active. If you do take a Vitamin D supplement, do not take more than you need; 2.5µg a day is enough for most adults. Three eggs or five helpings of margarine will provide this amount, but one kipper contains five times the recommended intake.

Foods containing Vitamin D include herrings, tuna, mackerel, salmon, sardines, pilchards, eggs, liver, butter and margarine.

Recommended intakes of Vitamin D (µg per day)

Babies	Toddlers	Pregnant women	Breast-feeding women
8.5	7.0	10	10

There is no RDI for any other groups

Vitamin E or tocopherol

Vitamin E is found in all cell structures in the body and protects poly-unsaturated fatty acids both in food and in the body. It is found in many foods particularly vegetable oils and vegetable margarine. There is so much of it in our diet that most people do not suffer from a lack of Vitamin E, but anyone who cannot digest fat might need to take extra. The amount of Vitamin E we need depends on how much poly-unsaturated fat we eat. For most men this works out to be 7mg per day and 5mg per day for women (see RDI tables on pp. 10–11). Two tins of tomatoes, two helpings of tuna, one avocado pear or a tablespoon of sunflower seeds would all individually supply this amount. The average intake in the UK is 6mg daily, most of which comes from vegetable oils, vegetables and cereals. The USA recommends 8mg per day for women and 10mg for men.

Vitamin E has often been used to treat a variety of other problems including infertility, skin disease, prevention of ageing and improvement of athletic performance. There is no real evidence that it is of any benefit, but the therapy is safe and some people might really feel it helps.

Foods high in Vitamin E include poly-unsaturated margarine, fish (particularly tuna and salmon), almonds, hazelnuts, sunflower seeds, avocado pear and tomatoes.

WATER-SOLUBLE VITAMINS

Vitamin B_1 or thiamin

Vitamin B_1 is involved in the breakdown of carbohydrate and release of energy. The body cannot store more Vitamin B_1 than it needs, so any excess is lost in the urine. Vitamin B_1 is found in all plant and animal foods, but the best sources in our diet are cereals, nuts, peas, beans and yeast. Refined carbohydrates, such as white rice and white bread, often lose their Vitamin B_1 which is present in the husk of the cereal. For this reason breakfast cereals often have Vitamin B_1 added. Vitamin B_1 is water-soluble, and large amounts can be lost if food is cooked in water which is then thrown away. The same is true of many B vitamins, which is why you should try to steam or microwave vegetables, or use their cooking water to make the gravy or sauce. The addition of baking powder to vegetable cooking water increases the amount destroyed, but luckily the practice of adding this ingredient to spring greens to preserve their colour has largely died out. A lack of Vitamin B_1 is rare in the western world, where the average intake of 1.29mg is greater than the highest requirement. However Vitamin B_1 deficiency, or beriberi, still occurs where people have a poorly balanced diet.

Foods high in Vitamin B_1 include pork, potatoes, wholegrain cereals, pulses and beans

Recommended intakes of Vitamin B_1 (mg per day – see also RDI tables on pp. 10–11)

Babies	Toddlers	4–10	Pregnant women	Breast-feeding women
0.2	0.5	0.7	0.9	1.0

Vitamin B_2 or riboflavin

Vitamin B_2 is essential to substances in the body known as enzymes and is involved in cell respiration. Like Vitamin B_1, Vitamin B_2 is not stored in the body and is soluble in water. It is present in many foods, especially liver, milk, cheese, eggs and green vegetables. Cereals which have been refined will have lost most of their Vitamin B_2, but it is often added back artificially. Milk left on the doorstep will have its Vitamin B_2 destroyed by ultraviolet light if it is in a clear glass or plastic bottle. The same is true of other foods exposed to sunshine. Yeast is a good natural source of Vitamin B_2, and it is also found in beer.

A lack of the vitamin is rare, but even people with severe deficiency do not suffer major symptoms. The main one is a sore mouth. There are groups of people in the UK who are more likely to have a low intake, such as those who have a restricted diet either medically or self-imposed. However, the average intake of 1.61mg a day is well above that recommended for all age groups.

Foods high in Vitamin B_2 include liver, kidney, beef extract, yeast extract, wholegrain cereals, milk, eggs, fatty fish, meat and green vegetables.

Recommended intakes of Vitamin B_2 (mg per day – see also RDI tables on pp. 10–11)

Babies	Toddlers	4–6	7–10	Pregnant women	Breast-feeding women
0.4	0.6	0.8	1.0	1.4	1.6

Niacin or nicotinic acid

Niacin plays an important role in the body's metabolism, and the amount we need depends on the amount of energy we use. Niacin is found in many foods, but in cereals such as maize it is present in a form our bodies cannot absorb. If these cereals are treated with an alkali, the bound niacin is freed and becomes available to the body. In bygone days, people in many parts of the world suffered from pellagra, the disease caused by a lack of this vitamin. The Mexican people did not have a problem because they treated their maize tortillas with lime water (an alkali), and so avoided illness. The human body is not solely dependent on the niacin in food to prevent pellagra: it can make niacin from other foods by changing an amino acid (see p. 12) called tryptophan into niacin. Despite this, pellagra is still endemic in some parts of Africa. Heat does not destroy it, but up to a quarter of all the niacin in the food we eat is lost during cooking. Currently we consume about 25mg of niacin a day, which is well above the recommended amount. Taking excess is of no benefit and can be harmful.

Foods high in niacin include fatty fish, liver, meat, chicken, yeast, peanuts and wholegrain cereals.

Recommended intakes of niacin (mg per day – see also RDI tables on pp. 10–11)

0–6 months	7–12 months	1–3 years	4–6 years	7–10 years	Breast-feeding women
3	4.5	8	11	12	15

Vitamin B_6 or pyridoxine

Vitamin B_6 plays an important role in protein metabolism. Like other vitamins, it is found in so many foods that a deficiency is rare, and is usually the result of a drug treatment or severe illness. The best source of this vitamin is liver, but cereal, meat, fruit and vegetables all contain some Vitamin B_6. Processed foods contain none unless it has been added back artificially. This vitamin is often used to help women who suffer from pre-menstrual tension (PMT), or to overcome side-effects from the oral contraceptive. It is known that oral contraceptives can reduce the amount of Vitamin B_6 in the body, but it is not clear whether taking extra is of any benefit. High intakes have been known to affect the nervous system and should not be taken without good advice. The average intake in the UK is 1.9mg, and no more than 10mg should be consumed per day.

Foods high in Vitamin B_6 include fish, liver, meat, bananas, fortified breakfast cereals, beans, lentils, leeks and spinach.

Recommended intakes of Vitamin B_6 (mg per day – see also RDI tables on pp. 10–11)

0–6 months	7–12 months	1–3 years	4–6 years	7–10 years
0.2	0.35	0.7	0.9	1.0

Vitamin B_{12}

Vitamin B_{12}, essential for making normal blood cells, also maintains the fatty covering of the nerves. It is unusual in that the body can store any excess in the liver. Another unique feature is that it is only found in animal foods. People who eat no animal foods, such as vegans, risk developing a type of anaemia and might need to take supplements (see p. 48). Vitamin B_{12} is absorbed only in the presence of a special substance called intrinsic factor which is found in the stomach. People who lack intrinsic factor cannot use the B_{12} in their food and develop pernicious anaemia. This lack of intrinsic factor can be inherited or it can occur when the body's immune system has been damaged due to infection or disease. In the last century, pernicious anaemia was a feared and fatal disease. By the 1920s doctors could treat the disease, but only by making their patients eat lots of raw liver, typically 8 ounces daily, and a pint of raw meat juice! The purification of Vitamin B_{12} in 1948 meant that such diets could be abandoned, and injections of B_{12} given instead. Unless you are a vegan, you are unlikely to develop a deficiency of B_{12}, especially as the average intake in the UK is 4.8µg a day, more than twice the highest recommended intake.

Foods high in Vitamin B_{12} include liver, kidney, fatty fish, meat and eggs. Milk contains a small amount.

Recommended intakes of Vitamin B_{12} (μg per day – see also RDI tables on pp. 10–11)

0–6 months	7–12 months	1–3 years	4–6 years	Breast-feeding women
0.3	0.4	0.5	0.8	2.0

Folate or folic acid

Folate is another B vitamin involved in the production of healthy blood. Too little folate results in megaloblastic anaemia, a disease similar to pernicious anaemia. This type of anaemia is quite common in under-developed countries, but rare in the western world. It occurs most often in pregnant women, or in groups of people who are eating very poorly. Folate is found in a number of foods, but there are not many naturally rich sources, the main ones being green vegetables and liver. Unfortunately, not only does cooking destroy quite a lot of the vitamin, but not all the folate we eat is absorbed and used by the body. The amount of folate in foods decreases the longer they are stored, so it is important to eat vegetables when they are as fresh as possible. The average intake of folate in the UK is 241μg a day, which is more than most of us need. However, two important groups of people need more: pregnant women and women who are planning to become pregnant. This is because folate plays a major role in the prevention of neural tube defects such as spina bifida. Women who are trying to conceive or who are in the first twelve weeks of pregnancy should take 400μg a day more than the recommended intake. Half of this amount can be achieved by eating one bowl of cornflakes, a portion of spinach and a portion of peas. It can be difficult for women to get enough folate, especially as liver is not recommended for pregnant women. Consequently, many women will need to take a supplement.

Food high in folate include liver, spinach, Brussels sprouts, fortified breakfast cereals, cabbage, peas and eggs.

Recommended intakes of folate (g per day – see also RDI tables on pp. 10–11)

Babies	Toddlers	4–6 years	Planning a pregnancy	During pregnancy: 0–12 weeks	12–40 weeks	Breast-feeding women
50	70	100	600	600	300	260

Pantothenate/Pantothenic acid

Pantothenic acid is found in all living things, so a deficiency is unlikely in man. It is not destroyed by heat unless above boiling point, but it is lost from frozen food during thawing. Yeast, liver, kidney and egg yolks contain the most pantothenic acid. Although a deficiency in rats resulted in grey hair, pantothenic acid is not useful in the treatment of grey hair in man. A bottle of colour shampoo would be a better investment. There are no recommended daily intakes for this vitamin, but 1.7mg per day for infants and 3–7mg per day for adults are the suggested safe levels.

Biotin

Biotin is one of the most active biological substances known, and is involved in several different body functions. Luckily we only need a very small amount, and most of this is supplied by the bacteria which live in our intestines. However it is also present in liver, kidney, yeast extract, pulses, nuts and chocolate. A deficiency of biotin never occurs unless someone eats a diet which includes a large number of raw whole eggs or egg whites. Deficiency causes dermatitis, fatigue, nausea and depression. Raw egg white contains a protein called avidin which combines with biotin and makes it unavailable to the body. Cooking the egg destroys the avidin and releases the biotin. So as well as being a potential source of salmonella, raw eggs can also cause other problems, and are best avoided. There is no recommended intake of biotin, but a safe intake is thought to be 10–200µg per day.

Vitamin C or ascorbic acid

Vitamin C prevents scurvy, helps the healing of wounds and aids the absorption of iron from non-animal sources. It is also known as an antioxidant and prevents damage to internal tissues. It might protect against cancer, and is claimed to prevent the common cold. Good sources in the diet include fruit, green vegetables and liver. Although potatoes only contain moderate amounts of Vitamin C, for many people they are the best or only source of Vitamin C in their diet. Vitamin C cannot be stored and once there is a certain amount in the blood the rest is discarded in the urine. Losses during cooking can be minimised if the vegetable is put straight into the boiling water, and served straight away. You will get the most Vitamin C from fruit and vegetables that are bought and eaten when fresh.

The deficiency disease scurvy, once the scourge of seamen, is very rare these days. However people who are unable or unwilling to eat any fruit or vegetables may be at risk of low Vitamin C levels. People who have had surgery need a higher intake to help the wound to heal, and smokers, who use up more Vitamin C than non-smokers might also benefit from increasing their intake. In the UK the average intake is 60mg a day, but some people take more than 1000mg a day, twenty-five times the recommended level. There is probably no harm in doing this, but at very high doses Vitamin C can cause diarrhoea and kidney stones, so seek advice if you want to take a large dose.

Foods high in Vitamin C include blackcurrants, strawberries, oranges and other citrus fruits, kiwifruits, green peppers, spinach, broccoli, cauliflower, cabbage, melon, pineapple, tomatoes and liver.

Recommended intakes of Vitamin C (mg per day – see also RDI tables on pp. 10–11)

Babies	1–10	Pregnant women	Breast-feeding women
25	30	50	70

Vitamin K

Vitamin K is essential for the normal clotting of blood. We get some from food but the rest is made by the bacteria which live in the large intestine: a deficiency is therefore very rare. Babies are born with no bacteria in their gut and may therefore be at risk from a rare spontaneous bleeding complication. For this reason some maternity units routinely give a Vitamin K injection to all new-born babies. There are no recommended intakes for adults, but a safe daily intake is 1μg per kilogram body weight.

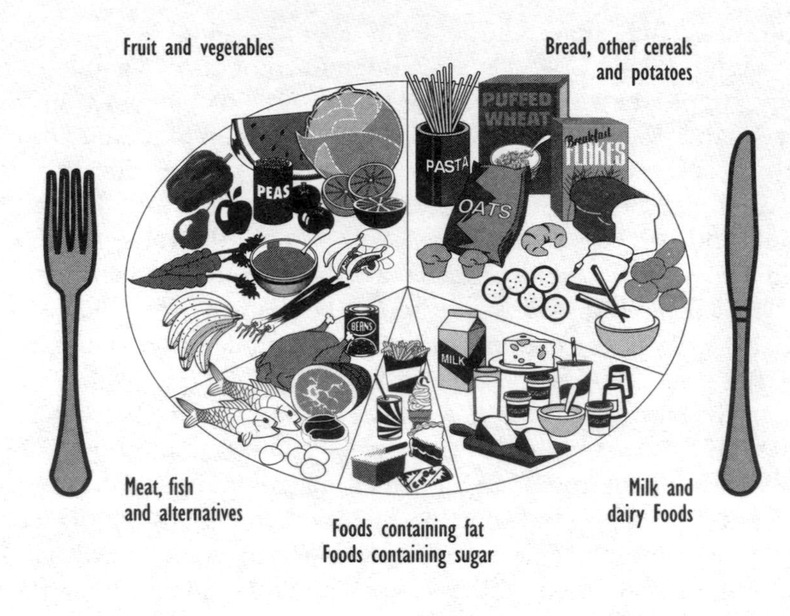

Balance of good health plate model

(based on material from the Health Education Authority)

The plate model (above) is a new national symbol and guide to healthy eating used by all those involved in advising on a healthy diet. It shows the amounts you should aim to eat in the different food groups. The foods in Section Three are grouped according to this model, so you will become familiar with it as you use the book.

How healthy is your diet?

This quiz is designed to help you discover how healthy your current diet is, and whether it needs to change. Remember, though, that if you have a specific dietary problem or concern you should ask your GP to refer you to a state-registered dietitian.

1. How many servings of starchy carbohydrate do you have each day? (One serving is equal to a bowl of cereal, one slice of bread or toast, or a portion of pasta, rice or potatoes.)

(a) 4–6 servings daily
(b) 2–3 servings daily
(c) less than 2 servings daily
(d) one serving or less daily

2. How often do you eat vegetables or salad (including canned and frozen products)?

(a) three times a day
(b) once or twice a day
(c) less than once a day
(d) less than three times a week

3. How much fruit do you eat? (One portion equals a whole apple/orange/pear etc., a handful of grapes or a serving of tinned fruit.)

(a) 3–5 portions daily
(b) 1–3 portions daily
(c) less than one portion daily
(d) less than 3 portions a week

4. Which vegetables do you eat? Tick all those you eat once a month, but any vegetable you eat at least once a week or more can have two ticks.

asparagus
aubergine
beansprouts
broccoli
white cabbage
cauliflower
carrots
celery
cress
cucumber
courgettes
green beans
leeks
lettuce
mushrooms
onions
parsnips
peas
peppers – green
peppers – red
potatoes
spinach
spring greens
swede
sweetcorn
tomatoes
turnips
vegetables – mixed

5. Which fruits do you eat? Tick all those you eat once a month, but any you eat at least once a week or more can have two ticks.

apples
apricots
bananas
clementines
cherries
grapefruit
grapes
kiwifruit
mango
melons – cantaloupe
melons – honeydew
nectarines
oranges
peaches
pears
pineapple
plums
raspberries
rhubarb
satsumas
strawberries
tangerines

6. How often do you eat fish (fresh, frozen or cured)?

(a) three times a week or more
(b) more than once a week
(c) less than once a week
(d) occasionally
(e) never

7. What sort of milk do you drink?

(a) Channel Island (gold top or breakfast) milk
(b) full-cream (silver top) milk – pasteurised/UHT/sterilized
(c) homogenised milk (red top)
(d) semi-skimmed milk (stripy top)
(e) skimmed milk (blue top)
(f) none

8. On your bread etc. do you use:

(a) thinly spread butter or margarine
(b) thickly spread butter
(c) thickly spread margarine
(d) low-fat spread
(e) nothing

9. How often do you eat the following foods?

	Daily	*2–4 times a week*	*Less than once a week*
Fried foods			
Pastry			
Cakes			
Chocolate			
Fizzy drinks			
Snacks, e.g. crisps and nuts			

How to Score

1. (a) 6; (b) 5; (c) 3; (d) 1

2. (a) 6; (b) 4; (c) 2; (d) 1

3. (a) 6; (b) 4; (c) 2; (d) 1

4. You score one for each tick. If the vegetable is in *italics*, double its score.

5. You score one for each tick. If the fruit is in *italics*, double its score.

6. (a) 6; (b) 4; (c) 2; (d) 1; (e) 0.

7. (a) 2; (b) 3; (c) 3; (d) 5; (e) 6; (f) 2.

8. (a) 4; (b) 1; (c) 1; (d) 4; (e) 3.

9.

	Daily	*2-4 times a week*	*Less than once a week*
Fried food	1	3	6
Pastry	1	3	6
Cakes	1	3	6
Chocolate	1	3	6
Fizzy drinks	0	3	6
Snacks	1	3	6

How did you do?

More than 95
Well done! You have a varied and healthy diet.

Between 50 and 95
There is room for improvement. Look back and see where you got low scores and try to do better.

Less than 50
Read this book carefully: it could do wonders for your diet!

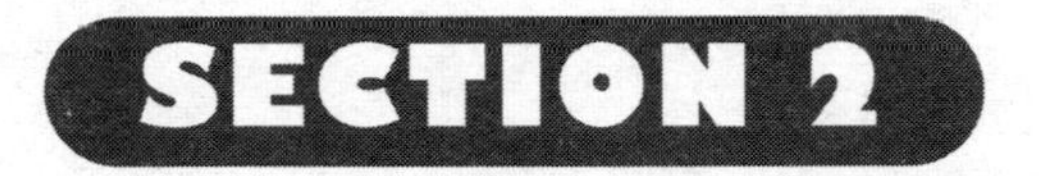

Food in Sickness and in Health

The food we eat plays a major role in our health, whether we are aged eight months or eighty years. Eating a balanced diet is important, particularly if you are cutting major food groups out of your diet or are at a vulnerable stage of life. Diet also has a part to play in the cause of and treatment for many diseases. This section will give an overview of the best diet for babies, toddlers and teenagers, mothers-to-be, and vegetarians and vegans. It also looks at the dietary factors involved in obesity, diabetes, heart disease, illness and convalescence, and food allergy.

Babies

It is beyond dispute that the best food for new-born babies is breast milk. Babies who are breast-fed for the first three to four months of life have greater protection against infection and allergic diseases such as asthma, and suffer fewer episodes of gastroenteritis. Bottle-feeding might seem a much easier option immediately after birth, especially if you have had a long or difficult labour. But, with practice, breast-feeding can be just as easy, as well as being cheaper, more convenient and better for your baby. Getting through those early days is hard – women do not instinctively know how to breast-feed. You will need advice and help in the beginning from a midwife, health visitor or trained breast-feeding counsellor. Although some new mothers find breast-feeding straightforward, enjoyable and immensely rewarding, it can be difficult, demanding and cause emotional conflict. What most people really need is encouragement to continue: if you are having problems, persevere for a week or two but get help!

If you are still struggling after giving it your best shot, you could think about changing to a formula milk. Try not to feel guilty if you stop breast-feeding: your baby will be better off if bottle-feeding means you are more confident, less tired and happier about what you are doing. Choosing a formula milk should not be difficult – any of those designed for babies up to six months will be fine. Find one that you both like and stick to it; there is no need to change to a follow-on milk at six months. All babies should have breast or formula milk until they are a year old, when they can change to full-cream cows' milk. Semi-skimmed milk should not be given before the age of two.

Starting solids is another milestone, but some find weaning more of a millstone! There is no magical starting date, but early weaning can cause problems and few babies need solids before the age of three months. Most babies are ready for weaning at around sixteen weeks and all babies should have started solids by the age of six months; by this age they need more energy and nutrients than milk alone provides. The best time to try solids is when your baby is not tired or hungry, so after or during the lunchtime milk feed is a good time. You will need a shallow plastic spoon, protective clothing and lots of patience. Some babies take to spoon-feeding straight away, but others take days or weeks. If your baby is really reluctant, try again in a week's time. Once your baby is accepting a reasonable amount, gradually cut down the volume and frequency of milk feeds.

Start weaning with a runny baby cereal, and add fruit or vegetable purée or first-stage baby foods (dried or in jars or tins). From the age of six months add meat, fish, eggs, cheese and cows' milk products such as custard and fromage frais. If you have a family history of allergy it is wise to delay eggs and cows' milk products until the baby is nine months or even a year old. Babies learn to swallow solids at about four to six months and need lumpier food from the age of six to seven months. To encourage their biting and chewing development, gradually increase the range of textures and tastes. By its first birthday your baby should be eating chopped family meals and you should be encouraging self-feeding.

Useful addresses

La Leche League, PO Box BM 3424, London WC1N 3XX.
Breast-feeding help and information

National Childbirth Trust, Breastfeeding Promotion Group,
Alexander House, Oldham Terrace, London W3 6NH

Good books

Rose Elliot's mother, baby and toddler book (HarperCollins, 1996)

Great Ormond Street new baby and childcare book (Vermilion, 1997)

Good Housekeeping's complete book of parenting
(Ebury Press, 1996)

Annabel Karmel, *Complete baby and toddler meal planner*
(Ebury Press, 1991)

Penelope Leach, *Baby and child* (Penguin, 1989)

Breast-feeding your baby (National Childbirth Trust, 1993)

Toddlers to teenagers

Food experiences should be fun for toddlers as they learn about eating and experiment with new tastes. Start at about ten to twelve months and let them explore with bits of banana or pear, cooked carrot, chips, grated mild cheese, chopped cold meat (e.g. ham), pieces of fish finger, cooked pasta shapes, bread or toast fingers and plain biscuits (e.g. rich tea fingers). Always supervise meals: it is safer and probably less messy. Splash mats and large plastic bibs are advisable and practical for most eaters under the age of two. Children learn by example and will eat what is in the house. If you want them to enjoy a healthy, well-balanced diet you must do so yourself. You cannot expect your child to eat breakfast if no-one else in the family does. However you also need to remember that children are growing, and a healthy diet for them is one not too low in fat or high in fibre.

Sensible use of convenience foods is often essential for the sanity of most mothers, especially if they are working or have a large and demanding family. Try to mix convenience foods with some homemade items by alternating pizza, fish fingers, fish cakes, sausages and chicken nuggets with homemade mince or burgers, fresh roast chicken or homemade pasta dishes such as spaghetti bolognaise, tuna pasta and macaroni cheese. Children often enjoy foods not thought to be child-friendly such as rice, cucumber and broccoli. Always offer new things, but remember that many under-fives are conservative by nature and stick to what they know. Do not worry if your child lives on sandwiches or baked beans; they will gradually eat other foods. The best way of changing them is not by being a nagging mum but by using peer pressure from friends and eventually schoolmates. No child will actively go hungry for long, so if they are not eating their meals do not give them snacks in between. This will encourage them to eat at mealtimes.

Drinking enough is also important. Encourage your child to have the equivalent of a pint of milk daily until they are four or five. It is easy to let them drink too much squash or fruit juice at the expense of food or milk. If your child is thin or a faddy eater, do not allow them more than a few sips of juice with meals. Fruit juices are acidic and can be very bad for children's teeth, especially if sipped through a straw or bottle. Dilute them and avoid giving children fizzy drinks daily. Eating a lot of sweets also contributes to tooth decay, but actively banning them may result in a child obsessed with having sweets and chocolates. Allowing them occasionally and leading by example is sensible and makes for a happier life for both of you. Never use sweets as a bribe or reward: other treats are just as effective.

Going to school often changes a child's outlook on food completely. They might have new foods for school dinners or see different foods in another child's lunchbox. Make the most of this by encouraging them to try new things. Children starting school will often be more tired at the end of the day, and also hungrier, so give them a small snack when they come home from school and their main meal by six. You are more likely to avoid arguments about food if they are eating regularly and getting enough sleep. Never let the school take all the responsibility for their diet. Look at the school menus, find out about meal supervision, and do not send them into school with sweets or chocolates (many schools do not allow them anyway).

If your child takes a packed lunch, make it healthy, varied and interesting. Sandwiches, rolls, breadsticks, cheese, ham, raw carrot and cucumber, apples and bananas, yoghurts and fromage frais should form the basis of the lunchbox. If these items are eaten regularly, crisps or other savoury snacks can be included several times a week. Cereal bars can be as high in sugar as other sweets, so only include them on an occasional basis. At school most children will learn about food and nutrition. Encourage them to put what they have learned into practice. You might even find out something new yourself! The most important message is that food should be healthy, tasty and fun to prepare. Get your children into the kitchen when they are young. Cooking your own tea occasionally is much more exciting than watching telly whilst mum opens a tin.

If your child has eating difficulties which have not improved on going to school, then these need to be sorted out as soon as possible. If you feel you need help, get it sooner rather than later, but first think carefully about the problem, decide whose problem it is and how much it is affecting your child's health. There may be things you can do to help. If your child eats better with friends or away from home, eating out or having friends round to tea could help. Children often eat more if they can serve themselves or have small portions of a number of different foods. If your child is a slow eater, try to be patient and avoid putting large helpings of food on the plate. Avoid confrontation. If you child eats nothing on the plate, take it away without comment. Do not substitute crisps, cake or biscuits for untouched meals. Give a dessert if you were going to anyway but nothing else. Try to eat as a family and discourage eating in front of the television or with toys at the table. If the lunchbox is coming home full or the evening meal untouched, cut out any between-meal snacks.

As they get older, children want to take more decisions about what they eat. You should let them do this but without giving them complete control over your freezer. So long as they are eating plenty of bread, rice, pasta, potatoes, some fruit and vegetables (frozen is fine), and some protein such as meat, fish, eggs or cheese, then you can turn a blind eye to other things. Many parents worry about the vast quantity of fast foods some teenagers eat but, as you will see from the food tables, not all fast foods are unhealthy. As with toddlers, the message is one of moderation and variation. Try to persuade them to eat vegetables two or three times a week and encourage them to drink milk.

Useful addresses

Child Poverty Action Group, 4th Floor, 1-5 Bath Street, London EC1V 9PY

Health Visitors Association, 50 Southwark Street, London SE1 1UN

Hyperactive Children's Support Group, c/o 71 Whyke Lane, Chichester, West Sussex, PO19 2LD

Good books

Suzanne Abraham and Derek Lewellyn-Jones, *Eating disorders: the facts* (Oxford University Press, 1996)

Dr John Court, *You and your teenager* (Collins/Angus and Robertson, 1996)

Dr David Haslam, *Food fights* (Cedar, 1995)

Anouchka Grose and Ruth Jones, *The teenage vegetarian survival guide* (Red Fox, 1992)

Petra Jackson, *Vegetarian baby and child* (Headline, 1995)

Pregnancy and diet

A healthy, well-balanced diet is never more important than before conception, so if you are planning a pregnancy, pay more attention to what you eat. The experts recommend a diet rich in folic acid (a B vitamin – see table on p. 31), as a diet poor in this vitamin is associated with an increased risk of conceiving a child born with spina bifida. As well as eating more foods high in folate, it is sensible to take extra in tablet form especially during the first three months of pregnancy.

People often talk about 'eating for two', but this is very much an old wives' tale. Pregnant women do need slightly more energy in the last three months of pregnancy, but only about 200kcal extra a day. It is sensible to avoid excessive weight gain as it can be very difficult to lose once the baby is born. A normal healthy diet high in starchy foods, fruit and vegetables is best during pregnancy. Pregnant women do need extra iron and calcium, but most are probably getting more than enough already to cover those extra needs. However, vegetarians and vegans, and people who are eating a very poor diet, or are avoiding certain foods for health reasons might need supplements. For good dietary sources of iron and calcium see pp. 19 and 21.

There are certain foods you should avoid when pregnant. The first is liver, which can contain very high levels of Vitamin A; sometimes as much as four times the recommended intake for pregnant women. Although it is crammed with other goodies such as folate and iron, too much Vitamin A is not healthy when you are pregnant; there might be a relationship between a high Vitamin A intake during pregnancy and an increase in birth defects. Other foods, especially soft, ripened cheeses such as brie, camembert, and goats' and sheep's milk cheeses, should be avoided because they might contain a bacteria called *Listeria monocytogenes*. This bug causes listeriosis, which can infect the unborn child and cause miscarriage, stillbirth or the delivery of a very ill baby. Hard cheese, butter and yoghurt are safe, as are processed cheese spreads and cottage cheese. It is also wise to avoid ready-prepared salads, pâté and raw or under-cooked meat. Always heat ready-prepared meals until piping hot, avoid reheating food more than once, and make sure your fridge is working at the correct temperature.

About half of all pregnant women experience nausea during pregnancy. Although popularly known as morning sickness, it can occur at any time of day and may be associated with tiredness. It often starts around four to six weeks into the pregnancy, usually diminishes by the twelfth week, but can continue well into the eighteenth week. Some women feel sick through their entire pregnancy. Not all those who feel sick actually are, and for some, eating prevents vomiting. The best way to relieve symptoms is by eating a starchy snack or meal every two hours. Plain dry foods are best, avoiding gravies, sauces, garlicky and fried foods. Sometimes the smell of cooking makes the nausea worse. In this case eat cold food, which can be just as nourishing. Sandwiches and salads are useful. Other quick snacks include breakfast cereals, biscuits, bread or toast, tinned pasta or a jacket potato (either plain or with baked beans). Some women go off certain foods; the common ones include coffee, tea, alcohol, eggs and fried foods. Others experience a metallic taste which taints all the food they eat. Food cravings are quite common, but much rarer are cravings for non-foods such as coal, although it has been known for women to eat this or to consume clay, rocks, earth and even matchboxes!

Useful addresses

Maternity Alliance, 45 Beech Street, London EC22 2OX

National Childbirth Trust, Alexandra House, Oldham Terrace, London W3 6NH

Good books

Sarah Brown's healthy pregnancy: a vegetarian approach (BBC Books, 1992)

Sheila Kitzinger, *The new pregnancy and childbirth* (Penguin, 1997)

Mary Nolan, *Being pregnant, giving birth* (HMSO, National Childbirth Trust Guide, 1996)

Glynnis Tucker, *Book of pregnancy, birth and parenthood* (Oxford University Press, 1996)

Vegetarian and vegan diets

Deciding to become a vegetarian has probably never been more popular, especially amongst young people. The number of people who have become vegetarian or vegan has increased by well over 120 per cent in the last ten years and probably between 6 and 10 per cent of people in the UK now avoid meat and animal products. BSE, livestock conditions, factory farming, the world economy, famines in Third World countries and a desire to live a healthier lifestyle are all factors which make people decide to change. Many people are semi-vegetarian and no longer eat red meat; others also avoid chicken but continue to eat fish. Someone who is fully vegetarian will eat no animal flesh or foods containing lard, gelatine or rennet. They normally drink milk and eat soft cheese, vegetarian hard cheese, yoghurt and eggs. Vegans usually avoid all animal foods including milk, eggs, honey and foods containing animal additives such as lecithin (from eggs). Common to vegetarian and vegan diets are fruit, vegetables, cereals, nuts and pulses.

Vegetarian and vegan diets are often lower in fat and higher in fibre than the normal western diet, and lifelong vegans are known to suffer less heart disease. The downside is that some people cut out all meat, fish, eggs and cheese without fully replacing the lost nutrients through eating other foods, and this can affect their health. In addition, very strict or unbalanced diets may not contain enough of certain nutrients for babies, teenagers, and pregnant and nursing women. If you, or someone you are close to, is already a vegetarian or vegan, or is thinking about becoming one, it is helpful to be well-informed about nutrition. Someone who eats foods from all food groups will usually get enough nutrients without having to think about it, but cutting out meat and other animal products can easily lead to insufficient intakes of iron, calcium, B vitamins and certain sorts of protein.

For most people, meat is the best source of iron in the diet, and iron from other foods is not as easily absorbed by the body. Non-meat sources of iron include eggs, dark green vegetables, wholemeal bread, breakfast cereals and chocolate (see p. 21). This iron will be better absorbed if you have some Vitamin C with it, so try to have fresh fruit juice with your main meals. Getting enough calcium is easy if you are drinking milk and eating cheese, but if you are avoiding these then try to drink fortified soya milk. Calcium is also found in pulses, nuts, pasta, bread and sesame seeds. If you are eating plenty of wholegrain cereals, green vegetables, and having eggs, milk or Marmite, you should be absorbing enough B vitamins. However, Vitamin B_{12} is only found in animal foods, so vegans will need to take a special supplement. Some breakfast cereals and soya milks are also fortified with this vitamin.

Vegetarians should be getting enough of all types of protein from milk and eggs, but people whose only sources of protein are pulses and cereals will need to be more careful. Since vegetable protein does not contain all essential amino acids, vegans need to eat a mixture of proteins to get all of their amino acids. Combine grains with pulses or nuts; for example, eating baked beans on toast, lentils with pasta, beans with rice, and peanut butter sandwiches will result in sufficient amino acids. It is worthwhile getting information from one of the relevant groups or societies, and investing in a good cookery book. In bygone days, vegetarians who could not cook were often condemned to a monotonous diet, but now there are many different types of animal-friendly fast foods and ready-made meals. However, be aware that some contain very little protein, and will need to be supplemented with other foods if eaten regularly.

Useful addresses

The Vegan Society, Donald Watson House, 7 Battle Road,
St Leonards-on-Sea, East Sussex, TN37 7AA

The Vegetarian Society, Parkdale, Dunham Road, Altrincham,
Cheshire, WA14 4QG

Good books

Rose Elliot's complete vegetarian cook book (HarperCollins, 1994)
(or any other Rose Elliot book)

Sarah Brown's fresh vegetarian cookery (BBC Books, 1995)

Frances Bissell, *'Times' book of vegetarian cookery*
(Chatto & Windus, 1994)

Obesity

The bottom line on obesity is that if we eat more energy than we use, the excess is stored as fat. We need energy for muscle movement, activity of essential organs such as the heart and liver, maintenance of the correct body temperature and the growth and repair of our body. How much energy you need depends on your sex, age and how active you are, but it is mainly dictated by your basal metabolic rate (BMR). BMR is the rate at which you use energy for your body's basic functions; it is the body's tickover rate. Your BMR accounts for 88 per cent of all your energy needs; only 12 per cent will be used for activity. People need different amounts of energy and there could be as much as 25 per cent difference even between individuals of the same age and sex. The amount of energy required for different activities is often overrated: you need to be doing something like swimming really to use a lot of energy. Housework is nothing like as energetic as it was in our grandmothers' day, and very few jobs these days are as physically strenuous as the manual work done by the majority in employment before the Second World War.

Our energy intake from food varies daily, but most of us naturally regulate our intake to suit our needs. Unfortunately, if our needs change or something affects our intake, the weight can start to pile on. It is a myth that fat people eat a lot; many overweight people eat a normal amount of food, and are overweight because they have been eating slightly more than they need over a number of years. Sometimes a bereavement, divorce or drastic change in social circumstances can change eating habits temporarily or permanently. This can cause weight gain which is then hard to lose. Everyone who is overweight has one thing in common: at some time in their lives they have eaten more than they needed. To lose weight they will need to eat less. Unfortunately, very low-calorie diets can lower the BMR, which means the dieter will eat fewer calories but will also need fewer. Every time you go on a diet it will be harder to lose weight and easier to regain it once off the diet because the amount of calories you need is getting less and less.

The message is clear: do not go on a crash diet; instead, make your first diet your last. It is much better to lose four pounds a month and keep it off than lose fifteen pounds in a month and regain the lot. Losing weight too quickly is bad for your health; as well as losing fat you also lose muscle, and the muscle could come from anywhere in the body. If you are trying to lose weight, it is worth taking some advice from a dietitian via your GP or going to a self-help group such as Weight Watchers. Wherever you go for help you will be advised to eat regularly and to try to follow the same meal pattern each day. It is a good idea to plan your diet so you have low-calorie foods in the house. Cut down on sugary, fatty food, and fill up on fruit, vegetables and starchy food. Most diets, however they are packaged, are based on the principle that if you take in less energy than you need, you will lose weight. However, no diet will work for long if you are not prepared to give it a good few months. You must actively want to lose weight, otherwise you will not have the stamina to continue with the diet in the face of temptation. You will also need help, so enlist the support of your relatives, friends and work colleagues.

Useful addresses

The British Dietetic Association, 7th Floor, Elizabeth House,
22 Suffolk Street Queensway, Birmingham B1 1LS

Health Education Authority, Hamilton House, Mabledon Place,
London WC1H 9TX

There are also many slimming clubs with UK networks, your local library or local hospital will have information on what is available in your area.

Good books

There are literally hundreds of very similar slimming books to choose from. Look for one which offers a balanced diet and avoid those with a calorie intake for the day of less than 1000kcals. If you want more help, ask your GP to refer you to a dietitian, or join a reputable slimming club. Your local hospital or health centre might also have some general information.

Eating for a healthy heart

In the UK, coronary heart disease (CHD) kills one out of every eleven men. It used to be almost exclusively a male disease, mainly affecting men over the age of forty-five, but now younger men and increasingly women especially those over the age of fifty are being affected. Although death rates from the disease are falling, they are still much higher than they were forty years ago. The disease is caused when the walls of blood vessels in the heart are damaged. The damaged walls then get deposits of fat in them which gradually become fibrous and eventually block the vessel. Most adults have got fatty deposits in their arteries but not all will get CHD; it depends on other factors such as age, sex and family medical history. If you smoke, have a stressful life, have diabetes, are overweight, had a parent with heart disease, are male, are over fifty, have high blood pressure, take no exercise, live in a soft water area or have one of the other 246 risk factors, you are more likely to develop CHD.

One of the most important risk factors is a high cholesterol level. It is normal to have cholesterol in the blood, but CHD is only common in countries where the average level is above 5.2mmol/litre (millimols per litre is a way of describing the number of cholesterol particles in a litre of blood). Research has also revealed that cutting levels to below 5mmol reduces the number of deaths from this disease. In men, cholesterol levels rise with age throughout their lives, but women's levels only start to increase after the menopause. Half of your level is inherited from your parents; if they had high cholesterol levels you are more likely to have them too. Genetic inheritance apart, diet is the most important factor governing cholesterol levels.

For a healthy person, a cholesterol level of 5mmol/litre or less is desirable. If you are going to get your level checked it is better to have it done by your GP who can then give you advice and refer you to a dietitian if your level is high.

Changing your diet can reduce your cholesterol level, but if it is very high you may also need drugs depending on your age, the number of risk factors you have and whether or not you already have heart disease.

A good diet for a healthy heart is one high in starchy foods, fresh fruit and vegetables, and low in fat. Try to have five helpings of fruit and vegetables every day. Carrots, broccoli, green, yellow, red and orange peppers, tomatoes, spinach, sprouts and other green yellow or red vegetables and fruit are rich in substances called antioxidants which are thought to help prevent the damage to the blood vessel walls. People who eat a lot of fruit and vegetables have low rates of heart disease. Greeks and Italians suffer far less from heart disease than the British. They also eat around 180–190kg of fruit and vegetables per person per year, compared to only 50kg per person in the UK.

Avoiding too much fat is important, but do not cut it out altogether; fat contains essential fatty acids and fat-soluble vitamins and has an important place in our diet. Eat different types of fat: have less saturated fat and more mono- and poly-unsaturated fat. Eat fish at least twice a week and avoid large portions of meat and full-fat cheese. Have fewer fried foods, use butter, margarine and cooking oils sparingly and avoid eating cream and mayonnaise regularly. Try incorporating foods such as low-fat spread, low-fat cheeses and reduced-fat salad dressings into your diet. If frying, use olive oil, rapeseed oil, sunflower oil, corn oil, or any other mono- or poly-unsaturated cooking oil and cook using shallow or stir-fry methods rather than deep-fat frying.

You should also eat lots of starchy foods such as bread, potatoes, pasta, rice and breakfast cereals as they are low in fat, and filling. Peas, beans, lentils and oats contain a special sort of fibre or non-starch polysaccharide (see p. 15) which helps reduce blood cholesterol levels.

Useful addresses

British Heart Foundation, 14 Fitzhardinge Street, London W1H 4DH

Coronary Prevention Group, 42 Store Street, London WC1E 9DB

Health Education Authority, Hamilton House, Mabledon Place, London WC1H 9TX

Good books

Professor John Yudkin and Sarah Stanner, *Eating for a healthy heart* (BBC Books, 1996)

All the associations listed above produce a variety of useful leaflets.

Diabetes

Diabetes occurs when the body's normal mechanism for controlling the amount of glucose in the blood is upset. Glucose is the end product of the digestion of starchy and sugary foods. After a meal the body's blood glucose level rises until the pancreas produces insulin. The insulin makes glucose levels return to normal, at which point insulin production is stopped. In diabetics, the pancreas does not produce enough or any insulin, or the insulin is prevented from working effectively, the blood glucose level continues to rise and becomes much higher than normal, a condition known as hyperglycaemia. At a critical level glucose appears in the urine, and this is often how DM is diagnosed. People with untreated DM will feel thirsty, go to the loo a lot, may lose weight, feel sick, and have frequent headaches or blurred vision.

When treating diabetes, blood glucose levels should be kept close to the normal level of 4–6mmol/litre (millimols per litre describes the number of glucose molecules in a litre of blood). Avoiding very high or very low blood sugars, or a level which fluctuates wildly between the two, is important.

Dietary treatment of diabetes is based on the effect of different foods on blood glucose levels. Sugar increases the level quite rapidly but the effect is short-lived. Bread and other starchy foods increase the level more slowly and maintain it for longer. The British Diabetic Association (BDA) recommends eating a diet high in starchy, fibre-rich carbohydrates, fruit and vegetables, and avoiding too much sugar and fat. This means eating lots of bread, potatoes, rice, pasta and breakfast cereals, and having five portions of fruit and vegetables every day. Oats, peas, beans and lentils should be included regularly if not daily, and large helpings of meat and cheese should be avoided. The BDA also advises eating regular meals, with starchy snacks between meals if insulin or tablets are taken. All diabetics should avoid eating large amounts of sugar, but unless you are overweight you can have up to an ounce a day. This should be taken as part of a meal, for example in a pudding, rather than as sweets or sugar in tea.

Good books

Dr Joan Gomez, *Living with diabetes* (Sheldon Press, 1995)

Asmina Govindji, *Quick and easy cooking for diabetes* (Thorsons, 1997)

Dr Rowan Hillson, *Diabetes: the complete guide* (Vermilion, 1996)

The British Diabetic Association, 10 Queen Anne Street, London W1M 0BD produces many different leaflets and books.

Illness and convalescence

It is important for everyone to eat a balanced diet. When people are ill or convalescing, they often need extra energy or protein to fight disease, help wounds to heal after surgery, or enable the body to respond better to medical treatments. Unfortunately, it is often just when they need to eat more that many people find they cannot face food. It is hard to eat if you have no appetite, feel sick or breathless, or are unable to swallow properly. Loss of appetite is often a serious problem and can be very upsetting both for the 'patient' and for the carer. Offering large meals to someone with little appetite or trying to tempt them with all their favourite foods may only make matters worse.

If you have lost your appetite, try eating very small meals or snacks. Forget about having proper 'knife and fork' meals if you cannot face them. Not only can the smell of hot food be offputting, but you are also under pressure to eat then and there. It may be easier to eat snacks such as sandwiches, cheese and biscuits, yoghurt, crisps, breakfast cereals, toast or scones every two hours. If you are okay with hot food, then tinned pasta, baked beans on toast or jacket potatoes with fillings are all nourishing and easy to make. When serving a main meal to someone with a poor appetite, put only a very small helping on the plate or better still, allow them to serve themselves. If you live alone, use ready-made meals when you don't feel up to cooking. UHT milk and sponge puddings, tinned fish, tinned pasta and packet rice are also useful items to keep in the cupboard.

If you drink alcohol, you may be able to stimulate your appetite by having an aperitif such as sherry or brandy before your meal. Avoid hot, spicy or greasy food if you feel very sick, and keep your meals fairly dry; avoid drinking with your meal. Slowly sipping a fizzy drink can sometimes help, as can eating dry biscuits or toast before getting up if you feel sick in the morning. Above all, try to relax about food and do not worry if you are not eating a conventionally healthy diet; a high-fibre low-fat diet is not healthy for people who are ill or convalescing. Exercise can also stimulate the appetite, so going for a short walk before a main meal may be helpful.

Sometimes illness can make swallowing difficult or affect your breathing. In both cases eating soft foods and adding extra sauces, gravy and butter helps food go down. New bread, chewy roast meats and plain grilled fish are best avoided. If you are taking a long time to eat your meal, keep it hot in a wide-necked thermos flask. If you are unable to eat any solid food at all, try to drink half a glass of liquid every hour. The best things to drink are milk and milkshakes, fruit juices with added glucose, or fizzy drinks. Try to rotate these but have as much milk as you can. Soups are often comforting, and cream soups or 'main-course' type soups are particularly nourishing; liquidise or sieve them if you cannot manage lumps.

When you are getting better and have regained some appetite, cram as much energy into your diet as you can. Eat three times a day and have snacks between every meal. In addition, try to drink about one to two pints of full-cream milk daily.

Useful addresses

Age Concern, Astral House, 1268 London Road, Norbury, London SW16 4ER

BACUP, 121–123 Charterhouse Street, London EC1M 6AA (British Association for Cancer United Patients and their families and friends)

Cancerlink, 11–21 Northdown Street, London N1 9BN

Carers' National Association, 20 Glasshouse Yard, London EC1

The Stroke Association, CHSA House, 123–127 Whitecross Street, London EC1Y 8JJ

Terrence Higgins Trust, 52–54 Grays Inn Road, London WC1 8JU

Good books

Clare Shaw and Maureen Hunter, *Special diet cookbooks – cancer* (2nd edition) (Thorsons, 1995)

St John Ambulance, St Andrew's Ambulance Association and The British Red Cross Society, *Caring for the sick* (Dorling Kindersley, 1995)

Food allergy

An allergy is the body's response to becoming sensitised to a food. The body's natural defence system, the immune system, reacts against foreign substances. Sensitisation occurs when the guardians of the immune system, the white blood cells, decide that a normally harmless food, such as milk protein, is an aggressor. The white blood cells then produce substances called antibodies. Antibodies are specific; in other words, they only recognise one aggressor. When the antibodies encounter that food again, they trigger a reaction in the body's mast cells. These are found in the mucous linings of the body and also on the skin. This reaction produces a substance called histamine, the cause of most of the problems which arise when an allergic reaction takes place. A food allergy is therefore an overreaction by the immune system.

The most helpful aid to diagnosis is a blood test called a RAST test which analyses the levels of the antibody IgE produced by different foods. Other tests are unreliable and often completely misleading. If you think you have a food allergy, ask your GP to refer you to an allergy clinic at a hospital where RAST testing and dietetic expertise are both available. The best way of finding out whether a particular food is causing the problem is to go on a diet avoiding the suspect food or food group and then challenge yourself with it. This should always be done under supervision, especially where children are the sufferers.

Some allergies, such as to peanuts and shellfish, are life-long and these tend to be the ones that cause life-threatening reactions. Foods which commonly cause allergies include eggs, milk, wheat, fish, shellfish, peanuts and nuts, but chocolate, peas, citrus fruits, soya beans, tomatoes, coffee, tea and meat have all been known to cause adverse reactions. Foods do not have to be eaten to cause a problem; food odours or contact with the skin can also give rise to an allergic reaction.

It is thought that up to 7.5 per cent of the population has an allergy to cows' milk. The antigens in cows' milk are the milk proteins, whey and casein. Goat, sheep and soya milk should all be avoided because they can also cause problems in a sensitive person, and must be tested separately. Heat treatment lowers the allergenicity of milk, so some milk-allergic people can drink evaporated milk or eat small amounts of cheese. People avoiding milk do not need to cut out beef, unless they are already doing so for other reasons. Dairy foods provide lots of nutrients; if they are removed from the diet, other sources of protein and calcium will need to be substituted, especially for children.

Egg allergy usually develops before the age of six months but is often gone by the time the child is three. The egg protein albumen in egg whites is the problem. Whole eggs and egg white can be hard to avoid because they are widely used in food production. Again, heat affects the allergenicity of the food, and cooking eggs makes them far less harmful. Children who are allergic to eggs can also be allergic to chicken, but cooked chicken does not cause a problem for most people.

Nut allergy is of major concern to all parents. Nuts are the food most commonly causing the life-threatening allergy symptom known as anaphylaxis. An allergy to peanuts is the commonest nut allergy, but sufferers should avoid all nuts. Peanuts are not a true nut, but belong to the legume family which includes peas, beans, sweetcorn and lentils. Most supermarkets now label foods containing nuts, and will send lists of own-brand foods to sufferers on request. People with nut allergies need expert help and advice.

Food additives are not a very common cause of food allergy, the vast majority being completely harmless. Most food additives have a number and are easily spotted on the label. The main additives which might cause a problem include the azo dye group of food colourings, a flavour enhancer called monosodium glutamate, and preservatives such as benzoates, sulphites and nitrites. All of these are found in a variety of foods; if you are concerned, get expert help.

Useful addresses

Action Against Allergy, PO Box 278, Twickenham, Middlesex TW1 4QQ

Anaphylaxis Campaign, PO Box 149, Fleet Hampshire GU13 9XU

British Allergy Foundation, St Bartholomew's Hospital,
West Smithfield, London EC1A 7BE

Migraine Trust, 45 Great Ormond Street, London WC1N 3HD

National Asthma Campaign, Providence House, Providence Place,
London N1 0NT

National Eczema Society, 163 Eversholt Street, London NW1 1BU

Supermarkets: Many supermarkets and other national retail chains have a wealth of information to offer about their own-brand products.

Good books

David J. Atherton, *Eczema in childhood: the facts*
(Oxford University Press, 1994)

Maurice Hanssen, *'E' for additives* (2nd edition) (Thorsons, 1988)

Dr J. O. Hunter with Elizabeth Workman and Dr Virginia Alun Jones,
The allergy diet (Vermilion, 1996)

Mark Levy, Sean Hilton and Greta Barnes, *Asthma at your fingertips* (Class Publishing, 1997)

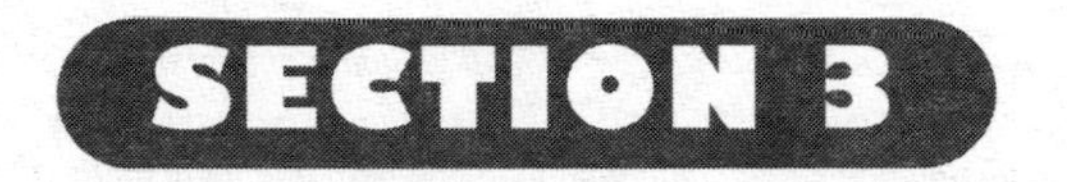

The Balance of Good Health

This section is the main part of the book and it is one you will want to dip in and out of. It is named after the balance of good health plate model now used by all health professionals to illustrate a healthy diet. The plate model was introduced by the Health Education Authority in 1995, and it is similar to the American food pyramid as it shows how much we should try to eat from different food groups at each meal.

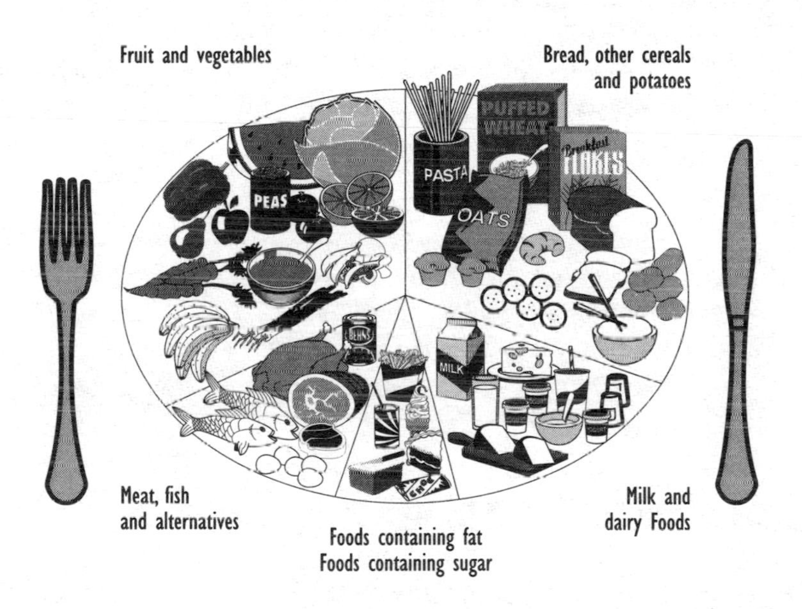

How to use the plate model

There are five basic food groups, and the plate model shows how much of each food group should contribute to meals or snacks. One third of our meal should come from the bread, other cereals and potatoes group, another third should come from the fruit and vegetable group, with the other three groups making up the last third. This last third should be subdivided so that just under one half of it comes from milk and dairy foods, just over one third of it from meat and fish and finally less than a quarter from foods containing fat and sugar.

This might all sound very confusing especially if you are not very good at fractions. However the easy way to remember is by looking at your own plate. If the amount of potatoes and vegetables is more than double the meat, fish or dairy products then you are doing very well. The good news is that although they should only make up less than 10 per cent of our everyday intake, some high fat or sugary foods can be eaten as part of a balanced diet.

How to use the tables

All the tables in this section are laid out in the same way, the abbreviations and symbols used are ones you are probably familiar with because they appear on many packets and tinned foods. In case you are not sure what they all mean, the explanation given below should help.

g	grams (1000 grams = 1 kilogram (kg))
mg	milligrams (1000 milligrams = 1 gram)
µg	micrograms (1000 micrograms = 1 milligram)
kcal	kilocalories – this is the same as calories and is a measurement of energy

How to find different foods

The tables are grouped according to the different segments of the plate model; each segment being subdivided in order to make it easier to find the food you are looking for. The segments and their subdivisions are as follows:

SEGMENT	SUBDIVISION
Bread, other cereals and potatoes	Bread, breakfast cereals, pasta, rice, flour and potatoes
Fruit and vegetables	Fruit, vegetables
Meat and fish	Meat, fish and seafood, eggs, pulses and nuts
Dairy foods	Cheese, cream, milk and yoghurt
Food high in fat and sugar	Cakes, biscuits, puddings, sweets, snacks, fats and oils, soups, sauces, savoury spreads and drinks

Most of the food groups fit easily into one of the segments, but some such as drinks and soups, spreads and sauces do not really fit easily anywhere. For this reason, they appear in the last segment. There are some foods such as chips and sugar-coated breakfast cereals which are high in fat or sugar, but because their nutritional value in other areas is good (and also to make it easier to find the food you are looking for), such foods will be listed with other similar dishes. Comparing the amount of fat and sugar a food contains with the fat content of a butter pat (8g fat), or a teaspoon of sugar (6g sugar), is a good way of finding out if it is a high-fat or high-sugar food.

Each food is given in the portion size normally eaten; usually the medium average adult portion of that food, but it might also be an entire food such as an apple. In most cases the amount is not displayed because most of us think about our food in its constituent portion and not its actual weight. However, for some foods, in order to make it easier to compare like with like, the portion weight has been included in the text. Since all foods have been calculated using a specific portion weight, the figures in the tables are very precise, even those foods in section four where the portion size of meals outside the home can be difficult to determine.

Most of the data has been calculated from McCance and Widdowson's *Composition of Foods*, 5th Edition and all supplements to that edition. The calculations were made using *Dietplan 5* (Forestfield software), based on portion sizes derived from *Food Portion Sizes*, 2nd Edition (MAFF). For some foods such as sweets, snacks, cakes and biscuits; the *Composition of Foods* provided very little other than basic information. In this case, manufacturer's data is reproduced with permission, to represent all similar products.

Segment One

Bread, other cereals and potatoes

The plate model shows that one third of our plate should be filled with starchy carbohydrate, preferably the low-fat types. With the wide variety of bread, rolls, baguettes, speciality breads and bagels around, it is easy to eat plenty of starchy carbohydrate. Some types of bread contain good amounts of calcium, iron and B vitamins. Breakfast cereals are also greatly underrated and are fortified with iron and vitamins and combined with milk provide most of the nutrients required, including good amounts of fibre. Pasta and rice (excellent low-fat high-carbohydrate foods) are replacing potatoes, but don't abandon the humble spud (an excellent source of Vitamin C, other vitamins, minerals and fibre). All fried potatoes are cooked in blended vegetable oil, unless otherwise stated. Similarly, all boiled potato dishes are cooked without salt. All portions sizes for breakfast cereals are 30g unless otherwise stated, and all values are for dry cereal or oats. Some manufacturer's data has been used in this segment:

[1] H J Heinz Co Ltd; [2] Kelloggs; [3] Nestlé; [4] Waitrose; [5] Weetabix.

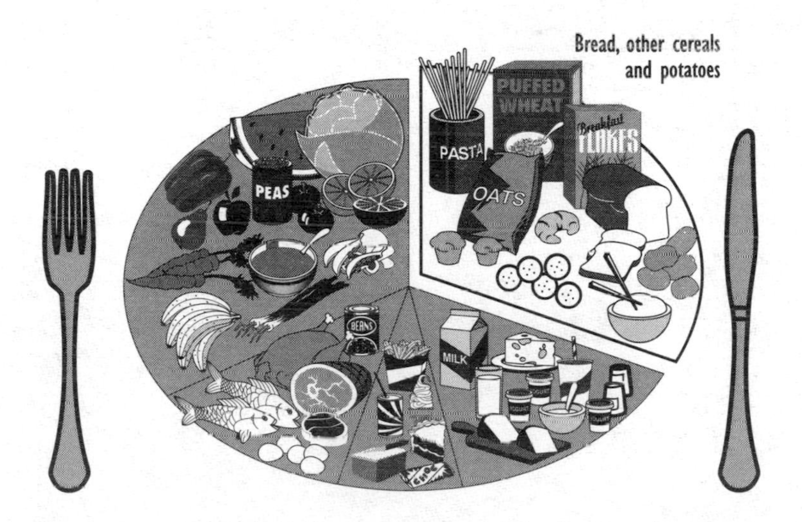

FOOD	Bagel[4]	Breadstick	Chapatis made without fat	Chapatis made with fat
PORTION SIZE	one	one	one	one
NUTRIENTS				
Energy (kcals)	228	27	111	197
Protein (g)	7.3	0.8	4.0	4.9
Total fat (g)	2.7	0.6	0.6	7.7
Saturated fat (g)	0.3	0.4	0.1	unknown
Mono-unsat. fat (g)	1.2	0.1	0.1	unknown
Poly-unsat. fat (g)	0.7	0.1	0.2	unknown
Carbohydrate (g)	43.7	5.1	24.0	29.0
Sugar (g)	3.2	0.3	0.9	1.1
Fibre (g)	1.8	0.2	unknown	unknown
Sodium (mg)	336	60	66	78
Potassium (mg)	84	11	83	96
Calcium (mg)	unknown	2	33	40
Magnesium (mg)	unknown	2	20	25
Phosphorus (mg)	unknown	8	66	78
Iron (mg)	unknown	0.08	1.15	1.38
Copper (mg)	unknown	0.01	0.11	0.12
Zinc (mg)	unknown	0.05	0.55	0.66
Selenium (µg)	unknown	unknown	0.66	0.84
Vitamin A (µg)	unknown	trace	nil	unknown
Vitamin D (µg)	unknown	nil	nil	unknown
Vitamin E (mg)	unknown	0.03	trace	unknown
Vitamin B_1 (mg)	unknown	0.01	0.13	0.16
Vitamin B_2 (mg)	unknown	0.01	0.02	0.02
Niacin (mg)	unknown	0.11	0.82	1.02
Vitamin B_6 (mg)	unknown	0.01	0.1	0.12
Vitamin B_{12} (µg)	unknown	trace	nil	nil
Folate (µg)	unknown	1	8	9
Pantothenate (mg)	unknown	0.04	0.11	0.12
Biotin (µg)	unknown	0.1	1.1	1.2
Vitamin C (mg)	unknown	nil	nil	nil

Cream cracker	Crispbread rye	Croissants	Crumpets toasted	FOOD
one	one	one	one	**PORTION SIZE**
				NUTRIENTS
31	32	216	80	Energy (kcals)
0.7	0.9	5.0	2.7	Protein (g)
1.1	0.2	12.2	0.4	Total fat (g)
unknown	trace	3.9	trace	Saturated fat (g)
unknown	trace	4.9	trace	Mono-unsat. fat (g)
unknown	0.1	2.9	0.2	Poly-unsat. fat (g)
4.8	7.1	23.0	17.4	Carbohydrate (g)
trace	6.7	0.6	0.8	Sugar (g)
0.2	1.2	1.0	0.8	Fibre (g)
43	22	234	324	Sodium (mg)
8	50	84	37	Potassium (mg)
8	5	48	48	Calcium (mg)
2	10	16	7	Magnesium (mg)
8	31	78	72	Phosphorus (mg)
0.12	0.35	1.2	0.44	Iron (mg)
0.01	0.04	0.16	0.08	Copper (mg)
0.05	0.3	0.54	0.24	Zinc (mg)
trace	trace	unknown	11	Selenium (µg)
nil	nil	13	nil	Vitamin A (µg)
nil	nil	0.12	nil	Vitamin D (µg)
0.09	0.05	trace	0.08	Vitamin E (mg)
0.02	0.03	0.11	0.07	Vitamin B_1 (mg)
trace	0.01	0.1	0.01	Vitamin B_2 (mg)
0.12	0.11	1.2	0.4	Niacin (mg)
0.01	0.03	0.07	0.02	Vitamin B_6 (mg)
nil	nil	trace	nil	Vitamin B_{12} (µg)
2	4	44	4	Folate (µg)
0.02	0.11	0.3	0.12	Pantothenate (mg)
0.1	0.7	5.4	1.6	Biotin (µg)
nil	nil	nil	nil	Vitamin C (mg)

FOOD	French bread	Granary bread large loaf	Muffin English	Naan bread plain served with ghee
PORTION SIZE	one 2-inch piece	one medium slice	one	one
NUTRIENTS				
Energy (kcals)	108	85	192	538
Protein (g)	3.8	3.3	6.9	14.2
Total fat (g)	1.1	1.0	4.3	20.0
Saturated fat (g)	0.2	unknown	unknown	unknown
Mono-unsat. fat (g)	0.2	unknown	unknown	unknown
Poly-unsat. fat (g)	0.3	unknown	unknown	unknown
Carbohydrate (g)	22.2	16.7	33.7	80.2
Sugar (g)	0.8	0.8	1.8	8.8
Fibre (g)	0.6	1.5	1.4	3.0
Sodium (mg)	228	209	88	608
Potassium (mg)	52	68	122	288
Calcium (mg)	52	28	95	256
Magnesium (mg)	11	21	20	45
Phosphorus (mg)	44	65	102	208
Iron (mg)	0.84	0.97	1.22	2.08
Copper (mg)	0.06	0.06	0.14	0.19
Zinc (mg)	0.28	0.54	0.61	1.28
Selenium (µg)	11	unknown	19	40
Vitamin A (µg)	nil	unknown	unknown	154
Vitamin D (µg)	nil	nil	0.29	0.32
Vitamin E (mg)	trace	unknown	0.46	2.21
Vitamin B_1 (mg)	0.08	0.11	0.14	0.3
Vitamin B_2 (mg)	0.03	0.04	0.11	0.16
Niacin (mg)	0.52	1.08	1.22	1.92
Vitamin B_6 (mg)	0.03	0.06	0.08	0.21
Vitamin B_{12} (µg)	nil	nil	trace	trace
Folate (µg)	10	32	31	22
Pantothenate (mg)	0.12	unknown	0.34	0.48
Biotin (µg)	0.4	unknown	4.8	3.2
Vitamin C (mg)	nil	nil	trace	trace

Oatcakes	Poppadums fried in oil	Paratha	Pitta bread	FOOD
one	one	one	one medium	PORTION SIZE
				NUTRIENTS
57	48	451	199	Energy (kcals)
1.3	2.3	11.2	6.9	Protein (g)
2.4	2.2	20.0	0.9	Total fat (g)
0.5	0.2	unknown	0.2	Saturated fat (g)
1.1	0.7	unknown	0.1	Mono-unsat. fat (g)
0.7	1.0	unknown	0.4	Poly-unsat. fat (g)
8.2	5.1	60.5	43.4	Carbohydrate (g)
0.4	trace	1.5	1.8	Sugar (g)
unknown	unknown	5.6	1.7	Fibre (g)
160	315	168	390	Sodium (mg)
44	98	224	83	Potassium (mg)
7	9	118	68	Calcium (mg)
13	22	71	18	Magnesium (mg)
55	33	210	69	Phosphorus (mg)
0.58	1.43	2.8	1.28	Iron (mg)
0.05	0.06	0.29	0.16	Copper (mg)
0.3	0.32	1.68	0.45	Zinc (mg)
unknown	unknown	unknown	unknown	Selenium (µg)
nil	unknown	unknown	nil	Vitamin A (µg)
nil	nil	0.17	nil	Vitamin D (µg)
0.28	unknown	0.98	unknown	Vitamin E (mg)
0.04	0.02	0.25	0.18	Vitamin B_1 (mg)
0.01	0.01	0.06	0.04	Vitamin B_2 (mg)
0.09	0.13	3.36	1.05	Niacin (mg)
0.01	unknown	0.2	unknown	Vitamin B_6 (mg)
nil	nil	nil	nil	Vitamin B_{12} (µg)
3	4	22	16	Folate (µg)
0.13	unknown	0.28	unknown	Pantothenate (mg)
2.2	unknown	2.8	unknown	Biotin (µg)
nil	nil	nil	nil	Vitamin C (mg)

FOOD	Pizza cheese and tomato	Rolls white soft	Rolls wholemeal	Rye bread
PORTION SIZE	one medium	one	one	one slice
NUTRIENTS				
Energy (kcals)	500	121	116	55
Protein (g)	15	4.1	4.3	2.1
Total fat (g)	21.4	1.9	1.4	0.4
Saturated fat (g)	8.6	unknown	unknown	0.1
Mono-unsat. fat (g)	7.2	unknown	unknown	0.1
Poly-unsat. fat (g)	3.8	unknown	unknown	0.2
Carbohydrate (g)	65.8	23.2	23.2	11.4
Sugar (g)	13.8	1.0	0.7	0.4
Fibre (g)	2.8	0.7	2.8	1.1
Sodium (mg)	1080	252	221	145
Potassium (mg)	340	54	110	48
Calcium (mg)	360	54	26	20
Magnesium (mg)	32	12	33	12
Phosphorus (mg)	260	45	82	40
Iron (mg)	2.0	0.99	1.68	0.63
Copper (mg)	0.22	0.06	0.12	0.05
Zinc (mg)	2.0	0.31	0.77	0.32
Selenium (µg)	8	13	17	unknown
Vitamin A (µg)	unknown	unknown	unknown	nil
Vitamin D (µg)	unknown	nil	nil	nil
Vitamin E (mg)	unknown	trace	0.1	0.3
Vitamin B_1 (mg)	0.32	0.13	0.14	0.07
Vitamin B_2 (mg)	0.28	0.02	0.04	0.01
Niacin (mg)	1.8	0.86	1.97	0.57
Vitamin B_6 (mg)	0.26	0.02	0.05	0.02
Vitamin B_{12} (µg)	trace	nil	nil	nil
Folate (µg)	40	11	30	6
Pantothenate (mg)	unknown	0.14	0.29	0.13
Biotin (µg)	unknown	0.4	2.9	unknown
Vitamin C (mg)	unknown	nil	nil	nil

Scotch pancakes	Slimmers bread	Soda bread	Water biscuits	FOOD
one average	one slice	one farl	one	**PORTION SIZE**
				NUTRIENTS
93	49	335	35	Energy (kcals)
1.8	1.8	10	0.9	Protein (g)
3.7	0.4	3.3	1.0	Total fat (g)
unknown	unknown	unknown	unknown	Saturated fat (g)
unknown	unknown	unknown	unknown	Mono-unsat. fat (g)
unknown	unknown	unknown	unknown	Poly-unsat. fat (g)
13.9	10.2	71	6.1	Carbohydrate (g)
2.8	0.4	3.8	0.2	Sugar (g)
0.4	0.4	2.7	0.2	Fibre (g)
137	112	546	38	Sodium (mg)
96	22	325	11	Potassium (mg)
38	26	182	10	Calcium (mg)
5.12	4	26	2	Magnesium (mg)
30	19	143	7	Phosphorus (mg)
0.3	0.34	1.82	0.13	Iron (mg)
0.02	0.03	0.13	0.01	Copper (mg)
0.1	0.12	0.78	0.06	Zinc (mg)
0.6	unknown	4	unknown	Selenium (µg)
unknown	unknown	unknown	unknown	Vitamin A (µg)
0.29	nil	0.01	nil	Vitamin D (µg)
0.35	trace	0.31	unknown	Vitamin E (mg)
0.04	0.06	0.22	0.01	Vitamin B_1 (mg)
0.02	0.01	0.1	trace	Vitamin B_2 (mg)
0.25	0.3	1.43	0.07	Niacin (mg)
0.02	0.01	0.12	trace	Vitamin B_6 (mg)
trace	nil	trace	nil	Vitamin B_{12} (µg)
1.92	8	12	unknown	Folate (µg)
0.09	unknown	0.39	unknown	Pantothenate (mg)
0.3	unknown	1.3	unknown	Biotin (µg)
trace	nil	trace	nil	Vitamin C (mg)

FOOD	Wheatmeal (brown) bread large unsliced	Wheatmeal (brown) bread large sliced	White bread large unsliced
PORTION SIZE	medium slice (38g)	medium slice (36g)	medium slice (35g)
NUTRIENTS			
Energy (kcals)	85	76	85
Protein (g)	3.3	2.9	3.1
Total fat (g)	0.9	0.6	0.7
Saturated fat (g)	unknown	unknown	unknown
Mono-unsat. fat (g)	unknown	unknown	unknown
Poly-unsat. fat (g)	unknown	unknown	unknown
Carbohydrate (g)	16.9	15.9	17.7
Sugar (g)	0.9	1.3	1.0
Fibre (g)	1.3	1.3	0.5
Sodium (mg)	209	194	186
Potassium (mg)	68	58	39
Calcium (mg)	35	40	39
Magnesium (mg)	22	17	9
Phosphorus (mg)	61	50	32
Iron (mg)	0.87	0.76	0.63
Copper (mg)	0.08	0.04	0.05
Zinc (mg)	0.46	0.36	0.24
Selenium (μg)	unknown	unknown	10
Vitamin A (μg)	unknown	unknown	unknown
Vitamin D (μg)	nil	nil	nil
Vitamin E (mg)	trace	trace	trace
Vitamin B_1 (mg)	0.11	0.09	0.08
Vitamin B_2 (mg)	0.04	0.03	0.02
Niacin (mg)	1.14	1.08	0.63
Vitamin B_6 (mg)	0.06	0.04	0.02
Vitamin B_{12} (μg)	nil	nil	nil
Folate (μg)	17	12	10
Pantothenate (mg)	0.11	0.11	0.11
Biotin (μg)	1.1	1.1	0.3
Vitamin C (mg)	nil	nil	nil

White bread large sliced	**Wholemeal bread** large unsliced	**Wholemeal bread** large sliced	**FOOD**
medium slice (36g)	medium slice (38g)	medium slice (36g)	**PORTION SIZE**
			NUTRIENTS
78	82	74	Energy (kcals)
2.7	3.5	3.3	Protein (g)
0.5	0.9	0.7	Total fat (g)
0.1	0.2	unknown	Saturated fat (g)
0.1	0.2	unknown	Mono-unsat. fat (g)
0.1	0.3	unknown	Poly-unsat. fat (g)
16.8	15.8	14.5	Carbohydrate (g)
1.1	0.7	0.6	Sugar (g)
0.5	2.2	2.1	Fibre (g)
191	209	205	Sodium (mg)
36	87	83	Potassium (mg)
36	21	23	Calcium (mg)
7	29	28	Magnesium (mg)
28	76	72	Phosphorus (mg)
0.5	1.03	1.04	Iron (mg)
0.05	0.1	0.1	Copper (mg)
0.18	0.68	0.68	Zinc (mg)
10	13	13	Selenium (µg)
nil	nil	unknown	Vitamin A (µg)
nil	nil	nil	Vitamin D (µg)
trace	0.08	0.07	Vitamin E (mg)
0.07	0.13	0.14	Vitamin B_1 (mg)
0.02	0.03	0.03	Vitamin B_2 (mg)
0.54	1.56	1.48	Niacin (mg)
0.03	0.05	0.04	Vitamin B_6 (mg)
nil	nil	nil	Vitamin B_{12} (µg)
6	15	15	Folate (µg)
0.11	0.23	0.22	Pantothenate (mg)
0.4	2.3	2.2	Biotin (µg)
nil	nil	nil	Vitamin C (mg)

FOOD	All-Bran[2]	Alpen[5]	Alpen no added sugar[5]	Tropical Alpen[5]
PORTION SIZE	average (40g)	average (50g)	average (50g)	average (50g)
NUTRIENTS				
Energy (kcals)	108	182	178	184
Protein (g)	5.2	5	6	5.4
Total fat (g)	1.4	3.3	3.5	3.5
Saturated fat (g)	0.2	0.6	0.6	1.4
Mono-unsat. fat (g)	unknown	unknown	unknown	unknown
Poly-unsat. fat (g)	unknown	unknown	unknown	unknown
Carbohydrate (g)	18	33	30.6	32.7
Sugar (g)	7.0	10.7	8	12.4
Fibre (g)	11.2	3.8	4.5	3.8
Sodium (mg)	400	100	100	100
Potassium (mg)	unknown	unknown	unknown	unknown
Calcium (mg)	24	unknown	unknown	unknown
Magnesium (mg)	88	unknown	unknown	unknown
Phosphorus (mg)	280	unknown	unknown	unknown
Iron (mg)	3.5	unknown	unknown	unknown
Copper (mg)	unknown	unknown	unknown	unknown
Zinc (mg)	2.3	unknown	unknown	unknown
Selenium (μg)	unknown	unknown	unknown	unknown
Vitamin A (μg)	unknown	unknown	unknown	unknown
Vitamin D (μg)	1.2	unknown	unknown	unknown
Vitamin E (mg)	unknown	unknown	unknown	unknown
Vitamin B_1 (mg)	0.4	unknown	unknown	unknown
Vitamin B_2 (mg)	0.4	unknown	unknown	unknown
Niacin (mg)	4.5	unknown	unknown	unknown
Vitamin B_6 (mg)	0.5	unknown	unknown	unknown
Vitamin B_{12} (μg)	0.26	unknown	unknown	unknown
Folate (μg)	50	unknown	unknown	unknown
Pantothenate (mg)	unknown	unknown	unknown	unknown
Biotin (μg)	unknown	unknown	unknown	unknown
Vitamin C (mg)	unknown	unknown	unknown	unknown

Alpen Nutty Crunch[5]	Bran Buds[2]	Bran Flakes[2]	Clusters[3]	FOOD
average (50g)	average (40g)	average	average	**PORTION SIZE**
				NUTRIENTS
190	112	96	115	Energy (kcals)
4.7	5.2	3.0	3.1	Protein (g)
4.75	1.2	0.6	2.4	Total fat (g)
0.87	0.2	0.1	0.7	Saturated fat (g)
unknown	unknown	unknown	unknown	Mono-unsat. fat (g)
unknown	unknown	unknown	unknown	Poly-unsat. fat (g)
32.3	20	20	20.4	Carbohydrate (g)
9.75	9	7	7.35	Sugar (g)
4.25	10.4	4.8	2.5	Fibre (g)
200	200	300	150	Sodium (mg)
unknown	unknown	unknown	unknown	Potassium (mg)
unknown	24	12	unknown	Calcium (mg)
unknown	88	39	unknown	Magnesium (mg)
unknown	260	120	unknown	Phosphorus (mg)
unknown	3.5	3.5	unknown	Iron (mg)
unknown	unknown	unknown	unknown	Copper (mg)
unknown	2.4	0.8	unknown	Zinc (mg)
unknown	unknown	unknown	unknown	Selenium (μg)
unknown	unknown	unknown	unknown	Vitamin A (μg)
unknown	unknown	1.3	unknown	Vitamin D (μg)
unknown	unknown	unknown	unknown	Vitamin E (mg)
unknown	0.4	0.4	unknown	Vitamin B_1 (mg)
unknown	0.4	0.4	unknown	Vitamin B_2 (mg)
unknown	4.5	4.5	unknown	Niacin (mg)
unknown	0.5	0.5	unknown	Vitamin B_6 (mg)
unknown	0.26	0.2	unknown	Vitamin B_{12} (μg)
unknown	50	50	unknown	Folate (μg)
unknown	unknown	unknown	unknown	Pantothenate (mg)
unknown	unknown	unknown	unknown	Biotin (μg)
unknown	unknown	15	unknown	Vitamin C (mg)

FOOD	Cinnamon Toast Crunch[3]	Coco Pops[2]	Common Sense Oat Bran Flakes[2]	Cornflakes[1]
PORTION SIZE	average	average	average	average
NUTRIENTS				
Energy (kcals)	124	114	108	111
Protein (g)	1.38	1.5	3.3	2.4
Total fat (g)	3.27	0.3	1.5	0.2
Saturated fat (g)	0.6	0.1	0.3	0.1
Mono-unsat. fat (g)	unknown	unknown	unknown	unknown
Poly-unsat. fat (g)	unknown	unknown	unknown	unknown
Carbohydrate (g)	22.5	26	20	25
Sugar (g)	10.1	11	5	2
Fibre (g)	1.26	0.5	3.6	0.9
Sodium (mg)	200	200	200	300
Potassium (mg)	unknown	unknown	unknown	unknown
Calcium (mg)	unknown	3	15	2
Magnesium (mg)	unknown	15	33	3
Phosphorus (mg)	unknown	36	105	15
Iron (mg)	unknown	2.4	2.4	2.4
Copper (mg)	unknown	unknown	unknown	unknown
Zinc (mg)	unknown	0.3	0.7	0.1
Selenium (μg)	unknown	unknown	unknown	unknown
Vitamin A (μg)	unknown	unknown	unknown	unknown
Vitamin D (μg)	unknown	unknown	unknown	unknown
Vitamin E (mg)	unknown	unknown	unknown	unknown
Vitamin B_1 (mg)	unknown	0.4	0.4	0.4
Vitamin B_2 (mg)	unknown	0.4	0.4	0.4
Niacin (mg)	unknown	4.5	4.5	4.5
Vitamin B_6 (mg)	unknown	0.5	0.5	0.5
Vitamin B_{12} (μg)	unknown	0.26	0.26	0.26
Folate (μg)	unknown	50	50	100
Pantothenate (mg)	unknown	unknown	unknown	unknown
Biotin (μg)	unknown	unknown	unknown	unknown
Vitamin C (mg)	unknown	unknown	unknown	unknown

Country Store[2]	Crunchy Bran[5]	Crunchy Nut Cornflakes[2]	Fibre 1[3]	FOOD
average (40g)	average (40g)	average	average (40g)	PORTION SIZE
				NUTRIENTS
144	121	117	105	Energy (kcals)
3.2	4.6	2.1	4.3	Protein (g)
1.8	1.9	1.1	1.0	Total fat (g)
0.4	0.4	0.2	0.1	Saturated fat (g)
unknown	unknown	unknown	unknown	Mono-unsat. fat (g)
unknown	unknown	unknown	unknown	Poly-unsat. fat (g)
28	21.3	25	19.6	Carbohydrate (g)
9	7.4	10	6.3	Sugar (g)
2.4	9.1	0.8	12.7	Fibre (g)
200	300	200	200	Sodium (mg)
unknown	unknown	unknown	unknown	Potassium (mg)
24	unknown	3	unknown	Calcium (mg)
28	unknown	6	unknown	Magnesium (mg)
100	unknown	15	unknown	Phosphorus (mg)
2.8	4.8	2.4	unknown	Iron (mg)
unknown	unknown	unknown	unknown	Copper (mg)
0.6	unknown	0.1	unknown	Zinc (mg)
unknown	unknown	unknown	unknown	Selenium (μg)
unknown	unknown	unknown	unknown	Vitamin A (μg)
unknown	unknown	unknown	unknown	Vitamin D (μg)
unknown	unknown	unknown	unknown	Vitamin E (mg)
0.2	0.5	0.4	unknown	Vitamin B_1 (mg)
0.4	0.5	0.4	unknown	Vitamin B_2 (mg)
3.6	6.1	4.5	unknown	Niacin (mg)
trace	0.7	0.5	unknown	Vitamin B_6 (mg)
trace	0.4	0.26	unknown	Vitamin B_{12} (μg)
trace	68	50	unknown	Folate (μg)
unknown	2.0	unknown	unknown	Pantothenate (mg)
unknown	unknown	unknown	unknown	Biotin (μg)
unknown	unknown	unknown	unknown	Vitamin C (mg)

FOOD	Frosted Chex[5]	Frosties[2]	Fruit 'n' Fibre[2]	Golden Grahams[3]
PORTION SIZE	average	average	average (40g)	average
NUTRIENTS				
Energy (kcals)	114	114	140	114
Protein (g)	1.7	1.5	3.2	1.6
Total fat (g)	0.5	0.2	2.4	1.0
Saturated fat (g)	0.1	trace	1.2	0.7
Mono-unsat. fat (g)	unknown	unknown	unknown	unknown
Poly-unsat. fat (g)	unknown	unknown	unknown	unknown
Carbohydrate (g)	25.7	26	27	24.4
Sugar (g)	9.7	11	8	10.2
Fibre (g)	0.7	0.6	3.6	0.9
Sodium (mg)	200	200	200	200
Potassium (mg)	unknown	unknown	unknown	unknown
Calcium (mg)	unknown	2	16	unknown
Magnesium (mg)	unknown	3	28	unknown
Phosphorus (mg)	unknown	12	96	unknown
Iron (mg)	3.6	2.4	3.5	unknown
Copper (mg)	unknown	unknown	unknown	unknown
Zinc (mg)	unknown	0.1	0.6	unknown
Selenium (μg)	unknown	unknown	unknown	unknown
Vitamin A (μg)	unknown	unknown	unknown	unknown
Vitamin D (μg)	unknown	unknown	unknown	unknown
Vitamin E (mg)	unknown	unknown	unknown	unknown
Vitamin B_1 (mg)	0.4	0.4	0.4	unknown
Vitamin B_2 (mg)	0.4	0.4	0.4	unknown
Niacin (mg)	4.6	4.5	4.5	unknown
Vitamin B_6 (mg)	0.5	0.5	0.5	unknown
Vitamin B_{12} (μg)	0.3	0.26	0.26	unknown
Folate (μg)	51.0	50	50	unknown
Pantothenate (mg)	1.5	unknown	unknown	unknown
Biotin (μg)	unknown	unknown	unknown	unknown
Vitamin C (mg)	unknown	unknown	unknown	unknown

Grapenuts	Honey Nut Loops[2]	Muesli Swiss-style	Multi Cheerios[3]	FOOD
average (40g)	average (50g)	average	average	**PORTION SIZE**
				NUTRIENTS
138	111	182	110	Energy (kcals)
4.2	2.1	5.3	2.3	Protein (g)
0.2	1.2	3.0	1.1	Total fat (g)
unknown	0.2	unknown	0.4	Saturated fat (g)
unknown	unknown	unknown	unknown	Mono-unsat. fat (g)
unknown	unknown	unknown	unknown	Poly-unsat. fat (g)
32.0	23	35.5	22.7	Carbohydrate (g)
4.8	11	11.9	6.7	Sugar (g)
unknown	1.8	3.0	1.8	Fibre (g)
236	200	190	200	Sodium (mg)
124	unknown	220	unknown	Potassium (mg)
15	15	60	unknown	Calcium (mg)
38	15	43	unknown	Magnesium (mg)
100	60	140	unknown	Phosphorus (mg)
3.8	2.4	2.8	unknown	Iron (mg)
0.18	unknown	0.05	unknown	Copper (mg)
1.68	0.4	1.25	unknown	Zinc (mg)
unknown	unknown	unknown	unknown	Selenium (µg)
unknown	unknown	unknown	unknown	Vitamin A (µg)
1.76	unknown	nil	unknown	Vitamin D (µg)
0.68	unknown	1.6	unknown	Vitamin E (mg)
0.52	0.4	0.25	unknown	Vitamin B_1 (mg)
0.6	0.4	0.35	unknown	Vitamin B_2 (mg)
7.04	4.5	3.25	unknown	Niacin (mg)
0.72	0.5	0.8	unknown	Vitamin B_6 (mg)
2.0	0.26	nil	unknown	Vitamin B_{12} (µg)
140	50	70	unknown	Folate (µg)
unknown	unknown	0.6	unknown	Pantothenate (mg)
unknown	unknown	7.5	unknown	Biotin (µg)
nil	unknown	trace	unknown	Vitamin C (mg)

FOOD	Nesquick[3]	Porridge Oats	Raisin Wheats[2]	Ready Brek[5]
PORTION SIZE	average	medium (30g raw oats)	average (40g)	average (30g dry cereal)
NUTRIENTS				
Energy (kcals)	114	120	128	107
Protein (g)	1.5	3.7	3.6	3.5
Total fat (g)	0.7	2.6	0.6	2.5
Saturated fat (g)	0.4	unknown	0.1	0.6
Mono-unsat. fat (g)	unknown	unknown	unknown	unknown
Poly-unsat. fat (g)	unknown	unknown	unknown	unknown
Carbohydrate (g)	25.4	21.8	28	17.6
Sugar (g)	11.9	trace	7	0.5
Fibre (g)	0.8	2.0	3.6	2.7
Sodium (mg)	100	10	10	0.1
Potassium (mg)	unknown	111	unknown	unknown
Calcium (mg)	unknown	17	16	360
Magnesium (mg)	unknown	33	28	unknown
Phosphorus (mg)	unknown	114	100	unknown
Iron (mg)	unknown	1.23	2.4	3.6
Copper (mg)	unknown	0.07	unknown	unknown
Zinc (mg)	unknown	0.99	0.6	unknown
Selenium (µg)	unknown	1	unknown	unknown
Vitamin A (µg)	unknown	unknown	unknown	unknown
Vitamin D (µg)	unknown	nil	unknown	unknown
Vitamin E (mg)	unknown	0.51	unknown	unknown
Vitamin B_1 (mg)	unknown	0.15	0.4	0.4
Vitamin B_2 (mg)	unknown	0.03	0.4	0.4
Niacin (mg)	unknown	0.3	4.5	4.6
Vitamin B_6 (mg)	unknown	0.04	0.5	0.5
Vitamin B_{12} (µg)	unknown	nil	0.26	0.3
Folate (µg)	unknown	18	50	51.0
Pantothenate (mg)	unknown	0.3	unknown	1.5
Biotin (µg)	unknown	6.0	unknown	unknown
Vitamin C (mg)	unknown	nil	unknown	unknown

Rice Krispies[2]	Ricicles[2]	Shredded Wheat[3]	Shreddies[3]	FOOD
average	average	two	average (45g)	PORTION SIZE
				NUTRIENTS
111	114	156	158	Energy (kcals)
1.8	1.4	4.9	4.4	Protein (g)
0.3	0.2	0.9	0.8	Total fat (g)
0.1	0.1	0.1	0.1	Saturated fat (g)
unknown	unknown	unknown	unknown	Mono-unsat. fat (g)
unknown	unknown	unknown	unknown	Poly-unsat. fat (g)
26	27	31.8	33.3	Carbohydrate (g)
3	11	0.2	6.8	Sugar (g)
0.5	0.2	4.2	3.7	Fibre (g)
300	200	trace	200	Sodium (mg)
unknown	unknown	unknown	unknown	Potassium (mg)
3	2	unknown	unknown	Calcium (mg)
15	9	unknown	unknown	Magnesium (mg)
42	27	unknown	unknown	Phosphorus (mg)
2.4	2.4	unknown	unknown	Iron (mg)
unknown	unknown	unknown	unknown	Copper (mg)
0.3	0.2	unknown	unknown	Zinc (mg)
unknown	unknown	unknown	unknow	Selenium (µg)
unknown	unknown	unknown	unknown	Vitamin A (µg)
1.3	unknown	unknown	unknown	Vitamin D (µg)
unknown	unknown	unknown	unknown	Vitamin E (mg)
0.4	0.4	unknown	unknown	Vitamin B_1 (mg)
0.4	0.4	unknown	unknown	Vitamin B_2 (mg)
4.5	4.5	unknown	unknown	Niacin (mg)
0.5	0.5	unknown	unknown	Vitamin B_6 (mg)
0.26	0.26	unknown	unknown	Vitamin B_{12} (µg)
100	50	unknown	unknown	Folate (µg)
unknown	unknown	unknown	unknown	Pantothenate (mg)
unknown	unknown	unknown	unknown	Biotin (µg)
unknown	unknown	unknown	unknown	Vitamin C (mg)

FOOD	Frosted Shreddies[3]	Coco Shreddies[3]	Special K[2]	Start[2]
PORTION SIZE	average (45g)	average (45g)	average	average (40g)
NUTRIENTS				
Energy (kcals)	163	163	111	148
Protein (g)	3.2	3.6	4.5	2.8
Total fat (g)	0.6	0.8	0.3	1.0
Saturated fat (g)	0.09	0.1	0.2	0.2
Mono-unsat. fat (g)	unknown	unknown	unknown	unknown
Poly-unsat. fat (g)	unknown	unknown	unknown	unknown
Carbohydrate (g)	36.2	35.3	23	32
Sugar (g)	16.6	15	5	10
Fibre (g)	2.7	2.9	0.8	2.4
Sodium (mg)	100	100	300	200
Potassium (mg)	unknown	unknown	unknown	unknown
Calcium (mg)	unknown	unknown	18	20
Magnesium (mg)	unknown	unknown	15	24
Phosphorus (mg)	unknown	unknown	60	80
Iron (mg)	unknown	unknown	7.0	4.7
Copper (mg)	unknown	unknown	unknown	unknown
Zinc (mg)	unknown	unknown	0.5	5.0
Selenium (µg)	unknown	unknown	unknown	unknown
Vitamin A (µg)	unknown	unknown	unknown	unknown
Vitamin D (µg)	unknown	unknown	2.5	1.7
Vitamin E (mg)	unknown	unknown	unknown	3.3
Vitamin B_1 (mg)	unknown	unknown	0.7	0.5
Vitamin B_2 (mg)	unknown	unknown	0.8	0.5
Niacin (mg)	unknown	unknown	9.0	6.0
Vitamin B_6 (mg)	unknown	unknown	1.0	0.7
Vitamin B_{12} (µg)	unknown	unknown	0.51	0.34
Folate (µg)	unknown	unknown	100	67
Pantothenate (mg)	unknown	unknown	unknown	unknown
Biotin (µg)	unknown	unknown	unknown	
Vitamin C (mg)	unknown	unknown	30	20

Sugar Puffs	Sultana Bran[2]	Sustain[2]	Weetabix[5]	FOOD
average (20g)	average (40g)	average (40g)	two	**PORTION SIZE**
				NUTRIENTS
65	124	144	127	Energy (kcals)
1.2	3.6	3.6	4.3	Protein (g)
0.2	0.8	1.2	1.0	Total fat (g)
unknown	0.1	0.6	0.3	Saturated fat (g)
unknown	unknown	unknown	unknown	Mono-unsat. fat (g)
unknown	unknown	unknown	unknown	Poly-unsat. fat (g)
16.9	26	29	25.2	Carbohydrate (g)
11.3	12	8	1.8	Sugar (g)
0.6	5.2	2.8	4.1	Fibre (g)
2000	300	100	unknown	Sodium (mg)
32	unknown	unknown	unknown	Potassium (mg)
3	16	12	unknown	Calcium (mg)
11	44	20	unknown	Magnesium (mg)
28	140	80	unknown	Phosphorus (mg)
0.42	3.5	3.5	4.5	Iron (mg)
0.05	unknown	unknown	unknown	Copper (mg)
0.3	0.9	3.8	unknown	Zinc (mg)
unknown	unknown	unknown	unknown	Selenium (μg)
unknown	unknown	136	unknown	Vitamin A (μg)
nil	1.2	1.2	nil	Vitamin D (μg)
0.07	unknown	2.5	unknown	Vitamin E (mg)
trace	0.4	0.4	0.4	Vitamin B_1 (mg)
0.01	0.4	0.4	0.5	Vitamin B_2 (mg)
0.5	4.5	4.5	5.7	Niacin (mg)
0.01	0.5	0.5	unknown	Vitamin B_6 (mg)
nil	0.26	0.26	nil	Vitamin B_{12} (μg)
2	50	50	63.8	Folate (μg)
unknown	unknown	unknown	unknown	Pantothenate (mg)
unknown	unknown	unknown	unknown	Biotin (μg)
nil	15	trace	nil	Vitamin C (mg)

FOOD	Cornflour	Couscous cooked	Custard Powder raw	Dumplings
PORTION SIZE	heaped tablespoon	average	heaped tablespoon	one average
NUTRIENTS				
Energy (kcals)	106	341	106	146
Protein (g)	0.2	8.5	0.2	2.0
Total fat (g)	0.2	1.5	0.2	8.2
Saturated fat (g)	unknown	unknown	unknown	4.5
Mono-unsat. fat (g)	unknown	unknown	unknown	2.9
Poly-unsat. fat (g)	unknown	unknown	unknown	0.3
Carbohydrate (g)	27.6	76.9	27.6	17.1
Sugar (g)	trace	unknown	trace	0.3
Fibre (g)	trace	unknown	trace	0.6
Sodium (mg)	16	unknown	96	280
Potassium (mg)	18	unknown	18	31
Calcium (mg)	5	29	5	36
Magnesium (mg)	2	unknown	2	6
Phosphorus (mg)	12	7.5	12	84
Iron (mg)	0.42	unknown	0.42	0.42
Copper (mg)	0.04	unknown	0.02	0.05
Zinc (mg)	0.09	unknown	0.09	0.14
Selenium (µg)	unknown	unknown	unknown	1
Vitamin A (µg)	unknown	trace	unknown	6
Vitamin D (µg)	nil	nil	nil	trace
Vitamin E (mg)	trace	unknown	trace	0.06
Vitamin B_1 (mg)	trace	0.3	trace	0.04
Vitamin B_2 (mg)	trace	0.09	trace	0.01
Niacin (mg)	trace	1.2	trace	0.21
Vitamin B_6 (mg)	trace	unknown	trace	0.02
Vitamin B_{12} (µg)	nil	nil	nil	trace
Folate (µg)	trace	unknown	trace	2
Pantothenate (mg)	trace	unknown	trace	0.07
Biotin (µg)	trace	unknown	trace	trace
Vitamin C (mg)	nil	nil	nil	nil

Flour white	Flour wholemeal	Macaroni boiled	Macaroni in cheese sauce	FOOD
heaped tablespoon	heaped tablespoon	medium average	medium average	**PORTION SIZE**
				NUTRIENTS
102	93	198	292	Energy (kcals)
2.8	3.7	6.9	16.1	Protein (g)
0.45	0.6	1.1	23.8	Total fat (g)
unknown	0.1	0.2	12.3	Saturated fat (g)
unknown	0.1	trace	7.5	Mono-unsat. fat (g)
unknown	0.3	0.5	2.6	Poly-unsat. fat (g)
23	19.2	42.5	29.9	Carbohydrate (g)
0.45	0.6	0.7	6.4	Sugar (g)
0.9	2.7	2.1	1.1	Fibre (g)
1.5	1.5	2	682	Sodium (mg)
45	102	58	242	Potassium (mg)
42	12	14	374	Calcium (mg)
6	36	32	37	Magnesium (mg)
33	96	97	330	Phosphorus (mg)
0.6	1.17	1.15	0.88	Iron (mg)
0.04	0.13	0.21	0.11	Copper (mg)
0.18	0.87	1.15	1.76	Zinc (mg)
1.5	16	9	9	Selenium (µg)
unknown	nil	nil	269	Vitamin A (µg)
nil	nil	nil	0.79	Vitamin D (µg)
0.09	0.42	trace	0.99	Vitamin E (mg)
0.09	0.13	0.07	0.09	Vitamin B_1 (mg)
0.01	0.03	trace	0.35	Vitamin B_2 (mg)
0.5	1.7	1.15	0.66	Niacin (mg)
0.04	0.15	0.02	3.74	Vitamin B_6 (mg)
nil	nil	nil	0.9	Vitamin B_{12} (µg)
6	16.5	7	11	Folate (µg)
0.09	0.24	trace	0.57	Pantothenate (mg)
0.3	2.1	trace	3.5	Biotin (µg)
nil	nil	nil	trace	Vitamin C (mg)

FOOD	Noodles egg, boiled	Oatmeal quick cook raw	Pasta shapes in tomato sauce[1]	Pot Noodles
PORTION SIZE	one packet made up	one tablespoon	one small tin	one snack pot
Nutrients				
Energy (kcals)	174	56	135	309
Protein (g)	6.2	1.7	4.3	9.9
Total fat (g)	1.4	1.4	0.8	9.3
Saturated fat (g)	0.3	0.2	trace	unknown
Mono-unsat. fat (g)	0.6	0.5	0.2	unknown
Poly-unsat. fat (g)	0.3	0.6	0.4	unknown
Carbohydrate (g)	36.4	9.9	29	50.1
Sugar (g)	0.6	0.2	11.3	6.9
Fibre (g)	1.7	1.1	1.5	unknown
Sodium (mg)	42	1	832	1110
Potassium (mg)	64	53	425	540
Calcium (mg)	14	8	25	153
Magnesium (mg)	22	17	34	66
Phosphorus (mg)	87	57	75	177
Iron (mg)	0.84	0.57	2.5	3.6
Copper (mg)	0.17	0.07	0.23	0.3
Zinc (mg)	0.84	0.5	0.6	1.2
Selenium (μg)	unknown	trace	nil	unknown
Vitamin A (μg)	6	nil	69	unknown
Vitamin D (μg)	trace	nil	nil	nil
Vitamin E (mg)	unknown	0.22	1.8	unknown
Vitamin B_1 (mg)	0.03	0.13	0.25	unknown
Vitamin B_2 (mg)	0.03	0.01	0.3	unknown
Niacin (mg)	0.56	0.12	3.2	unknown
Vitamin B_6 (mg)	0.03	0.05	0.1	unknown
Vitamin B_{12} (μg)	trace	nil	nil	nil
Folate (μg)	3	9	12.9	unknown
Pantothenate (mg)	unknown	0.18	0.2	unknown
Biotin (μg)	unknown	3.2	1.2	unknown
Vitamin C (mg)	nil	nil	4	nil

Rice brown boiled	Rice egg fried	Rice packet savoury	Rice white	FOOD
medium average	medium average	medium average	medium average	PORTION SIZE
				NUTRIENTS
254	374	256	248	Energy (kcals)
4.7	7.6	5.2	4.7	Protein (g)
2.0	19.1	6.3	2.3	Total fat (g)
unknown	2.7	2.0	0.5	Saturated fat (g)
unknown	7.4	2.3	0.5	Mono-unsat. fat (g)
unknown	7.6	1.1	0.9	Poly-unsat. fat (g)
57.8	46.3	47.3	55.6	Carbohydrate (g)
0.9	1.6	2.2	trace	Sugar (g)
1.4	0.7	2.5	0.2	Fibre (g)
2	49	882	2	Sodium (mg)
178	130	198	97	Potassium (mg)
7	23	45	32	Calcium (mg)
77	9	27	20	Magnesium (mg)
216	121	121	97	Phosphorus (mg)
0.9	0.9	0.9	0.36	Iron (mg)
0.59	0.13	0.09	0.23	Copper (mg)
1.26	1.26	0.72	1.26	Zinc (mg)
trace	9	unknown	7	Selenium (µg)
unknown	63	unknown	nil	Vitamin A (µg)
nil	0.56	trace	nil	Vitamin D (µg)
0.54	0.36	unknown	trace	Vitamin E (mg)
0.25	0.05	0.18	0.02	Vitamin B_1 (mg)
0.04	0.14	0.02	trace	Vitamin B_2 (mg)
2.34	0.54	1.98	1.62	Niacin (mg)
unknown	0.11	0.13	0.13	Vitamin B_6 (mg)
nil	0.7	trace	nil	Vitamin B_{12} (µg)
18	14	7	7	Folate (µg)
unknown	0.7	unknown	0.18	Pantothenate (mg)
unknown	8.1	unknown	1.8	Biotin (µg)
nil	trace	nil	nil	Vitamin C (mg)

FOOD	Salad pasta homemade	Salad rice homemade	Spaghetti boiled
PORTION SIZE	one tub	one tub	medium average
NUTRIENTS			
Energy (kcals)	254	332	229
Protein (g)	5.2	6.2	7.9
Total fat (g)	14.8	15	1.5
Saturated fat (g)	2.2	2.2	unknown
Mono-unsat. fat (g)	3.2	6	unknown
Poly-unsat. fat (g)	8.6	5.8	unknown
Carbohydrate (g)	26.6	46.2	48.8
Sugar (g)	4.4	9.6	1.1
Fibre (g)	3.2	1.4	2.6
Sodium (mg)	102	380	trace
Potassium (mg)	168	360	53
Calcium (mg)	28	42	15
Magnesium (mg)	22	48	33
Phosphorus (mg)	74	148	97
Iron (mg)	1.2	2	1.1
Copper (mg)	0.12	0.4	0.22
Zinc (mg)	0.8	1.6	1.1
Selenium (µg)	trace	8	trace
Vitamin A (µg)	469	45	unknown
Vitamin D (µg)	trace	nil	nil
Vitamin E (mg)	3.9	2.38	trace
Vitamin B_1 (mg)	0.8	0.1	0.02
Vitamin B_2 (mg)	0.04	0.04	0.02
Niacin (mg)	0.8	1.8	1.1
Vitamin B_6 (mg)	0.18	0.24	0.04
Vitamin B_{12} (µg)	trace	nil	nil
Folate (µg)	32	36	9
Pantothenate (mg)	unknown	0.28	trace
Biotin (µg)	unknown	2.4	trace
Vitamin C (mg)	42	24	nil

Spaghetti canned in tomato sauce	Stuffing packet mix reconstituted	Yorkshire Pudding	FOOD
small can	one helping	one individual	PORTION SIZE
			NUTRIENTS
134	49	166	Energy (kcals)
4.0	1.4	5.3	Protein (g)
0.8	0.8	7.9	Total fat (g)
0.2	0.4	4.2	Saturated fat (g)
0.2	0.3	2.9	Mono-unsat. fat (g)
0.4	trace	0.5	Poly-unsat. fat (g)
29.6	9.6	19.8	Carbohydrate (g)
11.6	0.6	3.0	Sugar (g)
1.5	0.6	0.7	Fibre (g)
882	210	472	Sodium (mg)
231	35	128	Potassium (mg)
25	140	104	Calcium (mg)
21	6	15	Magnesium (mg)
61	19	96	Phosphorus (mg)
0.63	0.75	0.72	Iron (mg)
0.13	0.03	0.04	Copper (mg)
0.63	0.1	0.48	Zinc (mg)
unknown	unknown	2	Selenium (µg)
unknown	nil	53	Vitamin A (µg)
nil	nil	0.24	Vitamin D (µg)
unknown	unknown	0.3	Vitamin E (mg)
0.15	0.16	0.08	Vitamin B_1 (mg)
0.02	0.11	0.13	Vitamin B_2 (mg)
1.26	0.25	0.4	Niacin (mg)
0.15	unknown	0.06	Vitamin B_6 (mg)
trace	nil	0.8	Vitamin B_{12} (µg)
11	unknown	7	Folate (µg)
trace	unknown	0.32	Pantothenate (mg)
trace	unknown	4.0	Biotin (µg)
trace	nil	1	Vitamin C (µg)

FOOD	Boiled potatoes old	Boiled potatoes new	Potato cake fried in oil	Croquette potatoes fried in oil
PORTION SIZE	average	average	one	one
NUTRIENTS				
Energy (kcals)	126	131	168	193
Protein (g)	3.1	2.6	3.1	3.3
Total fat (g)	0.2	0.5	6.8	11.8
Saturated fat (g)	trace	0.2	1.7	1.5
Mono-unsat. fat (g)	trace	trace	2.2	2.9
Poly-unsat. fat (g)	0.2	0.2	2.5	6.8
Carbohydrate (g)	29.8	31.1	25.1	19.4
Sugar (g)	1.2	1.9	1	0.4
Fibre (g)	2.1	1.9	1.3	1.2
Sodium (mg)	12	16	136	378
Potassium (mg)	490	438	192	324
Calcium (mg)	9	9	39	40
Magnesium (mg)	25	21	13	17
Phosphorus (mg)	54	49	46	44
Iron (mg)	0.7	0.53	0.64	0.81
Copper (mg)	0.12	0.1	0.07	0.07
Zinc (mg)	0.53	0.17	0.32	0.27
Selenium (µg)	2	2	2	unknown
Vitamin A (µg)	trace	trace	19.5	unknown
Vitamin D (µg)	nil	nil	trace	nil
Vitamin E (mg)	0.1	0.1	1.28	unknown
Vitamin B_1 (mg)	0.31	0.23	0.13	0.07
Vitamin B_2 (mg)	0.02	0.04	0.02	0.07
Niacin (mg)	0.88	0.7	0.64	1.26
Vitamin B_6 (mg)	0.58	0.58	0.16	0.2
Vitamin B_{12} (µg)	nil	nil	trace	nil
Folate (µg)	46	33	8	2
Pantothenate (mg)	0.66	0.66	0.29	unknown
Biotin (µg)	0.5	0.5	0.5	unknown
Vitamin C (mg)	11	16	2	2

Chips French fries – retail e.g. burger bar	Chips fresh, retail e.g. fish and chip shop	Chips frozen, straight cut cooked at home	Chips home-made	FOOD
restaurant serving	chip shop serving	average	average	**PORTION SIZE**
				NUTRIENTS
308	502	450	312	Energy (kcals)
3.6	6.7	6.8	6.4	Protein (g)
17	26	22.3	11.1	Total fat (g)
6.4	2.3	2	1.0	Saturated fat (g)
7.6	13	11.1	5.4	Mono-unsat. fat (g)
2.3	9.4	8.1	4.0	Poly-unsat. fat (g)
37.4	64.1	59.4	49.7	Carbohydrate (g)
1.4	3.6	1.2	1	Sugar (g)
2.3	4.6	4.0	3.6	Fibre (g)
341	74	48	20	Sodium (mg)
715	1386	1172	1089	Potassium (mg)
15	23	25	18	Calcium (mg)
29	65	54	51	Magnesium (mg)
143	130	198	102	Phosphorus (mg)
1.1	1.89	1.49	1.32	Iron (mg)
0.19	0.29	0.4	0.23	Copper (mg)
0.55	1.26	0.99	0.99	Zinc (mg)
unknown	4	3	3	Selenium (µg)
trace	trace	trace	trace	Vitamin A (µg)
nil	nil	nil	nil	Vitamin D (µg)
1.1	unknown	unknown	8.09	Vitamin E (mg)
0.09	0.17	0.26	0.4	Vitamin B_1 (mg)
0.05	0.02	0.13	0.03	Vitamin B_2 (mg)
2.53	1.47	3.46	1.15	Niacin (mg)
0.4	0.67	1.76	0.53	Vitamin B_6 (mg)
nil	nil	nil	nil	Vitamin B_{12} (µg)
unknown	unknown	50	71	Folate (µg)
unknown	0.52	unknown	0.41	Pantothenate (mg)
unknown	0.8	unknown	0.7	Biotin (µg)
4	19	26	15	Vitamin C (mg)

FOOD	**Jacket potato**	**Jacket potato**	**Mashed potatoes** homemade with butter	**Mashed potatoes** instant powder made with water
PORTION SIZE	one medium with skin	one medium without skin	one scoop	one scoop
NUTRIENTS				
Energy (kcals)	245	123	62	34
Protein (g)	7.0	3.5	1.1	0.9
Total fat (g)	0.4	0.2	9.3	0.1
Saturated fat (g)	trace	trace	1.7	trace
Mono-unsat. fat (g)	trace	trace	0.6	trace
Poly-unsat. fat (g)	0.2	0.2	0.1	0.1
Carbohydrate (g)	57.1	28.8	9.3	8.1
Sugar (g)	2.2	1.1	0.6	0.4
Fibre (g)	4.9	2.2	0.7	0.6
Sodium (mg)	22	11	29	120
Potassium (mg)	1134	576	156	156
Calcium (mg)	20	11	7	8
Magnesium (mg)	58	29	8	7
Phosphorus (mg)	122	64	20	25
Iron (mg)	1.26	0.64	0.24	0.24
Copper (mg)	0.25	0.13	0.04	0.02
Zinc (mg)	0.9	0.48	0.18	0.12
Selenium (µg)	4	2	1	unknown
Vitamin A (µg)	trace	trace	28	0.3
Vitamin D (µg)	nil	nil	0.23	nil
Vitamin E (mg)	0.2	0.1	0.27	0.03
Vitamin B_1 (mg)	0.67	0.34	0.1	0.01
Vitamin B_2 (mg)	0.04	0.02	0.01	0.02
Niacin (mg)	1.98	0.96	0.3	0.72
Vitamin B_6 (mg)	0.97	0.5	0.18	0.09
Vitamin B_{12} (µg)	nil	nil	trace	nil
Folate (µg)	79	40	14	1
Pantothenate (mg)	0.83	0.42	0.22	unknown
Biotin (µg)	0.9	0.5	0.2	unknown
Vitamin C (mg)	25	13	3	14

Roast potato in oil	**Potato salad** retail	**Sweet potato** baked	**Potato waffles** frozen, baked	**FOOD**
average	one tub	two medium	one	**PORTION SIZE**
				NUTRIENTS
298	244	150	90	Energy (kcals)
5.8	1.3	2.1	1.4	Protein (g)
9	22.5	0.5	3.7	Total fat (g)
0.8	3.3	0.3	0.4	Saturated fat (g)
4.4	5.2	trace	0.9	Mono-unsat. fat (g)
3.2	13.1	0.1	2.1	Poly-unsat. fat (g)
51.8	9.7	36.3	13.6	Carbohydrate (g)
1.2	0.9	18.9	0.3	Sugar (g)
3.6	0.7	4.3	1	Fibre (g)
18	136	68	194	Sodium (mg)
1140	153	624	216	Potassium (mg)
16	5	40	14	Calcium (mg)
50	8	30	9	Magnesium (mg)
110	25	85	54	Phosphorus (mg)
1.4	0.34	1.17	0.22	Iron (mg)
0.22	0.04	0.23	trace	Copper (mg)
0.8	0.17	0.52	0.14	Zinc (mg)
2	unknown	1	unknown	Selenium (μg)
trace	31	1113	trace	Vitamin A (μg)
nil	0.09	nil	nil	Vitamin D (μg)
unknown	5.68	7.75	unknown	Vitamin E (mg)
0.46	0.1	0.12	unknown	Vitamin B_1 (mg)
0.04	0.03	trace	unknown	Vitamin B_2 (mg)
1.4	0.25	0.65	unknown	Niacin (mg)
0.62	0.18	0.09	unknown	Vitamin B_6 (mg)
nil	0.2	nil	nil	Vitamin B_{12} (μg)
72	15	12	unknown	Folate (μg)
0.5	unknown	0.77	unknown	Pantothenate (mg)
0.6	unknown	unknown	unknown	Biotin (μg)
16	3	30	16	Vitamin C (mg)

Segment Two

Fruit and vegetables

As you can see from the plate model below, about one third of all the food you eat should come from the fruit and vegetable group. Current recommendations say we all need to eat five portions of fruit and vegetables daily, to make sure we get enough vitamins, minerals and fibre. Some vegetables, such as spinach, are much more nutritious than others, but it is important to conserve as much of their nutritional value as possible by buying them fresh, storing them correctly and either eating them raw or cooked in a way which preserves their nutritional value. The values for cooked vegetables in this section are for vegetables cooked without added salt except where it is is stated that salt was added to the cooking water. All fried vegetables are fried in blended vegetable oil unless otherwise stated.

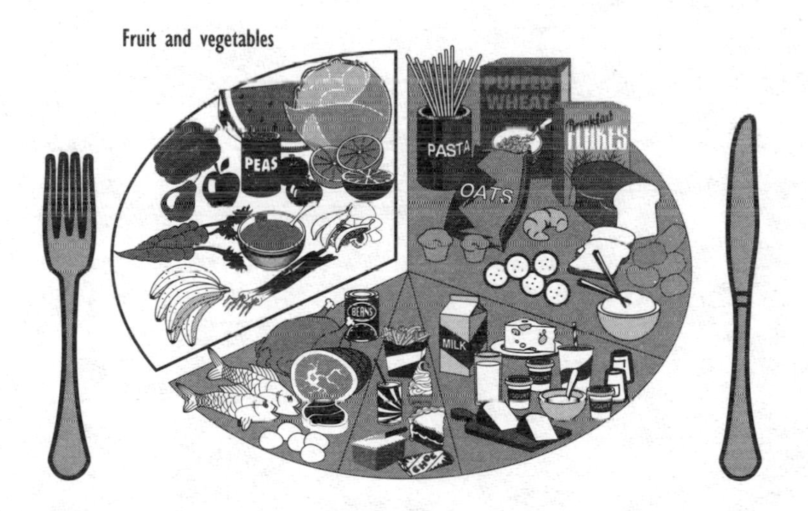

FOOD	Apple eating	Apple baked with sugar	Apple stewed with sugar	Apricot raw
PORTION SIZE	one	one	average	one
NUTRIENTS				
Energy (kcals)	47	141	81	12
Protein (g)	0.4	0.9	0.3	0.4
Total fat (g)	0.1	0.2	0.1	trace
Saturated fat (g)	trace	trace	trace	trace
Mono-unsat. fat (g)	trace	trace	trace	trace
Poly-unsat. fat (g)	0.1	trace	0.1	trace
Carbohydrate (g)	11.8	36.5	21	2.9
Sugar (g)	11.8	36.5	21	2.9
Fibre (g)	1.8	3.4	1.3	0.7
Sodium (mg)	3	6	4	1
Potassium (mg)	120	184	154	108
Calcium (mg)	4	15	4	6
Magnesium (mg)	5	8	3	4
Phosphorus (mg)	11	17	8	8
Iron (mg)	0.1	0.38	0.11	0.2
Copper (mg)	0.02	0.04	0.02	0.02
Zinc (mg)	0.1	unknown	trace	0.04
Selenium (µg)	trace	trace	trace	trace
Vitamin A (µg)	3	5	2.5	27
Vitamin D (µg)	nil	nil	nil	nil
Vitamin E (mg)	0.59	1.03	0.24	unknown
Vitamin B_1 (mg)	0.03	0.04	0.1	0.02
Vitamin B_2 (mg)	0.02	0.04	0.1	0.02
Niacin (mg)	0.1	0.19	0.11	0.2
Vitamin B_6 (mg)	0.06	0.08	0.05	0.03
Vitamin B_{12} (µg)	nil	nil	nil	nil
Folate (µg)	1	4	trace	2
Pantothenate (mg)	trace	trace	trace	0.1
Biotin (µg)	1.2	2.1	0.9	unknown
Vitamin C (mg)	6	29	11	2

Apricot dried	Avocado pear	Banana	Banana chips	FOOD
one	half	one medium	ten	**PORTION SIZE**
				NUTRIENTS
15	143	95	66	Energy (kcals)
0.4	1.4	1.2	0.1	Protein (g)
0.1	14.6	0.3	4.1	Total fat (g)
unknown	3.1	0.1	unknown	Saturated fat (g)
unknown	9.1	trace	unknown	Mono-unsat. fat (g)
unknown	1.7	0.1	unknown	Poly-unsat. fat (g)
3.5	1.4	23.2	7.8	Carbohydrate (g)
3.5	0.4	20.9	2.9	Sugar (g)
0.6	2.6	1.1	0.2	Fibre (g)
4	5	1	1	Sodium (mg)
150	338	400	61	Potassium (mg)
7	8	6	2	Calcium (mg)
5	19	34	9	Magnesium (mg)
10	29	28	8	Phosphorus (mg)
0.33	0.3	0.3	0.1	Iron (mg)
0.03	0.14	0.1	0.01	Copper (mg)
0.06	0.3	0.2	0.05	Zinc (mg)
1	trace	1	unknown	Selenium (µg)
8.6	2	3.5	unknown	Vitamin A (µg)
nil	nil	nil	nil	Vitamin D (µg)
unknown	2.4	0.27	unknown	Vitamin E (mg)
trace	0.08	0.04	0.01	Vitamin B_1 (mg)
0.02	0.14	0.06	0.01	Vitamin B_2 (mg)
0.24	0.83	0.7	0.1	Niacin (mg)
0.01	0.27	0.29	0.04	Vitamin B_6 (mg)
nil	nil	nil	nil	Vitamin B_{12} (µg)
1	8	14	2	Folate (µg)
0.06	0.83	0.36	0.05	Pantothenate (mg)
unknown	2.7	2.6	0.4	Biotin (µg)
trace	5	11	trace	Vitamin C (mg)

FOOD	Blackberries raw	Blackcurrants stewed with sugar	Cherries raw	Cherries glace
PORTION SIZE	ten	average	five	five
NUTRIENTS				
Energy (kcals)	13	81	10	63
Protein (g)	0.4	1	0.2	0.1
Total fat (g)	0.1	trace	trace	trace
Saturated fat (g)	trace	trace	trace	trace
Mono-unsat. fat (g)	0.1	trace	trace	trace
Poly-unsat. fat (g)	0.1	trace	trace	trace
Carbohydrate (g)	2.5	21	2.3	16.6
Sugar (g)	2.5	21	2.3	16.6
Fibre (g)	1.5	3.9	0.2	0.2
Sodium (mg)	1	3	trace	7.0
Potassium (mg)	80	406	42	6.0
Calcium (mg)	21	66	3	14
Magnesium (mg)	12	18	2	1.0
Phosphorus (mg)	16	46	4	2.0
Iron (mg)	0.35	1.4	0.04	0.22
Copper (mg)	0.05	0.15	0.01	0.02
Zinc (mg)	0.10	0.42	0.02	0.03
Selenium (μg)	trace	unknown	trace	trace
Vitamin A (μg)	6.6	18.1	0.8	trace
Vitamin D (μg)	nil	nil	nil	nil
Vitamin E (mg)	1.18	1.09	0.03	trace
Vitamin B_1 (mg)	0.01	0.03	0.01	trace
Vitamin B_2 (mg)	0.03	0.06	0.01	trace
Niacin (mg)	0.25	0.28	0.04	trace
Vitamin B_6 (mg)	0.03	0.07	0.01	trace
Vitamin B_{12} (μg)	nil	nil	nil	nil
Folate (μg)	17	unknown	1.0	trace
Pantothenate (mg)	0.13	0.32	0.05	trace
Biotin (μg)	0.2	2	0.1	trace
Vitamin C (mg)	8.0	161	2.0	trace

Currants dried	Date raw	Date dried	Fig raw	FOOD
heaped tablespoon	one without stone	one without stone	one	**PORTION SIZE**
				NUTRIENTS
67	31	41	24	Energy (kcals)
0.6	0.4	0.5	0.7	Protein (g)
0.1	trace	trace	0.2	Total fat (g)
unknown	trace	nil	0.1	Saturated fat (g)
unknown	trace	nil	0.1	Mono-unsat. fat (g)
unknown	trace	trace	0.1	Poly-unsat. fat (g)
17	7.8	10.2	5.2	Carbohydrate (g)
17	7.8	10.2	5.2	Sugar (g)
0.5	0.4	0.6	0.8	Fibre (g)
4	2	2	2	Sodium (mg)
180	103	105	110	Potassium (mg)
23	6	7	21	Calcium (mg)
8	6	6	8	Magnesium (mg)
18	7	9	8	Phosphorus (mg)
0.32	0.08	0.19	0.17	Iron (mg)
0.2	0.03	0.04	0.03	Copper (mg)
0.08	0.05	0.06	0.17	Zinc (mg)
unknown	trace	trace	trace	Selenium (µg)
0.3	0.8	1	13.8	Vitamin A (µg)
nil	nil	nil	nil	Vitamin D (µg)
unknown	unknown	unknown	unknown	Vitamin E (mg)
0.04	0.01	0.01	0.02	Vitamin B_1 (mg)
0.01	0.02	0.01	0.02	Vitamin B_2 (mg)
0.22	0.17	0.27	0.22	Niacin (mg)
0.06	0.03	0.03	0.04	Vitamin B_6 (mg)
nil	nil	nil	nil	Vitamin B_{12} (µg)
1	6	2	unknown	Folate (µg)
0.02	0.05	0.12	0.12	Pantothenate (mg)
1.2	unknown	unknown	unknown	Biotin (µg)
trace	4	trace	1	Vitamin C (mg)

FOOD	Fig dried	Fruit salad homemade	Gooseberries stewed with sugar	Grapes raw
PORTION SIZE	one	average serving	average serving	small bunch
NUTRIENTS				
Energy (kcals)	45	77	76	257
Protein (g)	0.7	1	1	0.4
Total fat (g)	0.3	0.1	0.4	0.1
Saturated fat (g)	unknown	trace	unknown	trace
Mono-unsat. fat (g)	unknown	trace	unknown	trace
Poly-unsat. fat (g)	unknown	trace	unknown	trace
Carbohydrate (g)	10.6	19.3	18.1	15.4
Sugar (g)	10.6	18.6	18.1	15.4
Fibre (g)	1.5	2.1	2.7	0.7
Sodium (mg)	12	3	10	2
Potassium (mg)	194	294	196	210
Calcium (mg)	50	22	27	13
Magnesium (mg)	16	17	8	7
Phosphorus (mg)	18	25	31	18
Iron (mg)	0.84	0.28	0.42	0.3
Copper (mg)	0.06	0.10	0.1	0.12
Zinc (mg)	0.14	0.14	0.14	0.1
Selenium (µg)	trace	1	trace	1
Vitamin A (µg)	2.1	4.6	9.5	2.8
Vitamin D (µg)	nil	nil	nil	nil
Vitamin E (mg)	unknown	0.45	0.41	trace
Vitamin B_1 (mg)	0.02	0.07	0.01	0.05
Vitamin B_2 (mg)	0.02	0.04	0.03	0.01
Niacin (mg)	0.16	0.42	0.28	0.2
Vitamin B_6 (mg)	0.05	0.15	0.01	0.1
Vitamin B_{12} (µg)	nil	nil	nil	nil
Folate (µg)	2	13	8	2
Pantothenate (mg)	0.10	0.24	0.24	0.05
Biotin (µg)	unknown	1.5	0.4	0.3
Vitamin C (mg)	trace	22	15	3

Grapefruit raw	Greengage raw	Kiwi fruit raw	Lemon raw	FOOD
half average	one without stone	one medium	one slice	PORTION SIZE
				NUTRIENTS
24	21	29	4	Energy (kcals)
0.6	0.4	0.7	0.2	Protein (g)
0.1	0.1	0.3	0.1	Total fat (g)
trace	trace	unknown	trace	Saturated fat (g)
trace	trace	unknown	trace	Mono-unsat. fat (g)
trace	trace	unknown	trace	Poly-unsat. fat (g)
5.4	4.8	6.4	0.6	Carbohydrate (g)
5.4	4.8	6.2	0.6	Sugar (g)
1	1	1.1	unknown	Fibre (g)
2	1	2	1	Sodium (mg)
160	155	174	30	Potassium (mg)
18	9	15	17	Calcium (mg)
7	4	9	2	Magnesium (mg)
16	12	19	4	Phosphorus (mg)
0.08	0.2	0.24	0.1	Iron (mg)
0.02	0.04	0.08	0.05	Copper (mg)
trace	0.05	0.06	0.02	Zinc (mg)
1	trace	unknown	trace	Selenium (µg)
2.3	8	3.6	0.6	Vitamin A (µg)
nil	nil	nil	nil	Vitamin D (µg)
0.15	0.35	unknown	unknown	Vitamin E (mg)
0.04	0.03	0.01	0.01	Vitamin B_1 (mg)
0.02	0.02	0.02	0.01	Vitamin B_2 (mg)
0.24	0.3	0.18	0.04	Niacin (mg)
0.02	0.03	0.09	0.02	Vitamin B_6 (mg)
nil	nil	nil	nil	Vitamin B_{12} (µg)
21	2	unknown	unknown	Folate (µg)
0.22	0.1	unknown	0.05	Pantothenate (mg)
0.8	trace	unknown	0.1	Biotin (µg)
29	3	35	12	Vitamin C (mg)

FOOD	Lychee raw	Mandarin oranges canned in syrup	Mango raw	Melon canteloupe raw
PORTION SIZE	one without stone	average serving	one slice	one slice
NUTRIENTS				
Energy (kcals)	9	60	23	29
Protein (g)	0.1	0.6	0.3	0.9
Total fat (g)	trace	trace	0.1	0.2
Saturated fat (g)	trace	trace	trace	trace
Mono-unsat. fat (g)	trace	trace	trace	trace
Poly-unsat. fat (g)	trace	trace	trace	trace
Carbohydrate (g)	2.1	15.4	5.6	6.3
Sugar (g)	2.1	15.4	5.5	6.3
Fibre (g)	0.1	0.2	1	1.5
Sodium (mg)	trace	7	1	12
Potassium (mg)	24	56	72	315
Calcium (mg)	1	20	5	30
Magnesium (mg)	1	8	5	17
Phosphorus (mg)	5	9	6	20
Iron (mg)	0.08	0.23	0.28	0.45
Copper (mg)	0.02	trace	0.05	trace
Zinc (mg)	0.05	trace	0.04	trace
Selenium (μg)	unknown	trace	unknown	trace
Vitamin A (μg)	nil	20	120	250
Vitamin D (μg)	nil	nil	nil	nil
Vitamin E (mg)	unknown	trace	0.42	0.15
Vitamin B_1 (mg)	0.01	0.07	0.02	0.06
Vitamin B_2 (mg)	0.01	0.01	0.02	0.03
Niacin (mg)	0.08	0.23	0.2	0.9
Vitamin B_6 (mg)	unknown	0.03	0.05	0.16
Vitamin B_{12} (μg)	nil	nil	nil	nil
Folate (μg)	unknown	14	unknown	8
Pantothenate (mg)	unknown	0.17	0.06	0.19
Biotin (μg)	unknown	0.9	unknown	unknown
Vitamin C (mg)	7	17	15	39

Melon honeydew raw	Melon watermelon raw	Nectarine raw	Olives in brine	FOOD
one slice	one slice	one medium	five	**PORTION SIZE**
				NUTRIENTS
56	62	60	15	Energy (kcals)
1.2	1.0	2.1	0.1	Protein (g)
0.2	0.6	0.2	1.6	Total fat (g)
trace	0.2	trace	0.3	Saturated fat (g)
trace	0.2	trace	0.9	Mono-unsat. fat (g)
trace	0.2	trace	0.2	Poly-unsat. fat (g)
13.2	14.2	13.5	trace	Carbohydrate (g)
13.2	14.2	13.5	trace	Sugar (g)
1.2	0.2	1.8	0.4	Fibre (g)
64	4	2	338	Sodium (mg)
420	200	255	14	Potassium (mg)
18	14	11	9.0	Calcium (mg)
20	16	15	3.0	Magnesium (mg)
32	18	33	3.0	Phosphorus (mg)
0.2	0.6	0.6	0.15	Iron (mg)
trace	0.06	0.09	0.03	Copper (mg)
trace	0.4	0.15	unknown	Zinc (mg)
trace	trace	2	unknown	Selenium (µg)
16	76	14.5	4.5	Vitamin A (µg)
nil	nil	nil	nil	Vitamin D (µg)
0.2	0.2	unknown	0.3	Vitamin E (mg)
0.06	0.1	0.03	trace	Vitamin B_1 (mg)
0.02	0.02	0.06	trace	Vitamin B_2 (mg)
0.6	0.2	0.9	trace	Niacin (mg)
0.12	0.28	0.04	trace	Vitamin B_6 (mg)
nil	nil	nil	nil	Vitamin B_{12} (µg)
4	4	trace	trace	Folate (µg)
0.42	0.42	0.2	trace	Pantothenate (mg)
unknown	2	0.3	trace	Biotin (µg)
18	16	56	nil	Vitamin C (mg)

FOOD	Orange raw	Passion fruit raw	Paw-paw raw	Peach raw
PORTION SIZE	one medium	one average	one slice	one medium
NUTRIENTS				
Energy (kcals)	59	5	50	36
Protein (g)	1.8	0.4	0.7	1.1
Total fat (g)	0.2	0.1	0.1	0.1
Saturated fat (g)	trace	trace	trace	trace
Mono-unsat. fat (g)	trace	trace	trace	trace
Poly-unsat. fat (g)	trace	trace	trace	trace
Carbohydrate (g)	13.6	0.9	12.3	8.4
Sugar (g)	13.6	0.9	12.3	8.4
Fibre (g)	2.7	0.5	3.1	1.6
Sodium (mg)	8	3	7	1
Potassium (mg)	240	30	280	176
Calcium (mg)	75	2	32	8
Magnesium (mg)	16	4	15	10
Phosphorus (mg)	34	10	18	24
Iron (mg)	0.16	0.19	0.7	0.44
Copper (mg)	0.08	unknown	0.11	0.07
Zinc (mg)	0.16	0.12	0.28	0.11
Selenium (μg)	2	unknown	unknown	1
Vitamin A (μg)	7.5	18.8	189	10.6
Vitamin D (μg)	nil	nil	nil	nil
Vitamin E (mg)	0.38	unknown	unknown	unknown
Vitamin B_1 (mg)	0.18	trace	0.04	0.02
Vitamin B_2 (mg)	0.06	0.02	0.06	0.04
Niacin (mg)	0.64	0.22	0.42	0.66
Vitamin B_6 (mg)	0.16	unknown	0.04	0.02
Vitamin B_{12} (μg)	nil	nil	nil	nil
Folate (μg)	50	unknown	1	3
Pantothenate (mg)	0.59	unknown	0.31	0.19
Biotin (μg)	1.6	unknown	unknown	0.2
Vitamin C (mg)	86	3	84	34

Peaches canned	Pear raw	Pineapple raw	Plum raw	FOOD
average serving	one medium	one large slice	one medium	**PORTION SIZE**
				NUTRIENTS
66	60	33	20	Energy (kcals)
0.6	0.5	0.3	0.3	Protein (g)
trace	0.2	0.2	0.1	Total fat (g)
trace	trace	trace	trace	Saturated fat (g)
trace	trace	0.1	trace	Mono-unsat. fat (g)
trace	trace	0.1	trace	Poly-unsat. fat (g)
16.8	15	8.1	4.8	Carbohydrate (g)
16.8	15	8.1	4.8	Sugar (g)
1.1	3.3	1	0.9	Fibre (g)
5	5	2	1	Sodium (mg)
132	225	128	132	Potassium (mg)
4	17	14	7	Calcium (mg)
6	11	13	4	Magnesium (mg)
13	20	8	13	Phosphorus (mg)
0.24	0.3	0.16	0.22	Iron (mg)
trace	0.09	0.09	0.05	Copper (mg)
trace	0.15	0.08	0.05	Zinc (mg)
trace	trace	trace	trace	Selenium (μg)
15	4.5	2.3	27	Vitamin A (μg)
nil	nil	nil	nil	Vitamin D (μg)
unknown	0.75	0.08	0.34	Vitamin E (mg)
0.01	0.03	0.06	0.03	Vitamin B_1 (mg)
0.01	0.04	0.02	0.02	Vitamin B_2 (mg)
0.72	0.3	0.24	0.61	Niacin (mg)
0.02	0.03	0.07	0.03	Vitamin B_6 (mg)
nil	nil	nil	nil	Vitamin B_{12} (μg)
8	3	4	2	Folate (μg)
0.06	0.11	0.13	0.08	Pantothenate (mg)
0.1	0.3	0.2	trace	Biotin (μg)
6	9	10	2	Vitamin C (mg)

FOOD	Prunes stewed with sugar	Raisins dried	Raspberries raw	Rhubarb stewed with sugar
PORTION SIZE	six	one tablespoon	fifteen	average serving
Nutrients				
Energy (kcals)	25	82	15	67
Protein (g)	0.3	0.6	0.8	1.3
Total fat (g)	trace	0.1	0.2	0.1
Saturated fat (g)	trace	unknown	0.1	trace
Mono-unsat. fat (g)	trace	unknown	0.1	trace
Poly-unsat. fat (g)	trace	unknown	0.1	trace
Carbohydrate (g)	6.1	20.8	2.8	16.1
Sugar (g)	6.1	20.8	2.8	16.1
Fibre (g)	0.7	0.6	1.5	1.7
Sodium (mg)	1	18	2	1
Potassium (mg)	98	306	102	294
Calcium (mg)	4	14	15	46
Magnesium (mg)	3	11	11	8
Phosphorus (mg)	9	23	19	25
Iron (mg)	0.34	1.14	0.42	0.14
Copper (mg)	0.02	0.12	0.06	0.03
Zinc (mg)	0.07	0.21	0.18	trace
Selenium (µg)	trace	2	unknown	trace
Vitamin A (µg)	3	0.6	0.6	6.5
Vitamin D (µg)	nil	nil	nil	nil
Vitamin E (mg)	unknown	unknown	0.29	0.24
Vitamin B_1 (mg)	0.01	0.04	0.02	0.04
Vitamin B_2 (mg)	0.02	0.02	0.03	0.03
Niacin (mg)	0.12	0.18	0.3	0.28
Vitamin B_6 (mg)	0.02	0.08	0.04	0.03
Vitamin B_{12} (µg)	nil	nil	nil	nil
Folate (µg)	trace	3	20	6
Pantothenate (mg)	0.04	0.05	0.14	0.11
Biotin (µg)	trace	0.6	1.1	unknown
Vitamin C (mg)	trace	trace	19	7

Strawberries raw	Sultanas dried	Tangerines raw	FOOD
average	one tablespoon	one medium	**PORTION SIZE**
			NUTRIENTS
27	83	25	Energy (kcals)
0.8	0.8	0.6	Protein (g)
0.1	0.1	0.1	Total fat (g)
trace	unknown	trace	Saturated fat (g)
trace	unknown	trace	Mono-unsat. fat (g)
trace	unknown	trace	Poly-unsat. fat (g)
6	20.8	5.6	Carbohydrate (g)
6	20.8	5.6	Sugar (g)
1.1	0.6	0.9	Fibre (g)
6	6	1	Sodium (mg)
160	318	112	Potassium (mg)
16	19	29	Calcium (mg)
10	9	8	Magnesium (mg)
24	26	12	Phosphorus (mg)
0.4	0.66	0.21	Iron (mg)
0.07	0.12	0.01	Copper (mg)
0.1	0.09	0.07	Zinc (mg)
trace	unknown	unknown	Selenium (µg)
1.3	0.6	11.3	Vitamin A (µg)
nil	nil	nil	Vitamin D (µg)
0.2	0.21	unknown	Vitamin E (mg)
0.03	0.03	0.05	Vitamin B_1 (mg)
0.03	0.02	0.01	Vitamin B_2 (mg)
0.6	0.24	0.14	Niacin (mg)
0.06	0.08	0.05	Vitamin B_6 (mg)
nil	nil	nil	Vitamin B_{12} (µg)
20	8	15	Folate (µg)
0.34	0.03	0.14	Pantothenate (mg)
1.1	1.4	unknown	Biotin (µg)
77	trace	21	Vitamin C (mg)

FOOD	**Artichoke** boiled	**Asparagus** boiled	**Aubergine** fried in blended oil	**Runner beans** fresh, boiled
PORTION SIZE	one heart	five spears	medium half	medium
NUTRIENTS				
Energy (kcals)	4	16	393	16
Protein (g)	0.6	2	1.6	1.1
Total fat (g)	0.1	0.5	41.5	0.4
Saturated fat (g)	trace	trace	3.5	0.17
Mono-unsat. fat (g)	trace	0.1	20.7	0.1
Poly-unsat. fat (g)	trace	0.1	15.2	trace
Carbohydrate (g)	0.6	0.9	3.6	2.1
Sugar (g)	0.3	0.9	3.4	1.8
Fibre (g)	unknown	0.9	3	1.7
Sodium (mg)	3	36	3	1
Potassium (mg)	70	138	221	117
Calcium (mg)	10	15	10	20
Magnesium (mg)	6	8	10	13
Phosphorus (mg)	9	30	33	19
Iron (mg)	0.1	0.38	0.65	0.9
Copper (mg)	0.02	0.05	0.04	0.01
Zinc (mg)	0.1	0.38	0.13	0.18
Selenium (μg)	trace	trace	1	unknown
Vitamin A (μg)	3.3	53	27	18
Vitamin D (μg)	nil	nil	nil	nil
Vitamin E (mg)	0.04	0.7	7.15	0.21
Vitamin B_1 (mg)	trace	0.07	nil	0.05
Vitamin B_2 (mg)	trace	0.04	trace	0.02
Niacin (mg)	0.2	0.5	trace	trace
Vitamin B_6 (mg)	trace	0.04	0.09	0.04
Vitamin B_{12} (μg)	nil	nil	nil	nil
Folate (μg)	11	93	7	38
Pantothenate (mg)	0.08	0.1	0.09	0.04
Biotin (μg)	0.9	0.3	unknown	0.4
Vitamin C (mg)	trace	6	1	9

Bean sprouts raw	**Beetroot** pickled	**Broccoli** fresh, boiled	**Brussels sprouts** fresh, boiled	**FOOD**
one tablespoon	average	one spear	medium (9)	**PORTION SIZE**
				NUTRIENTS
6	11	11	32	Energy (kcals)
0.6	0.5	1.4	2.6	Protein (g)
0.1	0.1	0.4	1.2	Total fat (g)
trace	trace	0.1	0.3	Saturated fat (g)
trace	trace	trace	0.1	Mono-unsat. fat (g)
trace	trace	0.2	0.6	Poly-unsat. fat (g)
0.8	2.2	0.5	3.2	Carbohydrate (g)
0.4	2.2	0.4	2.7	Sugar (g)
0.3	0.7	1	2.8	Fibre (g)
1	48	6	2.0	Sodium (mg)
15	76	77	279	Potassium (mg)
4	8	18	18	Calcium (mg)
4.0	5	6	12	Magnesium (mg)
10	7	26	55	Phosphorus (mg)
0.34	0.2	0.45	0.45	Iron (mg)
0.02	0.02	0.01	0.03	Copper (mg)
0.06	0.12	0.18	0.27	Zinc (mg)
unknown	trace	trace	unknown	Selenium (µg)
1	trace	35.6	48	Vitamin A (µg)
nil	nil	nil	nil	Vitamin D (µg)
unknown	trace	0.5	0.81	Vitamin E (mg)
0.02	0.01	0.02	0.06	Vitamin B_1 (mg)
0.01	0.01	0.02	0.08	Vitamin B_2 (mg)
0.1	0.04	0.31	trace	Niacin (mg)
0.02	0.02	0.05	0.17	Vitamin B_6 (mg)
nil	nil	nil	nil	Vitamin B_{12} (µg)
12	1	29	99	Folate (µg)
0.08	0.04	unknown	0.25	Pantothenate (mg)
unknown	trace	unknown	0.3	Biotin (µg)
1	unknown	20	54	Vitamin C (mg)

FOOD	**Bubble and squeak** fried in vegetable oil	**Cabbage (white)** fresh, boiled	**Cabbage (white)** raw	**Cabbage (red)** raw
PORTION SIZE	average	medium	one sixth of a cabbage	one sixth of a cabbage
NUTRIENTS				
Energy (kcals)	248	15	23	19
Protein (g)	2.8	0.9	1.5	1.0
Total fat (g)	18.2	0.4	0.4	0.3
Saturated fat (g)	19.6	0.1	0.1	trace
Mono-unsat. fat (g)	2	trace	trace	trace
Poly-unsat. fat (g)	6.4	0.3	0.3	0.2
Carbohydrate (g)	8.6	2.1	3.7	3.3
Sugar (g)	2.8	1.9	3.6	3.0
Fibre (g)	3.0	1.7	2.2	2.3
Sodium (mg)	14	8	5	7
Potassium (mg)	400	114	243	225
Calcium (mg)	38	31	47	54
Magnesium (mg)	18	4	7	8
Phosphorus (mg)	56	24	37	33
Iron (mg)	0.8	0.29	0.63	0.36
Copper (mg)	0.08	0.01	0.02	0.01
Zinc (mg)	0.4	0.09	0.27	0.09
Selenium (μg)	4	2.0	1	2
Vitamin A (μg)	35	33	57.8	2.3
Vitamin D (μg)	nil	nil	nil	nil
Vitamin E (mg)	4.5	0.19	0.18	0.18
Vitamin B_1 (mg)	0.22	0.08	0.14	0.02
Vitamin B_2 (mg)	0.02	0.01	0.02	0.01
Niacin (mg)	0.8	0.29	0.45	0.36
Vitamin B_6 (mg)	0.32	0.08	0.13	0.08
Vitamin B_{12} (μg)	nil	nil	nil	nil
Folate (μg)	24	28	68	35
Pantothenate (mg)	0.54	0.14	0.19	0.29
Biotin (μg)	0.4	trace	0.1	0.1
Vitamin C (mg)	18	19	44	50

Carrots (old) raw	Carrots (old) fresh, boiled	Cauliflower fresh, boiled	Cauliflower bhaji homemade	FOOD
medium	medium	medium	average	**PORTION SIZE**
				NUTRIENTS
21	14	25	300	Energy (kcals)
0.4	0.4	2.6	5.6	Protein (g)
0.2	0.2	0.8	28.7	Total fat (g)
0.1	0.06	0.2	3.1	Saturated fat (g)
trace	0.1	0.1	9.8	Mono-unsat. fat (g)
0.1	trace	0.4	13.9	Poly-unsat. fat (g)
4.7	2.9	1.9	5.6	Carbohydrate (g)
4.4	2.8	1.6	4.5	Sugar (g)
1.4	1.5	1.4	2.8	Fibre (g)
15	30	4	588	Sodium (mg)
102	72	108	602	Potassium (mg)
15	14	15	38	Calcium (mg)
2	2	11	31	Magnesium (mg)
9	10	47	102	Phosphorus (mg)
0.18	0.24	0.36	1.26	Iron (mg)
0.01	0.01	0.02	0.06	Copper (mg)
0.06	0.06	0.36	0.98	Zinc (mg)
1	1	trace	trace	Selenium (µg)
811	726	9	43	Vitamin A (µg)
nil	nil	nil	nil	Vitamin D (µg)
0.34	0.34	0.1	6.92	Vitamin E (mg)
0.06	0.05	0.06	0.22	Vitamin B_1 (mg)
0.01	trace	0.04	0.07	Vitamin B_2 (mg)
0.12	trace	0.36	0.84	Niacin (mg)
0.08	0.06	0.14	0.35	Vitamin B_6 (mg)
nil	nil	nil	nil	Vitamin B_{12} (µg)
7	10	46	49	Folate (µg)
0.15	0.11	0.38	0.71	Pantothenate (mg)
0.4	0.2	0.9	1.8	Biotin (µg)
4	1	24	32	Vitamin C (mg)

FOOD	Celery raw	Chicory raw	Chilli green, raw	Chinese leaves raw
PORTION SIZE	one stick	one head	one	one large leaf
NUTRIENTS				
Energy (kcals)	2	12	1	10
Protein (g)	0.2	0.5	0.1	1.4
Total fat (g)	0.1	0.6	trace	trace
Saturated fat (g)	trace	0.2	unknown	unknown
Mono-unsat. fat (g)	trace	trace	unknown	unknown
Poly-unsat. fat (g)	trace	0.3	unknown	unknown
Carbohydrate (g)	0.3	2.9	trace	1.4
Sugar (g)	0.3	0.7	trace	unknown
Fibre (g)	0.3	0.9	unknown	unknown
Sodium (mg)	18	1	trace	unknown
Potassium (mg)	96	179	11	unknown
Calcium (mg)	12	22	2	62
Magnesium (mg)	2	6	1	64
Phosphorus (mg)	6	28	4	unknown
Iron (mg)	0.12	0.42	0.06	1.16
Copper (mg)	trace	0.05	unknown	0.15
Zinc (mg)	0.03	0.21	0.02	unknown
Selenium (µg)	1	unknown	unknown	unknown
Vitamin A (µg)	2.5	21	1.5	436
Vitamin D (µg)	nil	nil	nil	nil
Vitamin E (mg)	0.06	unknown	unknown	unknown
Vitamin B_1 (mg)	0.02	0.15	trace	0.02
Vitamin B_2 (mg)	trace	trace	trace	0.09
Niacin (mg)	0.09	0.11	0.05	0.28
Vitamin B_6 (mg)	0.01	0.01	unknown	unknown
Vitamin B_{12} (µg)	nil	nil	nil	nil
Folate (µg)	5	15	1	34
Pantothenate (mg)	0.12	unknown	unknown	unknown
Biotin (µg)	trace	unknown	unknown	unknown
Vitamin C (mg)	2	5	6	9

Courgettes boiled	Cucumber raw	Garlic raw	Gherkins pickled	FOOD
medium	average in a salad	one clove	one	**PORTION SIZE**
				NUTRIENTS
17	2	6	4	Energy (kcals)
1.8	0.2	0.2	0.3	Protein (g)
0.4	trace	trace	trace	Total fat (g)
0.1	trace	unknown	trace	Saturated fat (g)
trace	trace	unknown	trace	Mono-unsat. fat (g)
0.2	trace	unknown	trace	Poly-unsat. fat (g)
1.8	0.3	1.3	0.8	Carbohydrate (g)
1.7	0.3	unknown	0.7	Sugar (g)
1.1	0.1	unknown	0.4	Fibre (g)
1	1	1	207	Sodium (mg)
189	32	19	33	Potassium (mg)
17	4	1	6	Calcium (mg)
15	2	trace	3	Magnesium (mg)
32	11	unknown	7	Phosphorus (mg)
0.54	0.07	0.08	0.21	Iron (mg)
0.01	trace	unknown	0.03	Copper (mg)
0.18	0.02	0.04	0.09	Zinc (mg)
1	trace	unknown	unknown	Selenium (µg)
66	2.3	trace	trace	Vitamin A (µg)
nil	nil	nil	nil	Vitamin D (µg)
unknown	0.02	unknown	unknown	Vitamin E (mg)
0.07	0.01	0.01	trace	Vitamin B_1 (mg)
0.02	trace	trace	0.01	Vitamin B_2 (mg)
0.18	0.05	0.02	0.03	Niacin (mg)
0.08	0.01	unknown	unknown	Vitamin B_6 (mg)
nil	nil	nil	nil	Vitamin B_{12} (µg)
28	2	trace	2	Folate (µg)
0.1	0.07	unknown	unknown	Pantothenate (mg)
unknown	0.2	unknown	unknown	Biotin (µg)
10	trace	1	trace	Vitamin C (mg)

FOOD	**Leeks** boiled	**Lettuce** round	**Marrow** boiled	**Mixed Vegetables** frozen, boiled in salted water
PORTION SIZE	average	average in a salad	average	average
NUTRIENTS				
Energy (kcals)	16	4	6	38
Protein (g)	0.9	0.2	0.3	3
Total fat (g)	0.5	0.2	0.1	0.4
Saturated fat (g)	0.1	trace	trace	unknown
Mono-unsat. fat (g)	trace	trace	trace	unknown
Poly-unsat. fat (g)	0.3	0.1	trace	unknown
Carbohydrate (g)	1.9	0.5	1	5.9
Sugar (g)	1.5	0.5	0.9	3.2
Fibre (g)	1.3	0.3	0.4	unknown
Sodium (mg)	5	1	1	86
Potassium (mg)	113	66	72	117
Calcium (mg)	15	8	9	32
Magnesium (mg)	2	2	5	14
Phosphorus (mg)	24	8	12	51
Iron (mg)	0.52	0.21	0.06	0.72
Copper (mg)	0.01	trace	0.01	0.02
Zinc (mg)	0.15	0.06	0.13	0.36
Selenium (µg)	1	1	unknown	unknown
Vitamin A (µg)	71	17	12	378
Vitamin D (µg)	nil	nil	nil	nil
Vitamin E (mg)	0.58	0.17	trace	unknown
Vitamin B_1 (mg)	0.01	0.04	0.05	0.11
Vitamin B_2 (mg)	0.01	0.01	trace	0.08
Niacin (mg)	0.3	0.12	0.13	0.72
Vitamin B_6 (mg)	0.04	0.01	0.01	0.1
Vitamin B_{12} (µg)	nil	nil	nil	nil
Folate (µg)	30	17	10	47
Pantothenate (mg)	0.08	0.05	0.05	unknown
Biotin (µg)	0.8	0.2	0.3	unknown
Vitamin C (mg)	5	2	2	12

Mushrooms raw	Mushrooms fried in oil	Mushroom bhaji homemade	Mustard and cress raw	FOOD
average (60g)	average (60g raw)	average	quarter of a punnet	**PORTION SIZE**
				NUTRIENTS
8	69	232	1	Energy (kcals)
1.1	1.1	2.4	0.2	Protein (g)
0.3	7.1	22.5	0.1	Total fat (g)
0.1	0.6	2.4	trace	Saturated fat (g)
trace	3.6	7.8	trace	Mono-unsat. fat (g)
0.2	2.6	10.9	trace	Poly-unsat. fat (g)
0.2	0.1	6.2	trace	Carbohydrate (g)
0.1	trace	4.2	trace	Sugar (g)
0.7	0.7	1.8	0.1	Fibre (g)
3	2	13	2	Sodium (mg)
192	150	392	11	Potassium (mg)
4	4	25	5	Calcium (mg)
5	8	11	2	Magnesium (mg)
48	44	87	3	Phosphorus (mg)
0.36	0.44	0.98	0.1	Iron (mg)
0.43	0.18	0.6	trace	Copper (mg)
0.24	0.22	0.56	0.03	Zinc (mg)
5	5	7	unknown	Selenium (µg)
nil	trace	24	21	Vitamin A (µg)
nil	nil	nil	nil	Vitamin D (µg)
0.07	unknown	5.6	0.07	Vitamin E (mg)
0.05	0.04	0.14	trace	Vitamin B_1 (mg)
0.19	0.15	0.2	trace	Vitamin B_2 (mg)
1.92	1.01	2.38	0.1	Niacin (mg)
0.11	0.08	0.22	0.02	Vitamin B_6 (mg)
nil	nil	nil	nil	Vitamin B_{12} (µg)
26	5	22	6	Folate (µg)
1.2	0.62	1.29	unknown	Pantothenate (mg)
7.2	3.5	7.8	unknown	Biotin (µg)
1	trace	3	3	Vitamin C (mg)

FOOD	**Okra** cooked bhaji-style with ghee	**Onions** raw	**Onions** fried in oil	**Spring onions** raw
PORTION SIZE	average	one average	average	one average
NUTRIENTS				
Energy (kcals)	238	54	66	2
Protein (g)	6.3	1.8	0.9	0.2
Total fat (g)	16	0.3	4.5	0.1
Saturated fat (g)	9.8	trace	0.4	trace
Mono-unsat. fat (g)	3.5	trace	2.2	trace
Poly-unsat. fat (g)	1	0.2	1.6	trace
Carbohydrate (g)	19	11.9	5.6	0.3
Sugar (g)	13.8	8.4	4	trace
Fibre (g)	8	2.1	1.2	0.2
Sodium (mg)	400	5	2	1
Potassium (mg)	775	240	148	26
Calcium (mg)	275	38	19	4
Magnesium (mg)	110	6	3	1
Phosphorus (mg)	143	45	18	3
Iron (mg)	2.5	0.45	0.32	0.19
Copper (mg)	0.28	0.08	0.02	0.01
Zinc (mg)	1.25	0.3	0.12	0.04
Selenium (µg)	3	2	1	unknown
Vitamin A (µg)	228	2.5	2.6	10
Vitamin D (µg)	0.25	nil	nil	nil
Vitamin E (mg)	unknown	0.47	unknown	unknown
Vitamin B_1 (mg)	0.43	0.19	0.03	trace
Vitamin B_2 (mg)	0.07	trace	trace	trace
Niacin (mg)	2.25	1.05	trace	0.05
Vitamin B_6 (mg)	0.52	0.3	0.04	0.01
Vitamin B_{12} (µg)	trace	nil	nil	nil
Folate (µg)	75	26	15	5
Pantothenate (mg)	0.43	0.16	0.05	0.01
Biotin (µg)	unknown	1.3	0.5	unknown
Vitamin C (mg)	23	8	1	3

Pickled onions raw	**Onion bhaji** retail	**Parsley** fresh	**Parsnip** boiled	**FOOD**
one average	one	one large sprig	medium average	**PORTION SIZE**
				NUTRIENTS
4	109	trace	4	Energy (kcals)
0.1	3	trace	1	Protein (g)
trace	7.5	trace	0.	Total fat (g)
trace	0.7	trace	0.1	Saturated fat (g)
trace	4.1	trace	0.3	Mono-unsat. fat (g)
trace	2.3	trace	0.1	Poly-unsat. fat (g)
0.7	7.8	trace	8.4	Carbohydrate (g)
0.5	2.7	trace	3.8	Sugar (g)
0.2	1.9	0.1	3.1	Fibre (g)
68	126	trace	3	Sodium (mg)
14	193	8	228	Potassium (mg)
3	34	2	33	Calcium (mg)
1	21	trace	15	Magnesium (mg)
3	60	1	49	Phosphorus (mg)
0.03	1.12	0.08	0.39	Iron (mg)
0.01	0.11	trace	0.03	Copper (mg)
0.02	0.52	0.1	0.2	Zinc (mg)
trace	trace	trace	unknown	Selenium (µg)
0.3	3	6	3.3	Vitamin A (µg)
nil	trace	nil	nil	Vitamin D (µg)
0.05	0.94	0.02	0.65	Vitamin E (mg)
trace	0.04	trace	0.05	Vitamin B_1 (mg)
trace	0.03	trace	0.01	Vitamin B_2 (mg)
0.02	0.42	0.01	0.45	Niacin (mg)
0.02	0.08	trace	0.06	Vitamin B_6 (mg)
nil	nil	nil	nil	Vitamin B_{12} (µg)
2	14	2	31	Folate (µg)
unknown	0.27	trace	0.23	Pantothenate (mg)
unknown	0.1	trace	trace	Biotin (µg)
trace	1	2	7	Vitamin C (mg)

FOOD	**Peppers green** raw	**Peppers red** raw	**Peppers yellow** raw	**Peppers stuffed** with rice homemade
PORTION SIZE	half a pepper	half a pepper	half a pepper	half a pepper
NUTRIENTS				
Energy (kcals)	12	26	21	149
Protein (g)	0.6	0.8	1	2.6
Total fat (g)	0.2	0.3	0.2	4.2
Saturated fat (g)	0.1	0.1	trace	0.7
Mono-unsat. fat (g)	trace	trace	trace	1.2
Poly-unsat. fat (g)	0.2	0.2	0.1	1.9
Carbohydrate (g)	2.1	5.1	4.2	26.9
Sugar (g)	1.9	4.9	4.1	10.2
Fibre (g)	1.3	1.3	1.4	2.3
Sodium (mg)	3	3	3	315
Potassium (mg)	96	128	176	333
Calcium (mg)	6	6	6	28
Magnesium (mg)	8	11	13	23
Phosphorus (mg)	15	18	21	63
Iron (mg)	0.32	0.24	0.32	1.05
Copper (mg)	0.02	0.01	0.02	0.14
Zinc (mg)	0.08	0.08	0.08	0.53
Selenium (μg)	trace	trace	unknown	4
Vitamin A (μg)	35	512	24	80
Vitamin D (μg)	nil	nil	nil	nil
Vitamin E (mg)	0.64	0.64	0.64	1.87
Vitamin B_1 (mg)	0.01	0.01	0.01	0.05
Vitamin B_2 (mg)	0.01	0.02	0.02	0.02
Niacin (mg)	0.08	1.04	0.56	0.88
Vitamin B_6 (mg)	0.21	0.29	0.26	0.31
Vitamin B_{12} (μg)	nil	nil	nil	nil
Folate (μg)	29	17	23	23
Pantothenate (mg)	0.06	0.06	0.06	0.17
Biotin (μg)	unknown	unknown	unknown	unknown
Vitamin C (mg)	96	112	104	60

Plantain boiled	**Radish** raw	**Ratatouille** homemade	**Salad coleslaw** retail	**FOOD**
average	one	average	one tub	**PORTION SIZE**
				NUTRIENTS
157	1	148	116	Energy (kcals)
1.1	0.1	2.3	0.5	Protein (g)
0.3	trace	12.6	11.9	Total fat (g)
0.1	trace	1.4	1.8	Saturated fat (g)
trace	trace	4.3	2.7	Mono-unsat. fat (g)
0.1	trace	6.1	6.9	Poly-unsat. fat (g)
39.9	0.2	6.8	1.9	Carbohydrate (g)
7.7	0.2	5.8	1.8	Sugar (g)
1.7	0.1	3.2	0.6	Fibre (g)
6	1	360	72	Sodium (mg)
560	19	504	68	Potassium (mg)
7	2	31	14	Calcium (mg)
46	trace	27	1	Magnesium (mg)
43	2	56	12	Phosphorus (mg)
0.7	0.05	0.9	0.18	Iron (mg)
0.11	trace	0.04	trace	Copper (mg)
0.28	0.02	0.36	0.09	Zinc (mg)
3	trace	2	unknown	Selenium (µg)
81	trace	112	78	Vitamin A (µg)
nil	nil	nil	0.05	Vitamin D (µg)
0.28	nil	3.73	3.03	Vitamin E (mg)
0.04	trace	0.13	0.04	Vitamin B_1 (mg)
0.06	trace	0.02	0.01	Vitamin B_2 (mg)
0.7	0.03	0.72	0.09	Niacin (mg)
0.34	0.01	0.25	0.05	Vitamin B_6 (mg)
nil	nil	nil	0.1	Vitamin B_{12} (µg)
31	3	27	9	Folate (µg)
0.35	0.01	0.22	unknown	Pantothenate (mg)
unknown	unknown	unknown	unknown	Biotin (µg)
13	1	25	9	Vitamin C (mg)

FOOD	Salad vegetable canned	Salad Greek	Salad Waldorf retail	Salad carrot retail
PORTION SIZE	one tub	one tub	one tub	one tub
NUTRIENTS				
Energy (kcals)	64	260	794	436
Protein (g)	0.7	5.4	4.2	4.2
Total fat (g)	4.4	25	79.2	35.2
Saturated fat (g)	0.6	6.6	10.8	3.4
Mono-unsat. fat (g)	0.9	14.4	17.6	18.4
Poly-unsat. fat (g)	2.7	2.6	47.2	11.6
Carbohydrate (g)	5.8	3.8	17.2	27.4
Sugar (g)	3.1	3.8	16.8	26.4
Fibre (g)	0.5	1.6	2	4.8
Sodium (mg)	239	720	440	260
Potassium (mg)	59	300	420	600
Calcium (mg)	10	122	50	76
Magnesium (mg)	5	18	34	46
Phosphorus (mg)	16	122	110	100
Iron (mg)	0.36	0.8	1.6	1.6
Copper (mg)	0.01	0.06	0.3	0.36
Zinc (mg)	0.09	0.4	0.8	0.6
Selenium (µg)	unknown	unknown	unknown	2
Vitamin A (µg)	57	146	95	1721
Vitamin D (µg)	0.05	0.2	0.4	nil
Vitamin E (mg)	1.54	2.24	17.8	5.9
Vitamin B_1 (mg)	0.01	0.08	0.14	0.24
Vitamin B_2 (mg)	0.01	0.08	0.1	0.06
Niacin (mg)	0.18	0.8	0.4	0.6
Vitamin B_6 (mg)	unknown	0.22	0.22	0.34
Vitamin B_{12} (µg)	0.1	0.4	0.4	nil
Folate (µg)	4	32	26	34
Pantothenate (mg)	unknown	0.42	unknown	0.64
Biotin (µg)	unknown	unknown	unknown	17
Vitamin C (mg)	1	52	10	8

Salad Florida retail	Sauerkraut	Spinach boiled	Spinach cannelloni	FOOD
one tub	one tablespoon	average	average	PORTION SIZE
				NUTRIENTS
448	3	17	449	Energy (kcals)
1.8	0.3	2	15.3	Protein (g)
41	trace	0.7	25.5	Total fat (g)
6	trace	0.1	7.8	Saturated fat (g)
9.4	trace	0.1	7.8	Mono-unsat. fat (g)
23.8	trace	0.4	7.8	Poly-unsat. fat (g)
19.4	0.3	0.7	42.8	Carbohydrate (g)
19.2	0.3	0.7	7.5	Sugar (g)
2	0.7	1.9	2.7	Fibre (g)
260	177	108	952	Sodium (mg)
240	54	207	374	Potassium (mg)
50	15	144	unknown	Calcium (mg)
10	3	31	58	Magnesium (mg)
40	7	25	286	Phosphorus (mg)
0.8	0.36	1.44	2.04	Iron (mg)
0.04	0.02	0.01	0.17	Copper (mg)
0.2	0.09	0.45	2.04	Zinc (mg)
unknown	trace	1	unknown	Selenium (µg)
65	0.8	576	504	Vitamin A (µg)
0.2	nil	nil	unknown	Vitamin D (µg)
10.44	unknown	1.54	4.49	Vitamin E (mg)
0.12	0.01	0.05	0.1	Vitamin B_1 (mg)
0.06	trace	0.05	0.24	Vitamin B_2 (mg)
0.4	0.06	0.81	1.36	Niacin (mg)
0.16	0.05	0.08	0.14	Vitamin B_6 (mg)
0.2	nil	nil	0.7	Vitamin B_{12} (µg)
26	5	81	31	Folate (µg)
0.22	0.07	0.19	0.48	Pantothenate (mg)
unknown	unknown	0.1	2.0	Biotin (µg)
28	3	7	3	Vitamin C (mg)

FOOD	Swede boiled	Sweetcorn on-the-cob, boiled	Sweetcorn canned kernels	Tomatoes raw
PORTION SIZE	medium	one average cob	one tablespoon	one medium
NUTRIENTS				
Energy (kcals)	7	83	7	14
Protein (g)	0.2	3.1	0.9	0.6
Total fat (g)	0.1	1.8	0.1	0.3
Saturated fat (g)	trace	0.3	unknown	0.1
Mono-unsat. fat (g)	trace	0.4	unknown	0.1
Poly-unsat. fat (g)	0.1	0.6	unknown	0.2
Carbohydrate (g)	1.4	14.5	0.6	2.6
Sugar (g)	1.3	1.8	0.4	2.6
Fibre (g)	0.4	1.6	0.4	0.9
Sodium (mg)	8	1	342	8
Potassium (mg)	52	175	54	213
Calcium (mg)	16	3	2	6
Magnesium (mg)	2	25	unknown	6
Phosphorus (mg)	7	60	unknown	20
Iron (mg)	0.06	0.38	0.36	0.43
Copper (mg)	trace	0.02	unknown	0.01
Zinc (mg)	0.06	0.25	unknown	0.09
Selenium (μg)	1	trace	unknown	trace
Vitamin A (μg)	16	14.8	7	90
Vitamin D (μg)	nil	nil	nil	nil
Vitamin E (mg)	trace	0.65	unknown	1.04
Vitamin B_1 (mg)	0.08	0.14	0.01	0.08
Vitamin B_2 (mg)	0.01	0.04	0.01	0.01
Niacin (mg)	0.6	1.5	0.03	0.85
Vitamin B_6 (mg)	0.02	0.11	unknown	0.12
Vitamin B_{12} (μg)	nil	nil	nil	nil
Folate (μg)	11	25	unknown	14
Pantothenate (mg)	0.04	0.46	unknown	0.21
Biotin (μg)	trace	unknown	unknown	1.3
Vitamin C (mg)	9	5	4	14

Tomatoes canned	Tomato cherry raw	Tomato puree tube	Turnip boiled	**FOOD**
contents of one medium can	one medium	one tablespoon	medium	**PORTION SIZE**
				NUTRIENTS
32	3	11	7	Energy (kcals)
2.0	0.1	0.8	0.4	Protein (g)
0.2	0.1	trace	0.1	Total fat (g)
trace	trace	trace	trace	Saturated fat (g)
trace	trace	trace	trace	Mono-unsat. fat (g)
trace	trace	trace	0.1	Poly-unsat. fat (g)
6	0.4	2.1	1.2	Carbohydrate (g)
5.6	0.4	2.1	1.1	Sugar (g)
1.4	0.2	0.4	1.1	Fibre (g)
78	2	36	17	Sodium (mg)
500	44	180	120	Potassium (mg)
24	2	5	27	Calcium (mg)
22	2	4	4	Magnesium (mg)
38	5	14	19	Phosphorus (mg)
0.8	0.06	0.21	0.12	Iron (mg)
0.14	0.01	0.44	0.01	Copper (mg)
0.2	0.03	0.08	0.06	Zinc (mg)
trace	trace	unknown	1	Selenium (µg)
73	12	16	2	Vitamin A (µg)
nil	nil	nil	nil	Vitamin D (µg)
2.44	0.18	0.81	trace	Vitamin E (mg)
0.1	0.01	0.06	0.03	Vitamin B_1 (mg)
0.04	0.01	0.03	0.01	Vitamin B_2 (mg)
1.4	0.15	0.6	0.12	Niacin (mg)
0.22	0.02	0.02	0.02	Vitamin B_6 (mg)
nil	nil	nil	nil	Vitamin B_{12} (µg)
22	3	3	5	Folate (µg)
0.4	0.04	0.15	0.08	Pantothenate (mg)
3	0.2	0.9	trace	Biotin (µg)
24	4	2	6	Vitamin C (mg)

FOOD	**Vegeburger** retail, grilled	**Vegetable curry** take-away	**Vegetable bake** homemade	**Vegetables** stir fried
PORTION SIZE	one	one serving	medium	average
NUTRIENTS				
Energy (kcals)	110	210	330	166
Protein (g)	9.3	5	10.9	5.2
Total fat (g)	6.2	14.8	1805	9.4
Saturated fat (g)	unknown	3	7.8	0.8
Mono-unsat. fat (g)	unknown	7.4	5.5	4.7
Poly-unsat. fat (g)	unknown	2.4	3.9	3.4
Carbohydrate (g)	4.5	15.2	32.2	16.6
Sugar (g)	2.0	6.2	11.7	10.1
Fibre (g)	2.4	unknown	2.9	unknown
Sodium (mg)	274	740	312	29
Potassium (mg)	342	unknown	598	598
Calcium (mg)	56	unknown	260	78
Magnesium (mg)	45	unknown	36	42
Phosphorus (mg)	134	unknown	231	120
Iron (mg)	2.52	5.4	1.3	1.3
Copper (mg)	0.22	unknown	0.1	0.29
Zinc (mg)	0.9	unknown	1.3	0.78
Selenium (µg)	4	unknown	8	trace
Vitamin A (µg)	unknown	213	917	unknown
Vitamin D (µg)	unknown	nil	1.04	nil
Vitamin E (mg)	unknown	1.84	0.57	unknown
Vitamin B_1 (mg)	1.34	0.06	0.23	0.18
Vitamin B_2 (mg)	0.24	0.1	0.21	0.34
Niacin (mg)	1.57	unknown	1.04	2.6
Vitamin B_6 (mg)	0.17	unknown	0.39	0.65
Vitamin B_{12} (µg)	unknown	nil	0.5	nil
Folate (µg)	53	unknown	26	42
Pantothenate (mg)	unknown	unknown	0.68	unknown
Biotin (µg)	unknown	unknown	2.6	unknown
Vitamin C (mg)	unknown	unknown	8	21

Vegetable lasagne	Vegetable pancake roll retail	Vegetable pasty	Vegetable pâté	FOOD
average	average	one	average as a starter	PORTION SIZE
				NUTRIENTS
428	131	425	138	Energy (kcals)
17.2	4.0	6.4	6.0	Protein (g)
18.5	7.5	23.1	10.7	Total fat (g)
9.2	2.1	5.7	unknown	Saturated fat (g)
5.0	3.6	7.1	unknown	Mono-unsat. fat (g)
2.9	1.5	9.0	unknown	Poly-unsat. fat (g)
52.1	12.6	51.6	4.7	Carbohydrate (g)
11.3	1.8	2.8	0.2	Sugar (g)
4.2	unknown	2.9	unknown	Fibre (g)
412	366	496	432	Sodium (mg)
756	unknown	217	240	Potassium (mg)
357	unknown	95	104	Calcium (mg)
59	unknown	20	22	Magnesium (mg)
344	unknown	87	152	Phosphorus (mg)
2.1	1.26	1.55	3.36	Iron (mg)
0.38	unknown	0.12	0.1	Copper (mg)
2.1	unknown	0.47	1.68	Zinc (mg)
13	unknown	3	unknown	Selenium (µg)
606	0.3	377	unknown	Vitamin A (µg)
0.42	nil	2.17	trace	Vitamin D (µg)
2.65	0.46	0.37	unknown	Vitamin E (mg)
0.21	0.05	0.2	1.68	Vitamin B_1 (mg)
0.29	0.03	0.02	1.04	Vitamin B_2 (mg)
2.1	unknown	1.09	3.76	Niacin (mg)
0.29	unknown	0.16	0.37	Vitamin B_6 (mg)
0.4	nil	nil	trace	Vitamin B_{12} (µg)
29	unknown	14	88	Folate (µg)
0.88	unknown	0.26	unknown	Pantothenate (mg)
5.0	unknown	0.8	unknown	Biotin (µg)
13	trace	3	trace	Vitamin C (mg)

FOOD	**Vegetable samosa** retail	**Vegetable shepherds pie**	**Watercress** raw	**Yam** boiled
PORTION SIZE	one average	average	quarter of a bunch	size of a medium potato
NUTRIENTS				
Energy (kcals)	163	350	4	173
Protein (g)	3.8	14.3	0.6	2.2
Total fat (g)	7	12.4	0.2	0.4
Saturated fat (g)	unknown	1.2	0.1	0.1
Mono-unsat. fat (g)	unknown	4.0	trace	trace
Poly-unsat. fat (g)	unknown	5.9	0.1	0.1
Carbohydrate (g)	22.5	49	0.1	42.9
Sugar (g)	2	4.3	0.1	0.9
Fibre (g)	1.9	7.4	0.3	1.8
Sodium (mg)	293	251	10	22
Potassium (mg)	113	1023	46	338
Calcium (mg)	49	50	34	16
Magnesium (mg)	14	68	3	16
Phosphorus (mg)	49	233	10	27
Iron (mg)	1.13	5.27	0.44	0.52
Copper (mg)	0.08	0.71	trace	0.04
Zinc (mg)	0.38	2.48	0.14	0.52
Selenium (µg)	unknown	53	unknown	unknown
Vitamin A (µg)	unknown	168	84	trace
Vitamin D (µg)	nil	nil	nil	nil
Vitamin E (mg)	unknown	3.29	0.29	unknown
Vitamin B_1 (mg)	0.09	0.4	0.03	0.18
Vitamin B_2 (mg)	0.06	0.16	0.01	0.01
Niacin (mg)	0.83	2.17	0.06	0.26
Vitamin B_6 (mg)	0.11	0.77	0.05	0.16
Vitamin B_{12} (µg)	nil	nil	nil	nil
Folate (µg)	33	47	unknown	8
Pantothenate (mg)	unknown	0.96	0.02	0.4
Biotin (µg)	unknown	3.1	0.1	unknown
Vitamin C (mg)	unknown	6	12	5

Segment Three

Meat, fish, eggs, pulses and nuts

Of our overall intake, foods from this group should account for less than an eighth of the space on our plate. Protein foods are good for us but most of us eat too much at the expense of starchy carbohydrate. The important thing about this group of foods is variety; try to get your protein from many different sources, not just meat. Fish and pulses are good sources of protein, but they are less fatty than meat, and pulses also contain fibre. Eggs are top quality protein and also an excellent source of iron. Mixing proteins such as meat and pulses means you get more protein for your money and you will also be eat ing less fat and more fibre. The problem with a lot of meat dishes is they have added fat, such as meat pies, curries, stir frys and some pasta dishes.

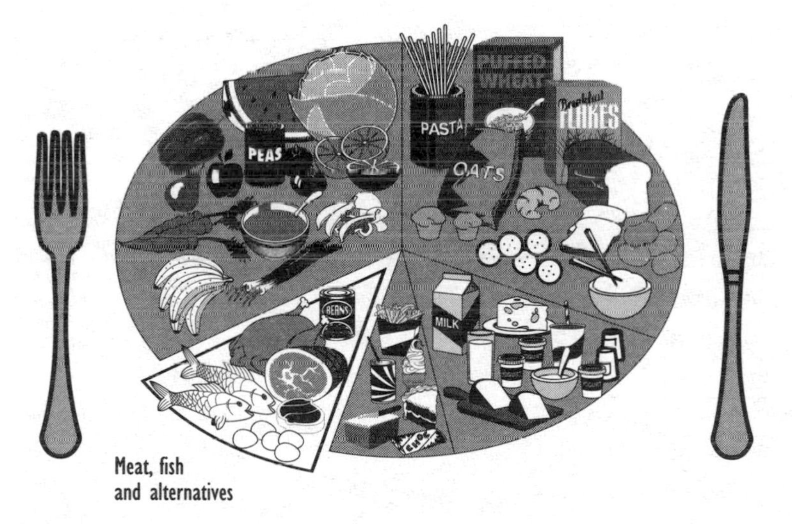

Meat, fish and alternatives

FOOD	**Bacon** back, dry fried	**Bacon** back, grilled	**Bacon** back, dry cured, grilled	**Bacon** back, fat trimmed, grilled
PORTION SIZE	one rasher	one rasher	one rasher	one rasher
NUTRIENTS				
Energy (kcals)	73	71	64	53
Protein (g)	6	5.8	7.1	6.4
Total fat (g)	5.5	5.4	3.9	3.0
Saturated fat (g)	2.0	2.0	1.5	1.1
Mono-unsat. fat (g)	2.3	2.25	1.6	1.3
Poly-unsat. fat (g)	0.7	0.7	0.5	0.4
Carbohydrate (g)	nil	nil	nil	nil
Sugar (g)	nil	nil	nil	nil
Fibre (g)	nil	nil	nil	nil
Sodium (mg)	477	470	535	482
Potassium (mg)	90	85	100	90
Calcium (mg)	1.5	1.7	2.2	2
Magnesium (mg)	5.2	5.2	6.5	5.7
Phosphorus (mg)	45	45	60	52
Iron (mg)	0.15	0.15	0.2	0.17
Copper (mg)	0.01	0.01	0.02	0.01
Zinc (mg)	0.47	0.42	0.6	0.55
Selenium (μg)	4.5	3	3.5	3.2
Vitamin A (μg)	trace	trace	trace	trace
Vitamin D (μg)	0.15	0.15	0.2	0.17
Vitamin E (mg)	0.01	0.01	0.02	0.01
Vitamin B_1 (mg)	0.21	0.29	0.27	0.24
Vitamin B_2 (mg)	0.03	0.03	0.04	0.04
Niacin (mg)	1.7	1.8	2.1	1.9
Vitamin B_6 (mg)	0.13	0.13	0.14	0.12
Vitamin B_{12} (μg)	0.25	0.25	0.25	0.25
Folate (μg)	0.5	1.2	0.7	0.7
Pantothenate (mg)	0.31	0.31	0.37	0.33
Biotin (μg)	1.25	0.75	1.5	1.25
Vitamin C (mg)	trace	trace	trace	trace

Bacon back, smoked, grilled	**Bacon** streaky, grilled	**Beefburger** chilled/frozen, fried	**Beefburger** chilled/frozen, grilled	**FOOD**
one rasher	one rasher	one average	one average	**PORTION SIZE**
				NUTRIENTS
73	61	118	117	Energy (kcals)
5.8	4.9	10.3	9.5	Protein (g)
5.5	5.3	8.6	8.8	Total fat (g)
2.0	1.9	3.9	3.9	Saturated fat (g)
4.6	2.3	3.9	4.0	Mono-unsat. fat (g)
0.7	0.7	0.3	0.3	Poly-unsat. fat (g)
nil	nil	trace	trace	Carbohydrate (g)
nil	nil	trace	trace	Sugar (g)
nil	nil	nil	nil	Fibre (g)
440	336	169	144	Sodium (mg)
82	66	151	137	Potassium (mg)
1.7	1.8	4	4	Calcium (mg)
5.2	4	9	8	Magnesium (mg)
47	36	86	76	Phosphorus (mg)
0.17	0.16	1.01	0.9	Iron (mg)
0.01	0.03	0.05	0.05	Copper (mg)
0.55	0.5	2.27	2.2	Zinc (mg)
3	2.2	4	3	Selenium (µg)
trace	trace	trace	trace	Vitamin A (µg)
0.15	0.14	0.68	0.65	Vitamin D (µg)
0.01	0.01	0.19	0.14	Vitamin E (mg)
0.22	0.14	trace	trace	Vitamin B_1 (mg)
0.04	0.03	0.08	0.07	Vitamin B_2 (mg)
1.7	1.26	1.98	1.84	Niacin (mg)
0.11	0.08	0.11	0.11	Vitamin B_6 (mg)
0.25	0.2	1.1	1.1	Vitamin B_{12} (µg)
0.5	0.6	3	4	Folate (µg)
0.3	0.24	0.31	0.3	Pantothenate (mg)
1.25	0.8	0.7	0.7	Biotin (µg)
trace	trace	nil	nil	Vitamin C (mg)

FOOD	Beef chow mein retail	Beef curry homemade	Beef pie chilled/frozen baked	Roast beef topside
PORTION SIZE	restaurant serving	medium	one individual	medium
NUTRIENTS				
Energy (kcals)	476	533	419	182
Protein (g)	23.4	35.4	10.2	32.6
Total fat (g)	21.0	41.6	29.1	5.7
Saturated fat (g)	4.5	8.8	11.9	2.3
Mono-unsat. fat (g)	10.8	16.1	12.6	2.5
Poly-unsat. fat (g)	4.9	13.8	2.9	0.3
Carbohydrate (g)	51.5	4.4	30.9	nil
Sugar (g)	8.4	3.4	2.8	nil
Fibre (g)	unknown	0.8	unknown	nil
Sodium (mg)	2065	468	644	56
Potassium (mg)	unknown	832	140	369
Calcium (mg)	unknown	57	67	7
Magnesium (mg)	unknown	60	15	24
Phosphorus (mg)	unknown	338	108	207
Iron (mg)	4.55	3.9	1.54	2.61
Copper (mg)	unknown	0.13	0.24	0.04
Zinc (mg)	unknown	9.36	0.98	5.85
Selenium (µg)	unknown	10	unknown	11
Vitamin A (µg)	trace	34	trace	1
Vitamin D (µg)	unknown	0.78	unknown	0.72
Vitamin E (mg)	1.5	0.96	unknown	0.07
Vitamin B_1 (mg)	0.1	0.16	0.35	0.08
Vitamin B_2 (mg)	0.1	0.39	0.08	0.26
Niacin (mg)	unknown	5.72	1.96	5.22
Vitamin B_6 (mg)	unknown	0.65	0.25	0.5
Vitamin B_{12} (µg)	trace	2.6	1.4	2.7
Folate (µg)	unknown	49	21	19
Pantothenate (mg)	unknown	0.91	unknown	0.54
Biotin (µg)	unknown	2.6	unknown	1.8
Vitamin C (mg)	trace	5	trace	nil

Beef stew homemade	**Beef stir fry** with green peppers and black bean sauce	**Beef stroganoff**	**Braised steak** braised	**FOOD**
medium	restaurant serving	medium	medium	**PORTION SIZE**
				NUTRIENTS
294	526	445	344	Energy (kcals)
31.5	42.5	40.0	46.1	Protein (g)
13.3	30.6	29.1	17.8	Total fat (g)
3.9	9.7	16.1	7.4	Saturated fat (g)
5.2	12.2	9.6	7.3	Mono-unsat. fat (g)
2.3	6.8	1.6	1.1	Poly-unsat. fat (g)
13.0	21.6	6.5	nil	Carbohydrate (g)
5.5	13.0	5.2	nil	Sugar (g)
1.8	2.9	1.3	nil	Fibre (g)
1014	972	494	84	Sodium (mg)
624	972	884	462	Potassium (mg)
44	58	73	11	Calcium (mg)
34	68	52	31	Magnesium (mg)
286	432	442	294	Phosphorus (mg)
3.38	5.4	4.16	3.64	Iron (mg)
0.1	0.14	0.42	trace	Copper (mg)
7.28	6.84	5.46	12.18	Zinc (mg)
10	unknown	18	14	Selenium (µg)
539	75	231	1.6	Vitamin A (µg)
1.04	0.72	0.78	0.98	Vitamin D (µg)
0.52	1.04	0.62	0.04	Vitamin E (mg)
0.16	0.18	0.29	0.07	Vitamin B_1 (mg)
0.29	0.4	0.6	0.36	Vitamin B_2 (mg)
4.68	8.28	8.06	6.86	Niacin (mg)
0.57	1.37	0.83	0.46	Vitamin B_6 (mg)
2.6	3.6	2.6	4.2	Vitamin B_{12} (µg)
10	47	29	73	Folate (µg)
0.83	1.12	2.44	0.8	Pantothenate (mg)
2.6	unknown	7.8	2.8	Biotin (µg)
3	97	3	nil	Vitamin C (mg)

FOOD	Fillet steak grilled	Rump steak grilled	Sirloin steak grilled	Black pudding fried
PORTION SIZE	8 oz	8 oz	8 oz	one slice
NUTRIENTS				
Energy (kcals)	336	362	427	92
Protein (g)	48.2	45.3	52.8	3.9
Total fat (g)	16	20.1	23.9	6.6
Saturated fat (g)	7.4	8.6	10.8	2.5
Mono-unsat. fat (g)	6.6	9.6	10.5	2.4
Poly-unsat. fat (g)	0.8	0.8	0.8	1.1
Carbohydrate (g)	nil	nil	nil	4.5
Sugar (g)	nil	nil	nil	trace
Fibre (g)	nil	nil	nil	unknown
Sodium (mg)	113	91	126	363
Potassium (mg)	655	631	730	42
Calcium (mg)	10	12	12	11
Magnesium (mg)	45	42	50	5
Phosphorus (mg)	4.3	365	432	33
Iron (mg)	3.86	5.64	4.15	6
Copper (mg)	unknown	0.3	0.07	0.11
Zinc (mg)	8.57	8.13	9.13	0.39
Selenium (µg)	17	5	17	unknown
Vitamin A (µg)	2	trace	2	12
Vitamin D (µg)	1.01	trace	1.16	trace
Vitamin E (mg)	0.1	0.53	0.13	0.07
Vitamin B_1 (mg)	0.2	0.13	0.23	0.03
Vitamin B_2 (mg)	0.44	0.53	0.50	0.02
Niacin (mg)	10.58	9.46	11.12	0.3
Vitamin B_6 (mg)	1.01	0.48	1.08	0.01
Vitamin B_{12} (µg)	3.4	3.3	5	0.3
Folate (µg)	29	25	35	2
Pantothenate (mg)	1.41	1.33	1.59	0.18
Biotin (µg)	3.4	trace	3.3	0.6
Vitamin C (mg)	nil	nil	nil	nil

Bolognese sauce	**Cannelloni** chilled, re-heated	**Chicken** roast - light and dark meat	**Chicken** breast grilled	**FOOD**
average	individual ready meal	medium	aveage breast	**PORTION SIZE**
				NUTRIENTS
247	315	148	191	Energy (kcals)
13.6	16.6	24.8	38.7	Protein (g)
18.9	13.0	5.4	4	Total fat (g)
5.3	5.2	1.6	1.2	Saturated fat (g)
8.0	5.2	2.5	1.7	Mono-unsat. fat (g)
4.4	1.6	1.0	0.8	Poly-unsat. fat (g)
6.3	35.1	nil	nil	Carbohydrate (g)
5.6	13.3	nil	nil	Sugar (g)
1.7	3.1	nil	nil	Fibre (g)
731	1196	81	78	Sodium (mg)
527	468	310	533	Potassium (mg)
39	169	9	9	Calcium (mg)
24	52	24	44	Magnesium (mg)
134	234	210	364	Phosphorus (mg)
2.38	3.12	0.8	0.65	Iron (mg)
0.19	0.42	0.12	0.08	Copper (mg)
2.89	1.82	1.5	1.04	Zinc (mg)
3	unknown	7	20	Selenium (µg)
361	unknown	trace	trace	Vitamin A (µg)
trace	unknown	trace	0.13	Vitamin D (µg)
3.28	unknown	0.11	0.16	Vitamin E (mg)
0.12	0.26	0.08	0.13	Vitamin B_1 (mg)
0.19	0.34	0.19	0.26	Vitamin B_2 (mg)
2.72	3.38	8.2	18.59	Niacin (mg)
0.27	0.75	0.26	0.55	Vitamin B_6 (mg)
1.4	trace	trace	trace	Vitamin B_{12} (µg)
12	34	10	7	Folate (µg)
0.56	unknown	1.2	2.16	Pantothenate (mg)
1.7	unknown	3	2.6	Biotin (µg)
7	trace	nil	nil	Vitamin C (mg)

FOOD	**Chicken** leg quarter, roasted	**Chicken** breaded, fried	**Chicken in breadcrumbs** stuffed with cheese and vegetables	**Chicken chasseur**
PORTION SIZE	average quarter	average	one breast	medium
NUTRIENTS				
Energy (kcals)	212	242	368	203
Protein (g)	18.8	18	25.9	33.3
Total fat (g)	15.2	12.7	22.2	4.9
Saturated fat (g)	4.1	2.1	6.6	0.8
Mono-unsat. fat (g)	7.0	5.3	7.2	1.6
Poly-unsat. fat (g)	2.9	4.7	6.9	1.8
Carbohydrate (g)	nil	14.8	17.3	6.8
Sugar (g)	nil	0.8	1.1	3.4
Fibre (g)	nil	0.7	1.4	0.8
Sodium (mg)	86	420	704	598
Potassium (mg)	207	320	400	702
Calcium (mg)	11	unknown	99	34
Magnesium (mg)	18	unknown	35	49
Phosphorus (mg)	162	unknown	352	338
Iron (mg)	0.72	unknown	0.96	1.56
Copper (mg)	0.05	unknown	0.06	0.34
Zinc (mg)	1.53	unknown	1.12	1.3
Selenium (µg)	14	unknown	unknown	18
Vitamin A (µg)	23	trace	96	4
Vitamin D (µg)	0.18	trace	0.8	0.26
Vitamin E (mg)	0.21	unknown	2.74	0.36
Vitamin B_1 (mg)	0.06	0.12	0.22	0.21
Vitamin B_2 (mg)	0.25	0.06	0.16	0.21
Niacin (mg)	4.5	8.2	8.96	12.22
Vitamin B_6 (mg)	0.36	0.53	0.61	0.62
Vitamin B_{12} (µg)	0.9	trace	trace	trace
Folate (µg)	10	unknown	14	18
Pantothenate (mg)	1.09	1.2	1.73	1.74
Biotin (µg)	2.7	2.0	6.4	5.2
Vitamin C (mg)	nil	nil	trace	trace

Chicken curry retail	Chicken fingers baked	Chicken fricassee retail	Chicken Kiev baked	FOOD
medium	one	medium	one breast	PORTION SIZE
				NUTRIENTS
387	31	278	375	Energy (kcals)
31.5	1.9	27.3	26.0	Protein (g)
23.1	1.4	16.1	23.7	Total fat (g)
10.4	0.4	6.2	9.9	Saturated fat (g)
7.5	0.8	5.5	7.7	Mono-unsat. fat (g)
3.9	0.5	3.1	4.9	Poly-unsat. fat (g)
14.0	2.8	6.8	15.5	Carbohydrate (g)
11.4	0.2	3.4	0.4	Sugar (g)
3.4	unknown	1.3	0.8	Fibre (g)
1170	96	936	476	Sodium (mg)
780	24	624	392	Potassium (mg)
unknown	4	55	60	Calcium (mg)
unknown	3	42	34	Magnesium (mg)
unknown	33	312	266	Phosphorus (mg)
unknown	0.17	1.56	1.12	Iron (mg)
unknown	0.02	0.26	0.11	Copper (mg)
unknown	0.12	1.56	0.84	Zinc (mg)
unknown	unknown	16	unknown	Selenium (μg)
160	trace	81	trace	Vitamin A (μg)
unknown	unknown	0.26	unknown	Vitamin D (μg)
3.38	unknown	unknown	1.25	Vitamin E (mg)
0.52	0.22	0.36	0.17	Vitamin B_1 (mg)
0.36	0.01	0.29	0.13	Vitamin B_2 (mg)
9.88	0.65	11.7	12.6	Niacin (mg)
0.62	0.07	0.75	0.66	Vitamin B_6 (mg)
unknown	trace	trace	trace	Vitamin B_{12} (μg)
unknown	1	34	15	Folate (μg)
2.65	unknown	1.9	2.09	Pantothenate (mg)
7.8	unknown	unknown	4.2	Biotin (μg)
3	nil	8	trace	Vitamin C (mg)

FOOD	Chicken korma homemade	Chicken and mushroom pie single crust	Chicken nuggets	Chicken pie chilled retail
PORTION SIZE	average	medium slice	average (6)	individual
NUTRIENTS				
Energy (kcals)	455	240	265	374
Protein (g)	53.2	16.1	18.7	11.7
Total fat (g)	20.3	12.4	13.0	23.0
Saturated fat (g)	6.0	5.4	3.3	9.1
Mono-unsat. fat (g)	6.7	4.4	6.8	9.6
Poly-unsat. fat (g)	6.3	1.7	2.2	3.1
Carbohydrate (g)	16.1	17.0	19.5	32.0
Sugar (g)	9.8	2.5	1.1	2.1
Fibre (g)	1.4	0.7	0.2	1.0
Sodium (mg)	595	336	510	559
Potassium (mg)	1155	300	280	182
Calcium (mg)	214	82	25	78
Magnesium (mg)	95	24	23	20
Phosphorus (mg)	595	180	210	117
Iron (mg)	2.8	0.72	0.6	1.04
Copper (mg)	0.21	0.2	trace	0.08
Zinc (mg)	2.45	0.72	0.5	0.78
Selenium (µg)	25	8	unknown	unknown
Vitamin A (µg)	71	74	14	trace
Vitamin D (µg)	0.35	0.48	unknown	unknown
Vitamin E (mg)	0.45	0.83	1.29	unknown
Vitamin B_1 (mg)	0.35	0.1	0.09	0.53
Vitamin B_2 (mg)	0.42	0.18	0.1	0.12
Niacin (mg)	17.5	4.8	6.3	1.95
Vitamin B_6 (mg)	0.98	0.26	0.29	0.16
Vitamin B_{12} (µg)	trace	trace	trace	trace
Folate (µg)	25	10	20	10
Pantothenate (mg)	2.41	0.86	1.3	0.83
Biotin (µg)	7.0	3.6	7.0	5.2
Vitamin C (mg)	4	trace	nil	unknown

Chicken risotto	Chicken roll	Chicken stir fry with mushrooms and cashew nuts	Chicken stir fry with peppers and black bean sauce	FOOD
average	one slice	average takeaway	average takeaway	PORTION SIZE
				NUTRIENTS
546	16	616	448	Energy (kcals)
30.6	2.1	78.8	70	Protein (g)
9.9	0.6	26	14	Total fat (g)
4.5	0.2	4.8	2.0	Saturated fat (g)
2.1	0.3	12.4	4.8	Mono-unsat. fat (g)
0.3	0.1	7.6	5.6	Poly-unsat. fat (g)
83.7	0.6	18.0	11.2	Carbohydrate (g)
unknown	nil	8.0	9.6	Sugar (g)
unknown	trace	2.8	3.2	Fibre (g)
1260	82	1200	1200	Sodium (mg)
690	23	1640	1280	Potassium (mg)
81	2	40	68	Calcium (mg)
45	2	188	112	Magnesium (mg)
360	26	880	680	Phosphorus (mg)
2.4	0.05	4.4	4.4	Iron (mg)
0.36	0.01	1.04	0.28	Copper (mg)
3.0	0.06	4.0	2.4	Zinc (mg)
unknown	unknown	48	32	Selenium (µg)
76	trace	563	55	Vitamin A (µg)
0.3	unknown	0.4	0.4	Vitamin D (µg)
unknown	unknown	1.08	1.04	Vitamin E (mg)
0.27	0.03	0.52	0.72	Vitamin B_1 (mg)
0.15	0.01	0.48	0.36	Vitamin B_2 (mg)
9.0	0.78	27.6	24.0	Niacin (mg)
unknown	0.04	1.6	1.44	Vitamin B_6 (mg)
trace	trace	trace	trace	Vitamin B_{12} (µg)
unknown	1	48	40	Folate (µg)
unknown	0.1	unknown	2.88	Pantothenate (mg)
unknown	0.2	unknown	unknown	Biotin (µg)
3	trace	60	64	Vitamin C (mg)

FOOD	Chicken tandoori retail	Chicken vindaloo	Chilli con carne homemade	Coq au vin
PORTION SIZE	restaurant portion	restaurant portion	medium	medium
NUTRIENTS				
Energy (kcals)	749	763	332	403
Protein (g)	95.9	64	24.2	28.9
Total fat (g)	37.8	52.9	18.7	28.6
Saturated fat (g)	11.6	6.3	6.6	11.2
Mono-unsat. fat (g)	17.5	19.9	8.4	11.4
Poly-unsat. fat (g)	7.0	23.1	2.4	4.2
Carbohydrate (g)	7.0	8.8	18.3	8.3
Sugar (g)	3.5	6.0	6.2	1.0
Fibre (g)	trace	1.1	5.1	0.8
Sodium (mg)	2065	735	550	676
Potassium (mg)	1645	1400	968	728
Calcium (mg)	203	144	64	42
Magnesium (mg)	126	130	73	49
Phosphorus (mg)	980	525	286	226
Iron (mg)	6.3	9.45	4.84	2.86
Copper (mg)	0.42	0.31	0.42	0.29
Zinc (mg)	5.25	4.2	4.84	2.34
Selenium (µg)	56	35	7	21
Vitamin A (µg)	122	70	53	126
Vitamin D (µg)	0.7	0.35	trace	0.78
Vitamin E (mg)	5.22	0.45	2.62	unknown
Vitamin B_1 (mg)	0.42	0.42	0.24	0.26
Vitamin B_2 (mg)	0.66	0.42	0.31	0.39
Niacin (mg)	35.7	17.5	4.18	6.76
Vitamin B_6 (mg)	2.13	0.95	0.46	0.42
Vitamin B_{12} (µg)	3.5	trace	1.8	trace
Folate (µg)	56	21	31	13
Pantothenate (mg)	7.8	2.52	0.81	1.56
Biotin (µg)	17.5	7.0	2.2	7.8
Vitamin C (mg)	7	4	20	3

Corned beef canned	**Cornish pasty**	**Cottage/ shepherd's pie**	**Duck** roasted, meat fat and skin	**FOOD**
one thin slice	one average	medium	breast and wing	**PORTION SIZE**
				NUTRIENTS
82	481	391	783	Energy (kcals)
10.2	11.6	19.8	37	Protein (g)
4.6	29.6	21.1	70.5	Total fat (g)
2.4	10.7	7.8	21.1	Saturated fat (g)
1.8	15.2	8.4	35.7	Mono-unsat. fat (g)
0.1	2.2	2.8	9.8	Poly-unsat. fat (g)
nil	45.1	32.2	nil	Carbohydrate (g)
nil	1.7	5.0	nil	Sugar (g)
nil	1.3	2.8	nil	Fibre (g)
361	856	899	161	Sodium (mg)
53	276	744	407	Potassium (mg)
5	87	53	41	Calcium (mg)
6	26	40	31	Magnesium (mg)
46	160	205	333	Phosphorus (mg)
1.1	2.17	2.17	3.14	Iron (mg)
0.09	0.51	0.12	0.43	Copper (mg)
2.13	1.45	3.72	4.07	Zinc (mg)
3	unknown	9	41	Selenium (µg)
trace	trace	455	unknown	Vitamin A (µg)
trace	trace	0.93	unknown	Vitamin D (µg)
0.3	1.88	1.21	unknown	Vitamin E (mg)
trace	0.14	0.28	0.33	Vitamin B_1 (mg)
0.09	0.09	0.09	0.94	Vitamin B_2 (mg)
0.95	2.32	3.72	7.03	Niacin (mg)
0.02	0.17	0.65	0.57	Vitamin B_6 (mg)
0.8	1.5	trace	3.7	Vitamin B_{12} (µg)
1	4	25	28	Folate (µg)
0.15	0.87	0.81	4.81	Pantothenate (mg)
0.8	1.5	3.1	12.9	Biotin (µg)
nil	nil	6	nil	Vitamin C (mg)

FOOD	**Faggots**	**Frankfurter sausages** (hot dogs)	**Game pie**	**Gammon** grilled
PORTION SIZE	two	one	average slice	average steak
NUTRIENTS				
Energy (kcals)	402	63	667	338
Protein (g)	16.7	2.2	21.4	46.8
Total fat (g)	27.8	5.8	39.4	16.8
Saturated fat (g)	unknown	unknown	13.8	5.8
Mono-unsat. fat (g)	unknown	unknown	15.8	7.0
Poly-unsat. fat (g)	unknown	unknown	7.0	2.9
Carbohydrate (g)	23.0	0.7	60.7	nil
Sugar (g)	trace	trace	6.0	nil
Fibre (g)	unknown	trace	2.3	nil
Sodium (mg)	1230	225	753	3281
Potassium (mg)	255	23	298	646
Calcium (mg)	83	8	112	14
Magnesium (mg)	27	2	32	44
Phosphorus (mg)	180	30	210	391
Iron (mg)	12.45	0.34	3.67	1.36
Copper (mg)	0.9	0.06	0.26	0.15
Zinc (mg)	2.4	0.32	2.1	3.74
Selenium (μg)	unknown	2	7	24
Vitamin A (μg)	705	trace	1090	trace
Vitamin D (μg)	0.3	trace	1.57	1.36
Vitamin E (mg)	unknown	0.06	1.68	0.14
Vitamin B_1 (mg)	0.21	0.02	0.37	1.97
Vitamin B_2 (mg)	0.74	0.03	0.42	0.31
Niacin (mg)	4.5	0.34	5.25	10.88
Vitamin B_6 (mg)	0.25	0.01	0.37	0.27
Vitamin B_{12} (μg)	7.5	0.2	5.3	1.7
Folate (μg)	33	trace	131	5
Pantothenate (mg)	1.65	0.09	1.09	2.43
Biotin (μg)	6.0	0.5	21.0	10.2
Vitamin C (mg)	trace	nil	2	trace

Goulash	Garlic sausage	Grouse roasted	Haggis	FOOD
medium	one small slice	one whole	half of one medium haggis	**PORTION SIZE**
				NUTRIENTS
216	12	205	232	Energy (kcals)
17.9	0.8	44.2	8.0	Protein (g)
8.8	1.0	3.2	16.2	Total fat (g)
2.1	0.4	0.8	5.7	Saturated fat (g)
3.1	0.5	0.3	5.1	Mono-unsat. fat (g)
2.1	0.1	1.9	1.05	Poly-unsat. fat (g)
17.2	trace	nil	14.4	Carbohydrate (g)
4.7	trace	nil	trace	Sugar (g)
2.1	trace	nil	0.1	Fibre (g)
988	47	176	577	Sodium (mg)
728	12	608	127	Potassium (mg)
34	1	72	21.7	Calcium (mg)
39	1	51	27	Magnesium (mg)
185	9	416	120	Phosphorus (mg)
2.6	0.04	7.36	3.6	Iron (mg)
0.16	trace	0.54	0.33	Copper (mg)
3.9	0.08	2.56	1.4	Zinc (mg)
5	unknown	32	unknown	Selenium (µg)
33	trace	unknown	1350	Vitamin A (µg)
0.52	unknown	unknown	0.07	Vitamin D (µg)
0.88	0.02	unknown	0.3	Vitamin E (mg)
0.21	0.03	0.3	0.12	Vitamin B_1 (mg)
0.18	0.01	1.28	0.26	Vitamin B_2 (mg)
3.12	0.2	11.2	1.1	Niacin (mg)
0.62	0.01	1.02	0.05	Vitamin B_6 (mg)
trace	0.1	1.6	1.5	Vitamin B_{12} (µg)
23	trace	59	6	Folate (µg)
0.68	0.05	unknown	0.3	Pantothenate (mg)
2.6	0.2	unknown	9	Biotin (µg)
21	unknown	nil	trace	Vitamin C (mg)

FOOD	Ham canned	Ham Parma	Ham premium (no added water)	Ham and pork chopped, canned
PORTION SIZE	one slice	restaurant serving	one slice	one slice
NUTRIENTS				
Energy (kcals)	37	105	37	39
Protein (g)	5.8	12.8	5.9	2.0
Total fat (g)	1.6	6.0	1.4	3.3
Saturated fat (g)	0.6	unknown	0.5	1.2
Mono-unsat. fat (g)	0.7	unknown	0.6	1.6
Poly-unsat. fat (g)	0.1	unknown	0.2	0.3
Carbohydrate (g)	trace	trace	0.1	0.2
Sugar (g)	trace	nil	0.1	trace
Fibre (g)	nil	trace	nil	trace
Sodium (mg)	515	940	294	153
Potassium (mg)	70	unknown	90	32
Calcium (mg)	11	unknown	2	2
Magnesium (mg)	6	unknown	6	2
Phosphorus (mg)	95	unknown	67	35
Iron (mg)	0.42	unknown	0.22	0.17
Copper (mg)	0.04	unknown	0.02	0.03
Zinc (mg)	0.7	unknown	0.59	0.41
Selenium (μg)	3	unknown	3	unknown
Vitamin A (μg)	trace	unknown	trace	trace
Vitamin D (μg)	unknown	unknown	unknown	trace
Vitamin E (mg)	0.03	unknown	0.01	0.02
Vitamin B_1 (mg)	0.1	unknown	0.08	0.03
Vitamin B_2 (mg)	0.08	unknown	0.06	0.03
Niacin (mg)	0.88	unknown	1.26	0.45
Vitamin B_6 (mg)	0.07	unknown	0.13	0.01
Vitamin B_{12} (μg)	trace	unknown	trace	0.1
Folate (μg)	1	unknown	2	trace
Pantothenate (mg)	0.21	unknown	unknown	0.06
Biotin (μg)	0.3	unknown	unknown	0.3
Vitamin C (mg)	7	unknown	trace	nil

Haslet	Heart lambs, roasted	Hot pot homemade	Irish stew homemade	FOOD
one slice	one average	medium	medium	PORTION SIZE
				NUTRIENTS
30	452	296	315	Energy (kcals)
1.9	50.6	24.4	19.8	Protein (g)
1.8	27.8	11.7	16.6	Total fat (g)
0.6	unknown	4.7	7.5	Saturated fat (g)
0.7	unknown	5.5	6.2	Mono-unsat. fat (g)
0.3	unknown	0.5	1.0	Poly-unsat. fat (g)
1.6	nil	26.3	23.1	Carbohydrate (g)
0.1	nil	7.3	4.9	Sugar (g)
trace	nil	3.1	2.6	Fibre (g)
134	168	1716	520	Sodium (mg)
31	420	910	728	Potassium (mg)
13	14	47	36	Calcium (mg)
2	42	47	36	Magnesium (mg)
29	480	211	213	Phosphorus (mg)
0.27	12.0	3.12	2.08	Iron (mg)
0.02	1.32	0.31	0.16	Copper (mg)
0.21	5.6	4.42	3.9	Zinc (mg)
unknown	unknown	5	3	Selenium (µg)
trace	trace	565	520	Vitamin A (µg)
unknown	unknown	trace	0.52	Vitamin D (µg)
0.09	unknown	0.68	0.34	Vitamin E (mg)
0.02	0.48	0.34	0.31	Vitamin B_1 (mg)
0.03	2.74	0.21	0.13	Vitamin B_2 (mg)
0.5	7.6	4.42	3.64	Niacin (mg)
0.03	0.52	0.73	0.57	Vitamin B_6 (mg)
0.4	12.0	2.1	trace	Vitamin B_{12} (µg)
2	4	29	21	Folate (µg)
0.12	7.6	0.94	1.01	Pantothenate (mg)
0.6	16.0	trace	2.6	Biotin (µg)
trace	4	8	8	Vitamin C (mg)

FOOD	Kebabs, doner meat, pitta bread and salad	Kebabs, shish meat only	Kidney lambs, fried	Lamb chump chops fried
PORTION SIZE	small takeaway	one skewer	one average	one medium
NUTRIENTS				
Energy (kcals)	587	175	66	216
Protein (g)	32.7	24.6	8.3	17.3
Total fat (g)	37.3	8.5	3.6	16.2
Saturated fat (g)	17.9	3.3	unknown	7.6
Mono-unsat. fat (g)	14.0	3.7	unknown	6.0
Poly-unsat. fat (g)	2.1	0.7	unknown	1.2
Carbohydrate (g)	32.2	nil	nil	nil
Sugar (g)	3.5	nil	nil	nil
Fibre (g)	1.8	nil	nil	nil
Sodium (mg)	1265	434	81	50
Potassium (mg)	598	357	98	252
Calcium (mg)	85	6	5	19
Magnesium (mg)	46	25	7	18
Phosphorus (mg)	299	213	123	161
Iron (mg)	3.68	2.21	3.92	1.47
Copper (mg)	0.25	0.12	0.2	0.07
Zinc (mg)	5.06	5.18	1.26	2.38
Selenium (µg)	7	3	31	3
Vitamin A (µg)	34	trace	39	5
Vitamin D (µg)	0.69	0.51	unknown	0.42
Vitamin E (mg)	1.08	0.57	0.14	unknown
Vitamin B_1 (mg)	0.32	0.12	0.18	0.11
Vitamin B_2 (mg)	0.32	0.24	1.08	0.17
Niacin (mg)	7.82	5.95	3.19	4.13
Vitamin B_6 (mg)	0.32	0.22	0.17	0.26
Vitamin B_{12} (µg)	2.3	2.5	18.9	1.4
Folate (µg)	37	8	25	1
Pantothenate (mg)	1.38	1.19	1.61	0.81
Biotin (µg)	2.3	2.5	25.5	1.4
Vitamin C (mg)	5	nil	2	nil

Lamb cutlets grilled	**Lamb** leg, roast	**Lamb biryani**	**Lamb rogan josh**	**FOOD**
one medium	medium	restaurant serving	restaurant serving	**PORTION SIZE**
				NUTRIENTS
185	239	800	553	Energy (kcals)
11.5	23.5	28.4	50.4	Protcin (g)
15.4	16.1	42.4	33.3	Total fat (g)
7.7	8.0	8.4	12.9	Saturated fat (g)
5.9	6.2	14.8	12.6	Mono-unsat. fat (g)
0.8	0.8	15.2	4.5	Poly-unsat. fat (g)
nil	nil	82.0	14.0	Carbohydrate (g)
nil	nil	7.6	10.5	Sugar (g)
nil	nil	2.4	2.8	Fibre (g)
36	59	unknown	595	Sodium (mg)
160	279	720	1330	Potassium (mg)
5	7	132	140	Calcium (mg)
12	23	56	84	Magnesium (mg)
100	180	328	420	Phosphorus (mg)
0.95	2.25	4.0	6.65	Iron (mg)
0.09	0.25	0.4	0.38	Copper (mg)
1.65	4.14	4.4	7.0	Zinc (mg)
1	1	20	4	Selenium (μg)
trace	trace	18	114	Vitamin A (μg)
trace	trace	0.4	1.05	Vitamin D (μg)
0.06	0.1	unknown	1.96	Vitamin E (mg)
0.05	0.11	0.24	0.35	Vitamin B_1 (mg)
0.1	0.28	0.2	0.35	Vitamin B_2 (mg)
2.4	4.86	4.4	8.4	Niacin (mg)
0.08	0.16	0.56	0.7	Vitamin B_6 (mg)
1.0	1.8	trace	3.5	Vitamin B_{12} (μg)
2	3	24	21	Folate (μg)
0.25	0.54	0.84	1.01	Pantothenate (mg)
0.5	0.9	4.0	3.5	Biotin (μg)
nil	nil	4	14	Vitamin C (mg)

FOOD	Lamb stir fry with vegetables	Lancashire hot-pot	Lasagne homemade	Lasagne frozen, cooked
PORTION SIZE	restaurant serving	medium	average	average ready meal for one
NUTRIENTS				
Energy (kcals)	857	289	668	296
Protein (g)	58.3	23.1	35.7	14.5
Total fat (g)	66.2	13.5	45.4	11.0
Saturated fat (g)	26.6	5.5	19.7	5.5
Mono-unsat. fat (g)	25.2	4.9	16.4	4.1
Poly-unsat. fat (g)	9.0	1.6	5.5	0.6
Carbohydrate (g)	7.2	19.5	31.1	37.1
Sugar (g)	6.1	3.6	10.5	6.1
Fibre (g)	2.2	2.3	2.1	unknown
Sodium (mg)	1332	520	1470	1247
Potassium (mg)	1332	676	798	435
Calcium (mg)	72	47	407	206
Magnesium (mg)	79	34	59	49
Phosphorus (mg)	576	200	504	241
Iron (mg)	6.48	1.82	2.94	2.03
Copper (mg)	0.29	0.16	0.25	0.49
Zinc (mg)	11.88	3.12	5.46	2.03
Selenium (μg)	unknown	3	17	unknown
Vitamin A (μg)	163	244	466	unknown
Vitamin D (μg)	1.44	0.52	1.26	unknown
Vitamin E (mg)	unknown	0.21	2.44	unknown
Vitamin B_1 (mg)	0.4	0.26	0.25	0.06
Vitamin B_2 (mg)	0.43	0.13	0.42	0.35
Niacin (mg)	10.08	3.38	5.88	2.32
Vitamin B_6 (mg)	0.65	0.55	0.5	0.14
Vitamin B_{12} (μg)	3.6	2.6	4.2	0.9
Folate (μg)	40	21	29	12
Pantothenate (mg)	2.12	0.65	1.3	unknown
Biotin (μg)	unknown	2.6	8.4	unknown
Vitamin C (mg)	18	8	4	trace

Liver calf, fried	**Liver** lambs, fried	**Liver** pigs, stewed	**Liver and onions**	**FOOD**
medium (40g)	medium (40g)	medium (70g)	average (142g)	**PORTION SIZE**
				NUTRIENTS
70	95	132	210	Energy (kcals)
8.9	12.0	17.9	21.0	Protein (g)
3.8	5.2	5.7	10.8	Total fat (g)
unknown	unknown	1.8	2.1	Saturated fat (g)
unknown	unknown	0.9	3.4	Mono-unsat. fat (g)
unknown	unknown	1.5	3.1	Poly-unsat. fat (g)
trace	trace	2.5	7.7	Carbohydrate (g)
nil	nil	nil	5.4	Sugar (g)
nil	nil	trace	1.4	Fibre (g)
28	33	91	398	Sodium (mg)
140	136	175	440	Potassium (mg)
3	3	8	31	Calcium (mg)
10	10	15	23	Magnesium (mg)
152	200	273	412	Phosphorus (mg)
4.88	4.36	11.9	7.67	Iron (mg)
9.54	5.42	1.75	9.47	Copper (mg)
6.36	2.36	5.74	4.12	Zinc (mg)
11	25	unknown	41	Selenium (µg)
10086	7884	15974	16913	Vitamin A (µg)
0.12	0.2	0.77	0.43	Vitamin D (µg)
0.2	0.13	0.11	0.84	Vitamin E (mg)
0.24	0.15	0.15	0.41	Vitamin B_1 (mg)
1.16	2.26	2.17	3.62	Vitamin B_2 (mg)
5.44	7.96	8.05	13.35	Niacin (mg)
0.36	0.21	0.45	0.53	Vitamin B_6 (mg)
23.2	33.2	18.2	42.6	Vitamin B_{12} (µg)
44	104	77	107	Folate (µg)
1.64	3.2	3.22	6.48	Pantothenate (mg)
20.0	13.2	23.8	36.9	Biotin (µg)
8	8	6	11	Vitamin C (mg)

FOOD	Liver pâté	Luncheon meat canned	Minced beef stewed	Minced beef extra lean, stewed
PORTION SIZE	average portion as a starter	one slice	medium	medium
NUTRIENTS				
Energy (kcals)	253	44	293	248
Protein (g)	10.5	1.8	30.5	34.6
Total fat (g)	23.1	3.8	18.9	12.2
Saturated fat (g)	6.7	1.4	8.3	5.3
Mono-unsat. fat (g)	8.1	1.7	8.3	5.3
Poly-unsat. fat (g)	2.2	0.5	0.7	0.4
Carbohydrate (g)	0.8	0.8	nil	nil
Sugar (g)	0.2	trace	nil	nil
Fibre (g)	trace	trace	nil	nil
Sodium (mg)	632	147	102	105
Potassium (mg)	128	20	294	392
Calcium (mg)	12	2	28	20
Magnesium (mg)	9	1	21	25
Phosphorus (mg)	392	28	210	238
Iron (mg)	5.68	0.15	3.08	3.22
Copper (mg)	0.47	0.05	0.14	0.11
Zinc (mg)	2.32	0.31	7	7.84
Selenium (µg)	unknown	1	10	11
Vitamin A (µg)	5881	trace	19	2
Vitamin D (µg)	unknown	trace	1.26	0.84
Vitamin E (mg)	unknown	0.02	0.48	0.42
Vitamin B_1 (mg)	0.1	0.01	0.04	0.04
Vitamin B_2 (mg)	0.88	0.02	0.27	0.18
Niacin (mg)	2.32	0.25	6.44	6.72
Vitamin B_6 (mg)	0.2	trace	0.39	0.22
Vitamin B_{12} (µg)	5.8	0.1	2.8	4.2
Folate (µg)	71	trace	24	28
Pantothenate (mg)	1.72	0.07	0.5	0.5
Biotin (µg)	8.0	trace	7	2.8
Vitamin C (mg)	unknown	nil	nil	nil

Minced lamb stewed	**Minced pork** stewed	**Moussaka** homemade	**Pheasant** roasted	**FOOD**
medium	medium	medium	half a bird	**PORTION SIZE**
				NUTRIENTS
291	267	403	473	Energy (kcals)
34.2	34.2	28.0	60	Protein (g)
17.2	14.6	26.1	25.8	Total fat (g)
8.1	5.46	11.9	8.8	Saturated fat (g)
6.7	5.5	9.2	12.05	Mono-unsat. fat (g)
0.8	5.9	2.6	3.45	Poly-unsat. fat (g)
nil	nil	14.9	nil	Carbohydrate (g)
nil	nil	9.2	nil	Sugar (g)
nil	nil	3.3	nil	Fibre (g)
83	85	660	142	Sodium (mg)
378	448	891	774	Potassium (mg)
21	18	208	60	Calcium (mg)
28	29	56	56	Magnesium (mg)
252	280	363	473	Phosphorus (mg)
2.94	1.96	2.97	4.73	Iron (mg)
0.15	0.14	0.2	0.21	Copper (mg)
6.44	4.9	4.62	2.79	Zinc (mg)
4	21	7	30	Selenium (µg)
7	trace	187	unknown	Vitamin A (µg)
0.7	1.26	1.32	unknown	Vitamin D (µg)
0.15	0.03	2.14	unknown	Vitamin E (mg)
0.13	1.36	0.23	0.04	Vitamin B_1 (mg)
0.29	0.31	0.33	0.62	Vitamin B_2 (mg)
7.28	8.68	4.62	19.7	Niacin (mg)
0.29	0.32	0.4	1.22	Vitamin B_6 (mg)
2.8	1.4	3.3	6.45	Vitamin B_{12} (µg)
13	3	23	43	Folate (µg)
1.26	2.21	1.32	2.06	Pantothenate (mg)
5.6	5.6	unknown	unknown	Biotin (µg)
nil	nil	7	nil	Vitamin C (mg)

FOOD	**Pork** leg, roasted	**Pork** steaks, grilled	**Pork** chump chops fried	**Pork and apple casserole**
PORTION SIZE	medium	one	one	medium
NUTRIENTS				
Energy (kcals)	233	238	498	257
Protein (g)	27.1	38.9	41.8	28.3
Total fat (g)	13.9	9.1	36.7	8.1
Saturated fat (g)	4.9	3.2	11.9	1.8
Mono-unsat. fat (g)	5.9	3.6	14.1	2.9
Poly-unsat. fat (g)	2.0	1.4	7.8	2.3
Carbohydrate (g)	nil	nil	nil	19.0
Sugar (g)	nil	nil	nil	10.9
Fibre (g)	nil	nil	nil	1.3
Sodium (mg)	64	91	102	676
Potassium (mg)	324	552	629	624
Calcium (mg)	8	10	22	39
Magnesium (mg)	23	38	41	39
Phosphorus (mg)	207	336	374	286
Iron (mg)	0.99	1.32	1.36	1.56
Copper (mg)	0.05	0.12	0.07	0.08
Zinc (mg)	2.52	3.24	3.23	2.34
Selenium (µg)	17	24	26	18
Vitamin A (µg)	trace	trace	trace	2
Vitamin D (µg)	0.9	1.08	1.53	0.52
Vitamin E (mg)	0.04	0.02	unknown	unknown
Vitamin B_1 (mg)	0.62	1.74	1.29	0.94
Vitamin B_2 (mg)	0.22	0.32	0.36	0.23
Niacin (mg)	6.21	10.92	12.92	7.28
Vitamin B_6 (mg)	0.33	0.82	0.65	0.62
Vitamin B_{12} (µg)	0.9	1.2	trace	trace
Folate (µg)	1	10	3	5
Pantothenate (mg)	1.74	2.51	4.56	1.51
Biotin (µg)	4.5	6.0	8.5	2.6
Vitamin C (mg)	nil	nil	nil	5

Pork and chicken chow mein	Pork spare ribs barbeque-style	Pork stir fry with vegetables	Pork pie	FOOD
average	restaurant serving	restaurant serving	individual	**PORTION SIZE**
				NUTRIENTS
284	350	378	526	Energy (kcals)
27.6	22.7	43.6	13.7	Protein (g)
10.2	26.6	16.9	37.8	Total fat (g)
2.5	7.0	4.7	14.3	Saturated fat (g)
3.9	10.1	5.8	17.5	Mono-unsat. fat (g)
2.8	7.3	5.0	3.8	Poly-unsat. fat (g)
21.4	5.3	14.0	34.9	Carbohydrate (g)
6.7	3.7	5.8	0.7	Sugar (g)
2.1	0.7	3.2	1.3	Fibre (g)
1540	1276	1188	1008	Sodium (mg)
700	462	936	210	Potassium (mg)
46	39	58	66	Calcium (mg)
53	31	86	22	Magnesium (mg)
294	198	504	168	Phosphorus (mg)
2.8	1.87	4.68	1.96	Iron (mg)
0.35	0.08	0.36	0.45	Copper (mg)
2.45	3.08	3.6	1.4	Zinc (mg)
unknown	unknown	unknown	unknown	Selenium (μg)
268	0.6	46	trace	Vitamin A (μg)
0.35	0.88	1.08	trace	Vitamin D (μg)
0.56	0.11	unknown	0.6	Vitamin E (mg)
0.45	0.75	1.73	0.22	Vitamin B_1 (mg)
0.28	0.18	0.5	0.13	Vitamin B_2 (mg)
7.0	5.17	9.0	2.52	Niacin (mg)
0.49	0.37	0.94	0.08	Vitamin B_6 (mg)
trace	1.1	trace	1.4	Vitamin B_{12} (μg)
25	6	58	4	Folate (μg)
unknown	1.44	2.52	0.84	Pantothenate (mg)
unknown	trace	unknown	1.4	Biotin (μg)
14	1	29	nil	Vitamin C (mg)

FOOD	Pork and egg (gala) pie	Rabbit stewed	Ravioli canned	Salami retail
PORTION SIZE	one slice	quarter of whole	average portion	one large slice
NUTRIENTS				
Energy (kcals)	414	145	154	52
Protein (g)	14.7	26.9	6.6	2.4
Total fat (g)	29.4	4.1	4.8	4.8
Saturated fat (g)	10.4	2.2	1.1	1.6
Mono-unsat. fat (g)	12.9	0.9	1.8	2.1
Poly-unsat. fat (g)	3.2	0.8	1.8	0.4
Carbohydrate (g)	24.4	nil	22.7	trace
Sugar (g)	1.8	nil	4.8	trace
Fibre (g)	unknown	nil	2.0	trace
Sodium (mg)	994	61	1078	216
Potassium (mg)	196	254	330	38
Calcium (mg)	46	50	35	2.4
Magnesium (mg)	15	23	26	2.4
Phosphorus (mg)	196	191	95	21.6
Iron (mg)	1.12	1.4	1.76	0.14
Copper (mg)	0.22	0.08	0.18	0.02
Zinc (mg)	1.12	2.16	1.1	0.36
Selenium (µg)	unknown	20	unknown	trace
Vitamin A (µg)	trace	unknown	unknown	trace
Vitamin D (µg)	unknown	unknown	nil	unknown
Vitamin E (mg)	unknown	unknown	unknown	0.02
Vitamin B_1 (mg)	0.2	0.03	0.11	0.07
Vitamin B_2 (mg)	0.15	0.2	0.09	0.02
Niacin (mg)	2.38	7.87	1.98	0.67
Vitamin B_6 (mg)	0.21	0.37	0.22	0.04
Vitamin B_{12} (µg)	trace	3.8	trace	0.24
Folate (µg)	32	6	7	trace
Pantothenate (mg)	unknown	1.02	unknown	0.19
Biotin (µg)	unknown	1.3	unknown	0.72
Vitamin C (mg)	unknown	nil	trace	unknown

Sausages and beans canned	**Sausage casserole** homemade	**Sausage roll** flaky pastry	**Sausages beef** grilled	**FOOD**
small can	medium	one regular	one	**PORTION SIZE**
				NUTRIENTS
239	429	286	106	Energy (kcals)
13.5	30.9	4.3	5.2	Protein (g)
10.1	28.3	21.8	6.9	Total fat (g)
unknown	9.1	8.0	2.7	Saturated fat (g)
unknown	11.7	9.4	3.3	Mono-unsat. fat (g)
unknown	5.2	3.2	0.5	Poly-unsat. fat (g)
24.8	13.3	19.4	6.1	Carbohydrate (g)
9.0	5.5	0.7	1.0	Sugar (g)
6.3	2.3	0.7	0.3	Fibre (g)
1215	1690	306	440	Sodium (mg)
563	650	66	76	Potassium (mg)
88	83	40	29	Calcium (mg)
61	47	7	7	Magnesium (mg)
209	364	58	84	Phosphorus (mg)
3.38	2.34	0.72	0.68	Iron (mg)
0.04	0.16	0.1	0.12	Copper (mg)
1.35	3.12	0.42	0.68	Zinc (mg)
unknown	16	1	unknown	Selenium (µg)
21	7	76	trace	Vitamin A (µg)
trace	1.3	0.66	trace	Vitamin D (µg)
unknown	unknown	0.79	0.09	Vitamin E (mg)
0.18	0.83	0.06	nil	Vitamin B_1 (mg)
0.16	0.26	0.02	0.06	Vitamin B_2 (mg)
0.23	7.02	1.02	2.16	Niacin (mg)
0.27	0.55	0.04	0.03	Vitamin B_6 (mg)
unknown	trace	0.2	0.4	Vitamin B_{12} (µg)
36	13	2	2	Folate (µg)
unknown	1.56	0.14	0.2	Pantothenate (mg)
unknown	5.2	0.6	0.8	Biotin (µg)
trace	trace	trace	unknown	Vitamin C (mg)

FOOD	Sausages low fat grilled	Sausages pepperami	Sausages premium (e.g. Cumberland) grilled	Sausages pork grilled
PORTION SIZE	one	one	one	one
NUTRIENTS				
Energy (kcals)	92	138	117	127
Protein (g)	6.5	5.6	6.7	5.3
Total fat (g)	5.5	12.8	9.0	9.8
Saturated fat (g)	2.0	4.9	3.3	3.8
Mono-unsat. fat (g)	2.4	5.8	3.8	4.4
Poly-unsat. fat (g)	0.9	1.3	1.3	1.1
Carbohydrate (g)	4.3	0.2	2.5	4.6
Sugar (g)	0.4	0.2	0.4	0.7
Fibre (g)	0.6	trace	unknown	0.3
Sodium (mg)	476	448	336	400
Potassium (mg)	88	83	88	80
Calcium (mg)	52	3	72	21
Magnesium (mg)	8	5	6	6
Phosphorus (mg)	92	45	72	88
Iron (mg)	0.52	0.55	0.48	0.6
Copper (mg)	0.03	0.03	0.03	0.14
Zinc (mg)	0.68	0.98	0.56	0.64
Selenium (µg)	unknown	unknown	unknown	unknown
Vitamin A (µg)	trace	trace	trace	trace
Vitamin D (µg)	trace	unknown	unknown	trace
Vitamin E (mg)	0.12	0.51	0.32	0.09
Vitamin B_1 (mg)	trace	0.07	0.02	0.01
Vitamin B_2 (mg)	0.05	0.04	0.04	0.06
Niacin (mg)	1.12	1.38	1.08	1.6
Vitamin B_6 (mg)	0.04	0.07	0.06	0.02
Vitamin B_{12} (µg)	0.4	0.5	0.4	0.4
Folate (µg)	1	trace	3	1
Pantothenate (mg)	0.42	0.3	0.3	0.24
Biotin (µg)	1.2	1.5	1.2	1.2
Vitamin C (mg)	unknown	unknown	3	unknown

Saveloy retail	**Scotch pie** mutton	**Spaghetti bolognaise** canned	**Steak and kidney pie** individual	**FOOD**
one	one individual	small can	one	**PORTION SIZE**
				NUTRIENTS
170	226	181	517	Energy (kcals)
6.4	8.3	6.9	14.6	Protein (g)
133	11.8	6.3	33.9	Total fat (g)
unknown	5.4	unknown	13.4	Saturated fat (g)
unknown	5.2	unknown	15.5	Mono-unsat. fat (g)
unknown	0.3	unknown	3.4	Poly-unsat. fat (g)
6.6	23.4	25.6	41.0	Carbohydrate (g)
trace	2.1	5.3	3.7	Sugar (g)
unknown	unknown	1.9	1.4	Fibre (g)
579	493	861	816	Sodium (mg)
104	134	294	224	Potassium (mg)
15	55	38	85	Calcium (mg)
6	18	29	29	Magnesium (mg)
137	84	95	176	Phosphorus (mg)
0.98	1.46	1.47	4.0	Iron (mg)
0.18	0.22	0.06	0.16	Copper (mg)
0.91	0.78	0.84	1.92	Zinc (mg)
unknown	unknown	unknown	unknown	Selenium (µg)
trace	trace	unknown	unknown	Vitamin A (µg)
trace	unknown	nil	unknown	Vitamin D (µg)
0.05	unknown	unknown	unknown	Vitamin E (mg)
0.09	0.11	0.15	0.19	Vitamin B_1 (mg)
0.06	0.08	0.06	0.24	Vitamin B_2 (mg)
1.24	1.23	1.68	2.72	Niacin (mg)
0.04	0.11	0.21	0.1	Vitamin B_6 (mg)
trace	trace	trace	3.2	Vitamin B_{12} (µg)
1	11	17	13	Folate (µg)
0.26	unknown	unknown	0.48	Pantothenate (mg)
trace	unknown	unknown	1.6	Biotin (µg)
unknown	trace	nil	nil	Vitamin C (mg)

FOOD	Turkey roast	Turkey roll	Veal escalope, fried
PORTION SIZE	medium	one slice	one
NUTRIENTS			
Energy (kcals)	149	18	294
Protein (g)	28.1	1.9	50.6
Total fat (g)	4.1	1.0	102
Saturated fat (g)	1.3	0.3	2.7
Mono-unsat. fat (g)	1.5	0.4	3.9
Poly-unsat. fat (g)	1.0	0.2	2.8
Carbohydrate (g)	nil	0.5	nil
Sugar (g)	nil	nil	nil
Fibre (g)	nil	unknown	nil
Sodium (mg)	81	76	129
Potassium (mg)	315	20	690
Calcium (mg)	10	2	9
Magnesium (mg)	24	2	48
Phosphorus (mg)	234	22	450
Iron (mg)	0.72	0.09	1.35
Copper (mg)	0.08	0.01	trace
Zinc (mg)	2.25	0.17	4.65
Selenium (μg)	15	unknown	17
Vitamin A (μg)	trace	trace	9
Vitamin D (μg)	0.27	unknown	2.10
Vitamin E (mg)	0.05	unknown	0.58
Vitamin B_1 (mg)	0.05	0..01	0.12
Vitamin B_2 (mg)	0.17	0.01	0.38
Niacin (mg)	9.27	0.57	11.7
Vitamin B_6 (mg)	0.44	0.03	1.05
Vitamin B_{12} (μg)	0.9	0.1	6.0
Folate (μg)	15	1	26
Pantothenate (mg)	0.88	0.04	1.53
Biotin (μg)	1.8	0.2	7.5
Vitamin C (mg)	nil	trace	nil

Venison roasted	**Venison** in port and red wine	**Weiner schnitzel**	**FOOD**
average	medium	one	**PORTION SIZE**
			NUTRIENTS
198	198	335	Energy (kcals)
42.7	25.5	31.3	Protein (g)
3.0	6.8	15.0	Total fat (g)
unknown	3.9	2.4	Saturated fat (g)
unknown	1.6	5.4	Mono-unsat. fat (g)
unknown	0.5	5.9	Poly-unsat. fat (g)
nil	9.1	19.7	Carbohydrate (g)
nil	4.2	0.6	Sugar (g)
nil	1.0	0.6	Fibre (g)
62	754	435	Sodium (mg)
348	520	465	Potassium (mg)
7	31	48	Calcium (mg)
32	36	39	Magnesium (mg)
288	257	330	Phosphorus (mg)
6.12	4.42	1.65	Iron (mg)
0.43	0.29	0.06	Copper (mg)
4.68	2.86	3.15	Zinc (mg)
unknown	10	12	Selenium (µg)
unknown	unknown	30	Vitamin A (µg)
unknown	unknown	1.8	Vitamin D (µg)
unknown	unknown	0.39	Vitamin E (mg)
0.19	unknown	0.16	Vitamin B_1 (mg)
0.83	0.23	0.28	Vitamin B_2 (mg)
6.6	unknown	7.65	Niacin (mg)
0.78	unknown	0.64	Vitamin B_6 (mg)
1.2	unknown	1.5	Vitamin B_{12} (µg)
7	unknown	21	Folate (µg)
unknown	unknown	1.1	Pantothenate (mg)
unknown	unknown	4.5	Biotin (µg)
nil	nil	nil	Vitamin C (mg)

FOOD	Anchovies canned in oil	Caviare bottled in brine	Cockles bottled in vinegar	Cod in batter frozen baked
PORTION SIZE	one	one tablespoon	average (6)	average
NUTRIENTS				
Energy (kcals)	8	17	18	211
Protein (g)	0.8	2.1	3	12.8
Total fat (g)	0.6	1	trace	11.8
Saturated fat (g)	unknown	0.2	trace	3.6
Mono-unsat. fat (g)	unknown	0.2	trace	5.9
Poly-unsat. fat (g)	unknown	0.3	trace	1.8
Carbohydrate (g)	nil	nil	trace	14.3
Sugar (g)	nil	nil	nil	0.1
Fibre (g)	nil	nil	nil	0.6
Sodium (mg)	118	403	156	650
Potassium (mg)	7	11	108	250
Calcium (mg)	9	2	18	42
Magnesium (mg)	2	1	6	21
Phosphorus (mg)	9	unknown	42	250
Iron (mg)	0.12	0.09	8	0.5
Copper (mg)	0.01	unknown	0.06	0.08
Zinc (mg)	0.09	0.21	0.36	0.5
Selenium (µg)	unknown	unknown	12	15
Vitamin A (µg)	2	trace	12	trace
Vitamin D (µg)	unknown	unknown	trace	trace
Vitamin E (mg)	unknown	unknown	unknown	unknown
Vitamin B_1 (mg)	trace	trace	trace	0.07
Vitamin B_2 (mg)	trace	0.02	trace	0.07
Niacin (mg)	0.11	trace	0.30	1.10
Vitamin B_6 (mg)	unknown	unknown	trace	0.21
Vitamin B_{12} (µg)	0.3	unknown	11.4	unknown
Folate (µg)	1	unknown	unknown	8
Pantothenate (mg)	unknown	unknown	0.06	0.34
Biotin (µg)	unknown	unknown	2.4	2
Vitamin C (mg)	trace	nil	trace	trace

Cod in batter fresh fried	Cod baked	Cod in parsley sauce boil in the bag	Cod roe hard, fried	FOOD
chip shop	medium	average	medium	**PORTION SIZE**
				NUTRIENTS
445	115	143	234	Energy (kcals)
29	25.7	20.4	24.2	Protein (g)
27.7	1.4	4.8	13.8	Total fat (g)
2.9	0.4	unknown	1.9	Saturated fat (g)
9.9	0.2	unknown	4.8	Mono-unsat. fat (g)
13.5	0.5	unknown	6.6	Poly-unsat. fat (g)
21.1	trace	4.8	3.5	Carbohydrate (g)
trace	trace	trace	trace	Sugar (g)
0.9	nil	0.2	0.1	Fibre (g)
288	408	442	139	Sodium (mg)
522	420	459	197	Potassium (mg)
121	13	87	15	Calcium (mg)
45	31	32	10	Magnesium (mg)
360	228	289	348	Phosphorus (mg)
0.9	0.12	0.17	1.16	Iron (mg)
0.07	0.02	0.07	0.26	Copper (mg)
0.9	0.6	0.68	3.83	Zinc (mg)
unknown	41	unknown	unknown	Selenium (µg)
unknown	2	trace	87	Vitamin A (µg)
trace	trace	trace	19.72	Vitamin D (µg)
unknown	0.71	unknown	unknown	Vitamin E (mg)
0.16	0.04	0.1	0.68	Vitamin B_1 (mg)
0.13	0.06	0.17	0.43	Vitamin B_2 (mg)
3.06	2.76	1.87	1.16	Niacin (mg)
0.23	0.23	0.22	0.32	Vitamin B_6 (mg)
3.6	2.4	unknown	12.8	Vitamin B_{12} (µg)
103	14	29	unknown	Folate (µg)
0.54	0.31	0.8	3.02	Pantothenate (mg)
5.4	1.2	3.4	17.4	Biotin (µg)
trace	trace	trace	trace	Vitamin C (mg)

FOOD	Conger eel grilled	Crab boiled	Crabstick	Eel jellied
PORTION SIZE	medium	one dressed crab	one	average
NUTRIENTS				
Energy (kcals)	158	166	12	69
Protein (g)	25	25.4	1.7	5.9
Total fat (g)	6.3	7.2	0.1	5
Saturated fat (g)	unknown	0.9	unknown	1.3
Mono-unsat. fat (g)	unknown	2	unknown	2.5
Poly-unsat. fat (g)	unknown	2.1	unknown	0.7
Carbohydrate (g)	nil	trace	1.1	trace
Sugar (g)	nil	trace	trace	nil
Fibre (g)	nil	nil	nil	nil
Sodium (mg)	69	546	119	462
Potassium (mg)	334	325	10	39
Calcium (mg)	98	unknown	2	43
Magnesium (mg)	28	75	1	4
Phosphorus (mg)	368	442	8	51
Iron (mg)	1.73	2.08	0.14	0.07
Copper (mg)	0.28	2.30	0.05	0.03
Zinc (mg)	1.26	7.15	0.63	0.63
Selenium (μg)	unknown	22	unknown	15
Vitamin A (μg)	unknown	trace	trace	77
Vitamin D (μg)	unknown	trace	trace	2.1
Vitamin E (mg)	unknown	unknown	unknown	1.82
Vitamin B_1 (mg)	0.07	0.09	trace	0.05
Vitamin B_2 (mg)	0.05	1.12	0.01	0.11
Niacin (mg)	5.4	1.95	0.03	0.56
Vitamin B_6 (mg)	unknown	0.21	trace	0.02
Vitamin B_{12} (μg)	4.6	trace	0.2	1.4
Folate (μg)	unknown	26	unknown	unknown
Pantothenate (mg)	0.31	1.24	unknown	0.24
Biotin (μg)	unknown	9.1	unknown	1.4
Vitamin C (mg)	trace	trace	trace	trace

Fish cakes fried	Fish fingers fried	Fish fingers grilled	Fish paste	FOOD
one	one	one	average spread on bread	PORTION SIZE
				NUTRIENTS
109	67	56	17	Energy (kcals)
4.3	3.7	4	1.5	Protein (g)
6.7	3.9	2.5	1.0	Total fat (g)
0.9	1.0	0.8	unknown	Saturated fat (g)
2.7	1.5	1.0	unknown	Mono-unsat. fat (g)
2.8	1.3	0.6	unknown	Poly-unsat. fat (g)
8.4	4.3	4.6	0.4	Carbohydrate (g)
trace	trace	trace	0.1	Sugar (g)
unknown	0.2	0.2	trace	Fibre (g)
255	126	123	60	Sodium (mg)
115	73	81	30	Potassium (mg)
55	24	26	28	Calcium (mg)
9	6	6	3	Magnesium (mg)
55	62	62	31	Phosphorus (mg)
0.4	0.22	0.22	0.9	Iron (mg)
0.01	0.01	0.01	0.06	Copper (mg)
0.2	0.08	0.11	0.2	Zinc (mg)
unknown	6	6	unknown	Selenium (μg)
trace	trace	trace	2	Vitamin A (μg)
trace	trace	trace	unknown	Vitamin D (μg)
unknown	unknown	unknown	0.09	Vitamin E (mg)
0.04	0.03	0.03	trace	Vitamin B_1 (mg)
0.07	0.02	0.02	0.02	Vitamin B_2 (mg)
0.8	0.45	0.48	0.41	Niacin (mg)
0.13	0.04	0.05	unknown	Vitamin B_6 (mg)
0.5	0.3	0.3	unknown	Vitamin B_{12} (μg)
unknown	4	4	unknown	Folate (μg)
0.17	0.09	0.1	unknown	Pantothenate (mg)
0.5	0.3	0.3	unknown	Biotin (μg)
trace	trace	trace	trace	Vitamin C (mg)

FOOD	Fish pie potato based	Haddock coated in crumbs, frozen, fried	Haddock smoked, poached	Hake grilled
PORTION SIZE	average	average purchased	average fillet	average steak
NUTRIENTS				
Energy (kcals)	298	235	201	113
Protein (g)	16.8	17.6	28.1	22.2
Total fat (g)	13.5	12	9.1	2.7
Saturated fat (g)	4.8	unknown	5.6	0.4
Mono-unsat. fat (g)	4.8	unknown	2.3	0.7
Poly-unsat. fat (g)	3.0	unknown	0.6	0.7
Carbohydrate (g)	28.8	15.1	1.7	nil
Sugar (g)	4	trace	1.7	nil
Fibre (g)	1.8	0.7	nil	nil
Sodium (mg)	250	348	1155	130
Potassium (mg)	650	276	525	340
Calcium (mg)	118	144	74	17
Magnesium (mg)	43	25	36	28
Phosphorus (mg)	233	240	285	240
Iron (mg)	1	0.96	0.15	0.6
Copper (mg)	0.1	0.06	0.04	0.04
Zinc (mg)	1	0.48	0.6	0.4
Selenium (μg)	28	22	41	unknown
Vitamin A (μg)	151	trace	100	unknown
Vitamin D (μg)	1	trace	0.15	trace
Vitamin E (mg)	1.13	unknown	0.21	unknown
Vitamin B_1 (mg)	0.28	0.1	0.06	unknown
Vitamin B_2 (mg)	0.2	0.1	0.23	unknown
Niacin (mg)	2.5	3.36	4.65	unknown
Vitamin B_6 (mg)	0.55	0.29	0.51	unknown
Vitamin B_{12} (μg)	nil	1.2	3	unknown
Folate (μg)	35	unknown	14	unknown
Pantothenate (mg)	1.02	0.31	0.39	unknown
Biotin (μg)	32.5	2.4	1.5	unknown
Vitamin C (mg)	8	trace	trace	trace

Halibut grilled	Herring grilled	Herring pickled rollmop	Hoki grilled	**FOOD**
average	medium filleted	one	average fillet	**PORTION SIZE**
				NUTRIENTS
175	215	188	230	Energy (kcals)
36.7	23.9	15	45.8	Protein (g)
3.2	13.3	10	5.1	Total fat (g)
0.6	3.3	unknown	0.9	Saturated fat (g)
1.0	5.6	unknown	1.3	Mono-unsat. fat (g)
0.7	2.7	unknown	101	Poly-unsat. fat (g)
nil	nil	9	nil	Carbohydrate (g)
nil	nil	9	nil	Sugar (g)
nil	nil	nil	nil	Fibre (g)
103	190	747	228	Sodium (mg)
711	512	56	1045	Potassium (mg)
49	94	12	40	Calcium (mg)
42	50	5	78	Magnesium (mg)
348	369	69	513	Phosphorus (mg)
0.87	1.9	0.63	1.9	Iron (mg)
0.07	0.23	0.11	0.08	Copper (mg)
0.73	1.43	0.27	1.14	Zinc (mg)
unknown	55	unknown	114	Selenium (µg)
unknown	40	33	trace	Vitamin A (µg)
unknown	19.16	14.4	trace	Vitamin D (µg)
1.45	0.76	0.58	unknown	Vitamin E (mg)
0.1	trace	trace	0.06	Vitamin B_1 (mg)
0.1	0.32	0.12	0.11	Vitamin B_2 (mg)
8.85	4.76	0.72	3.99	Niacin (mg)
0.58	0.42	0.1	unknown	Vitamin B_6 (mg)
1.5	17.9	unknown	unknown	Vitamin B_{12} (µg)
16	12	1	unknown	Folate (µg)
0.51	0.93	unknown	unknown	Pantothenate (mg)
5.8	8.3	unknown	unknown	Biotin (µg)
trace	trace	trace	trace	Vitamin C (mg)

FOOD	Kedgeree homemade	King prawn	Kipper boil in the bag	Lemon sole grilled
PORTION SIZE	average	one	average	one medium average
NUTRIENTS				
Energy (kcals)	513	8	403	105
Protein (g)	47.7	1.8	34	21.9
Total fat (g)	26.1	0.1	29.6	1.9
Saturated fat (g)	7.5	trace	unknown	0.3
Mono-unsat.	9.9	trace	unknown	0.3
Poly-unsat. fat (g)	5.4	trace	unknown	0.7
Carbohydrate (g)	23.4	nil	trace	nil
Sugar (g)	0.3	nil	trace	nil
Fibre (g)	0.3	nil	nil	nil
Sodium (mg)	1890	127	1190	121
Potassium (mg)	810	21	612	289
Calcium (mg)	93	9	148	22
Magnesium (mg)	66	4	66	22
Phosphorus (mg)	540	22	459	255
Iron (mg)	1.8	0.09	2.04	0.68
Copper (mg)	0.18	0.02	0.27	0.02
Zinc (mg)	2.1	0.18	2.55	0.51
Selenium (µg)	69	2	56	77
Vitamin A (µg)	324	trace	unknown	trace
Vitamin D (µg)	3	trace	13.43	trace
Vitamin E (mg)	unknown	unknown	0.53	unknown
Vitamin B_1 (mg)	0.15	trace	trace	0.1
Vitamin B_2 (mg)	0.63	0.01	0.7	0.09
Niacin (mg)	6.3	0.02	10.03	3.91
Vitamin B_6 (mg)	0.84	trace	0.44	unknown
Vitamin B_{12} (µg)	6	0.6	28.9	1.7
Folate (µg)	unknown	unknown	unknown	14
Pantothenate (mg)	1.56	0.01	1.75	0.36
Biotin (µg)	18	0.1	13.6	6.8
Vitamin C (mg)	trace	trace	trace	trace

Lobster boiled	**Mackerel** grilled	**Mackerel** smoked	**Mackerel pâté** smoked	**FOOD**
half a dressed lobster	average	one medium average	average as a starter	**PORTION SIZE**
				NUTRIENTS
93	382	531	147	Energy (kcals)
20.0	33.3	28.3	5.4	Protein (g)
1.5	27.7	46.3	13.8	Total fat (g)
0.3	5.6	9.5	unknown	Saturated fat (g)
0.3	13.6	22.7	unknown	Mono-unsat. fat (g)
0.5	5.6	9.5	unknown	Poly-unsat. fat (g)
trace	nil	nil	0.5	Carbohydrate (g)
trace	nil	nil	0.3	Sugar (g)
nil	nil	nil	trace	Fibre (g)
300	101	1125	292	Sodium (mg)
235	576	465	92	Potassium (mg)
55	19	30	11	Calcium (mg)
30	45	42	8	Magnesium (mg)
233	368	315	64	Phosphorus (mg)
0.75	1.28	1.8	0.4	Iron (mg)
1.23	0.14	0.14	0.04	Copper (mg)
2.25	1.12	1.65	0.28	Zinc (mg)
118	58	50	10	Selenium (µg)
trace	77	47	66	Vitamin A (µg)
trace	8.64	12	1.32	Vitamin D (µg)
1.32	0.74	0.38	0.44	Vitamin E (mg)
0.07	0.24	0.39	0.04	Vitamin B_1 (mg)
0.05	0.51	0.78	0.18	Vitamin B_2 (mg)
1.25	15.04	14.25	1.96	Niacin (mg)
0.07	0.72	0.75	0.11	Vitamin B_6 (mg)
2.5	1.6	9	7.2	Vitamin B_{12} (µg)
8	unknown	unknown	1	Folate (µg)
0.9	1.49	1.54	0.36	Pantothenate (mg)
5.0	9.6	4.5	2.4	Biotin (µg)
trace	trace	trace	unknown	Vitamin C (mg)

FOOD	**Monkfish** grilled	**Mullet red** grilled *with bones and skin*	**Oysters** raw	**Pilchards** canned in tomato sauce
PORTION SIZE	average	one average whole	one	one
NUTRIENTS				
Energy (kcals)	67	43	7	79
Protein (g)	15.9	7.2	1.1	9.2
Total fat (g)	0.4	1.6	0.1	4.5
Saturated fat (g)	0.1	unknown	trace	0.9
Mono-unsat. fat (g)	0.1	unknown	trace	1.2
Poly-unsat. fat (g)	0.1	unknown	trace	1.9
Carbohydrate (g)	nil	nil	0.3	0.6
Sugar (g)	nil	nil	trace	0.5
Fibre (g)	nil	nil	nil	trace
Sodium (mg)	18	38	51	160
Potassium (mg)	301	143	26	171
Calcium (mg)	8	27	14	138
Magnesium (mg)	21	12	4	16
Phosphorus (mg)	336	90	21	154
Iron (mg)	0.35	0.15	0.57	1.38
Copper (mg)	0.01	0.01	0.75	0.09
Zinc (mg)	0.49	0.15	5.92	0.71
Selenium (µg)	unknown	19	2	17
Vitamin A (µg)	trace	trace	8	16
Vitamin D (µg)	trace	0.3	0.1	7.7
Vitamin E (mg)	unknown	0.21	0.09	1.41
Vitamin B_1 (mg)	0.03	0.02	0.02	0.01
Vitamin B_2 (mg)	0.06	0.04	0.02	0.18
Niacin (mg)	unknown	1.5	0.18	3.25
Vitamin B_6 (mg)	unknown	0.14	0.02	0.15
Vitamin B_{12} (µg)	unknown	0.8	1.7	7.2
Folate (µg)	unknown	4	unknown	unknown
Pantothenate (mg)	unknown	0.17	0.04	0.47
Biotin (µg)	unknown	0.8	1	6.1
Vitamin C (mg)	trace	trace	trace	trace

Plaice in bread-crumbs	**Red snapper** fried, weighed with bones	**Prawns** boiled shelled	**Salmon** canned	**FOOD**
one medium	average whole	average	average	**PORTION SIZE**
				NUTRIENTS
342	128	59	155	Energy (kcals)
27	25	13.6	20.3	Protein (g)
20.5	3.2	0.5	8.2	Total fat (g)
2.3	0.6	0.1	1.5	Saturated fat (g)
7.4	0.8	0.1	3.5	Mono-unsat. fat (g)
10	1.2	0.1	2.4	Poly-unsat. fat (g)
12.9	nil	nil	nil	Carbohydrate (g)
0.5	nil	nil	nil	Sugar (g)
0.3	nil	nil	nil	Fibre (g)
330	118	954	570	Sodium (mg)
420	460	156	300	Potassium (mg)
101	54	66	93	Calcium (mg)
36	36	29	30	Magnesium (mg)
270	280	162	240	Phosphorus (mg)
1.2	0.4	0.66	1.4	Iron (mg)
0.03	0.04	0.12	0.09	Copper (mg)
1.05	0.4	1.32	0.9	Zinc (mg)
44	36	14	25	Selenium (μg)
trace	4	trace	35	Vitamin A (μg)
trace	3	trace	12.5	Vitamin D (μg)
4.97	1.38	unknown	1.5	Vitamin E (mg)
0.34	0.08	0.01	0.04	Vitamin B_1 (mg)
0.27	0.08	0.07	0.18	Vitamin B_2 (mg)
4.35	6.6	0.18	7	Niacin (mg)
0.23	0.46	0.02	0.45	Vitamin B_6 (mg)
1.5	2	4.8	4	Vitamin B_{12} (μg)
26	unknown	unknown	12	Folate (μg)
0.78	0.34	0.1	0.5	Pantothenate (mg)
45	2	0.6	5	Biotin (μg)
trace	trace	trace	trace	Vitamin C (mg)

FOOD	Salmon fresh, grilled	Salmon smoked	Rock salmon battered and fried	Sardines fresh, grilled
PORTION SIZE	average steak	average	medium average	six average
NUTRIENTS				
Energy (kcals)	215	80	590	102
Protein (g)	24.2	14.2	29.4	13.2
Total fat (g)	13.1	2.5	43.8	5.4
Saturated fat (g)	2.5	0.4	5.8	1.5
Mono-unsat. fat (g)	5.8	1	16	1.5
Poly-unsat. fat (g)	4.1	0.7	19.8	1.6
Carbohydrate (g)	nil	nil	20.6	nil
Sugar (g)	nil	nil	trace	nil
Fibre (g)	nil	nil	0.8	nil
Sodium (mg)	54	1053	320	73
Potassium (mg)	430	235	460	206
Calcium (mg)	25	11	88	65
Magnesium (mg)	32	18	36	18
Phosphorus (mg)	300	140	380	172
Iron (mg)	0.5	0.34	1	0.86
Copper (mg)	0.04	0.05	0.16	0.08
Zinc (mg)	0.7	0.22	0.8	0.77
Selenium (μg)	31	13	44	20
Vitamin A (μg)	16	unknown	188	unknown
Vitamin D (μg)	9.6	unknown	unknown	6.45
Vitamin E (mg)	2.29	unknown	unknown	0.17
Vitamin B_1 (mg)	0.25	0.09	0.14	trace
Vitamin B_2 (mg)	0.14	0.1	0.16	0.13
Niacin (mg)	7.7	4.93	6.4	3.61
Vitamin B_6 (mg)	0.81	0.16	0.42	0.22
Vitamin B_{12} (μg)	5	1.7	unknown	6
Folate (μg)	19	1	8	2
Pantothenate (mg)	1.16	0.49	1.14	0.46
Biotin (μg)	9	unknown	24	3.4
Vitamin C (mg)	trace	trace	trace	trace

Sardines canned in oil	**Scampi** breaded, fried	**Seafood pasta** retail	**Skate** fried in batter	**FOOD**
average (4)	average	ready meal for one	average	**PORTION SIZE**
				NUTRIENTS
220	403	303	286	Energy (kcals)
23.2	16	24.5	25	Protein (g)
14	23.1	13.2	17.2	Total fat (g)
2.8	2.4	7.7	1.8	Saturated fat (g)
4.8	8.7	3.3	5.8	Mono-unsat. fat (g)
5.2	10.9	0.8	8	Poly-unsat. fat (g)
nil	34.8	20.9	8.4	Carbohydrate (g)
nil	trace	4.4	0.2	Sugar (g)
nil	unknown	1.1	0.4	Fibre (g)
452	1122	468	240	Sodium (mg)
412	221	523	400	Potassium (mg)
500	357	105	86	Calcium (mg)
48	41	55	46	Magnesium (mg)
520	527	275	300	Phosphorus (mg)
3.0	2.89	1.1	1.8	Iron (mg)
0.12	0.27	0.19	0.16	Copper (mg)
2.2	1.02	1.38	1.6	Zinc (mg)
48	29	33	unknown	Selenium (µg)
8	trace	166	16	Vitamin A (µg)
5	trace	nil	unknown	Vitamin D (µg)
0.32	unknown	1.1	2.04	Vitamin E (mg)
trace	0.19	0.08	0.06	Vitamin B_1 (mg)
0.28	0.07	0.16	0.18	Vitamin B_2 (mg)
5.2	2.04	2.75	4	Niacin (mg)
0.20	0.15	0.25	unknown	Vitamin B_6 (mg)
15.2	1.7	2.8	unknown	Vitamin B_{12} (µg)
8	unknown	17	unknown	Folate (µg)
0.88	0.44	0.58	unknown	Pantothenate (mg)
5.2	1.7	2.8	unknown	Biotin (µg)
trace	trace	3	trace	Vitamin C (mg)

FOOD	Squid battered and fried	Swordfish grilled	Taramasalata	Trout rainbow grilled
PORTION SIZE	average	average steak	one tablespoon	one average without bones
NUTRIENTS				
Energy (kcals)	234	195	227	209
Protein (g)	13.8	32.1	1.4	33.3
Total fat (g)	12	7.3	23.8	8.4
Saturated fat (g)	2.5	1.7	1.8	1.7
Mono-unsat. fat (g)	4	2.9	13.2	3.1
Poly-unsat. fat (g)	4.4	2	7.5	2.6
Carbohydrate (g)	18.8	nil	1.8	nil
Sugar (g)	2.6	nil	trace	nil
Fibre (g)	0.6	nil	trace	nil
Sodium (mg)	106	238	293	85
Potassium (mg)	276	630	27	636
Calcium (mg)	97	7	9	33
Magnesium (mg)	28	48	3	40
Phosphorus (mg)	192	476	23	388
Iron (mg)	0.84	0.84	0.18	0.62
Copper (mg)	0.62	unknown	unknown	0.08
Zinc (mg)	1.08	unknown	0.18	0.77
Selenium (μg)	42	80	unknown	33
Vitamin A (μg)	57	unknown	unknown	45
Vitamin D (μg)	0.12	unknown	unknown	17.05
Vitamin E (mg)	2.82	unknown	unknown	1.57
Vitamin B_1 (mg)	0.12	0.27	0.04	0.31
Vitamin B_2 (mg)	0.16	0.28	0.05	0.19
Niacin (mg)	1.92	13.3	0.14	6.51
Vitamin B_6 (mg)	0.38	0.83	unknown	0.54
Vitamin B_{12} (μg)	2.4	7	1.4	7.8
Folate (μg)	18	unknown	2	16
Pantothenate (mg)	0.62	0.7	unknown	2.45
Biotin (μg)	unknown	unknown	unknown	4.7
Vitamin C (mg)	trace	trace	trace	trace

Tuna canned in oil	**Turbot** grilled	**Whelks** boiled	**Whitebait** floured and fried	**FOOD**
average portion in a salad	one average	average portion (4+)	average (20)	**PORTION SIZE**
				NUTRIENTS
174	195	27	420	Energy (kcals)
24.9	36.3	5.8	15.6	Protein (g)
8.3	5.6	0.4	38	Total fat (g)
1.4	1.4	0.1	unknown	Saturated fat (g)
2.1	1.3	0.1	unknown	Mono-unsat. fat (g)
4.4	1.1	0.1	unknown	Poly-unsat. fat (g)
nil	nil	nil	4.2	Carbohydrate (g)
nil	nil	nil	0.1	Sugar (g)
nil	nil	nil	0.2	Fibre (g)
267	14	84	184	Sodium (mg)
239	544	57	88	Potassium (mg)
11	99	25	688	Calcium (mg)
30	99	26	40	Magnesium (mg)
184	416	42	688	Phosphorus (mg)
1.47	0.96	0.99	4.08	Iron (mg)
0.18	0.08	1.98	unknown	Copper (mg)
1.01	0.48	3.63	unknown	Zinc (mg)
83	unknown	unknown	unknown	Selenium (µg)
unknown	trace	unknown	unknown	Vitamin A (µg)
2.76	trace	trace	unknown	Vitamin D (mg)
1.78	unknown	0.24	unknown	Vitamin E (mg)
0.02	0.1	0.01	unknown	Vitamin B_1 (mg)
0.11	0.22	0.05	unknown	Vitamin B_2 (mg)
14.81	3.84	0.39	unknown	Niacin (mg)
0.47	4.03	0.03	unknown	Vitamin B_6 (mg)
4.6	nil	6.3	unknown	Vitamin B_{12} (µg)
5	unknown	2	unknown	Folate (µg)
0.29	1.06	0.17	unknown	Pantothenate (mg)
2.8	unknown	1.8	unknown	Biotin (µg)
trace	trace	trace	trace	Vitamin C (mg)

FOOD	Boiled egg	Fried egg	Omelette cheese	Omelette plain
PORTION SIZE	one	one	two egg	two egg
NUTRIENTS				
Energy (kcals)	74	107	372	229
Protein (g)	6.3	8.2	22.2	13.1
Total fat (g)	5.4	8.3	31.6	19.7
Saturated fat (g)	1.5	2.4	17	8.9
Mono-unsat. fat (g)	2.3	3.6	10	7.0
Poly-unsat. fat (g)	0.6	0.9	1.6	1.6
Carbohydrate (g)	trace	trace	trace	trace
Sugar (g)	trace	trace	trace	trace
Fibre (g)	nil	nil	nil	nil
Sodium (mg)	70	96	1260	1236
Potassium (mg)	65	90	140	132
Calcium (mg)	29	39	392	61
Magnesium (mg)	6	8	26	19
Phosphorus (mg)	100	138	392	204
Iron (mg)	0.95	1.32	1.68	2.04
Copper (mg)	0.04	0.05	0.08	0.08
Zinc (mg)	0.65	0.9	2.1	1.32
Selenium (μg)	6	7	14	11
Vitamin A (μg)	95	129	394	289
Vitamin D (μg)	0.88	1.19	1.58	1.9
Vitamin E (mg)	0.56	unknown	1.28	1.36
Vitamin B_1 (mg)	0.04	0.04	0.08	0.08
Vitamin B_2 (mg)	0.17	0.19	0.44	0.4
Niacin (mg)	0.05	0.06	0.14	0.12
Vitamin B_6 (mg)	0.06	0.08	0.12	0.11
Vitamin B_{12} (μg)	0.6	1.0	2.5	2.6
Folate (μg)	20	24	37	36
Pantothenate (mg)	0.65	0.78	1.37	1.6
Biotin (μg)	8	10.8	17.3	20.8
Vitamin C (mg)	nil	nil	trace	nil

Omelette Spanish	**Poached egg**	**Quiche** cheese and egg	**Quiche** Lorraine	**FOOD**
two egg	one	medium slice	medium slice	**PORTION SIZE**
				NUTRIENTS
240	74	439	546	Energy (kcals)
11.4	6.3	17.5	22.5	Protein (g)
16.6	5.4	31	39.3	Total fat (g)
3.2	1.5	14.4	17.2	Saturated fat (g)
6.6	2.3	11	15.3	Mono-unsat. fat (g)
5.0	0.6	3.2	4.4	Poly-unsat. fat (g)
12.4	trace	24	27.7	Carbohydrate (g)
7.4	trace	2.2	3.2	Sugar (g)
2.8	nil	0.88	1.03	Fibre (g)
240	70	476	1078	Sodium (mg)
420	65	168	266	Potassium (mg)
62	29	364	322	Calcium (mg)
26	6	23.5	29	Magnesium (mg)
194	100	308	350	Phosphorus (mg)
2.2	0.95	1.4	1.68	Iron (mg)
0.12	0.04	0.08	0.14	Copper (mg)
1.2	0.65	1.54	2.24	Zinc (mg)
8	6	10.3	unknown	Selenium (µg)
668	95	282	245	Vitamin A (µg)
1.2	0.88	1.29	1.19	Vitamin D (µg)
1.76	0.56	1.26	1.26	Vitamin E (mg)
0.18	0.04	0.11	0.2	Vitamin B_1 (mg)
0.28	0.18	0.32	0.35	Vitamin B_2 (mg)
1.0	0.05	0.56	2.38	Niacin (mg)
0.28	0.06	0.11	0.2	Vitamin B_6 (mg)
1.8	0.5	1.32	1.32	Vitamin B_{12} (µg)
44	23	17.6	16.2	Folate (µg)
1.28	0.65	0.73	0.84	Pantothenate (mg)
14.2	7.5	9.2	9.1	Biotin (µg)
42	nil	trace	trace	Vitamin C (mg)

FOOD	Quiche mushroom	Scrambled egg with milk	Scrambled egg without milk
PORTION SIZE	medium slice	two egg	two egg
NUTRIENTS			
Energy (kcals)	397	296	192
Protein (g)	14	12.8	16.6
Total fat (g)	27.2	27.1	13.9
Saturated fat (g)	12.2	13.9	4.0
Mono-unsat. fat (g)	9.8	8.6	6.0
Poly-unsat. fat (g)	3.38	1.7	1.6
Carbohydrate (g)	25.6	0.7	trace
Sugar (g)	1.9	0.7	trace
Fibre (g)	1.32	nil	nil
Sodium (mg)	406	1236	180
Potassium (mg)	224	156	168
Calcium (mg)	280	76	73
Magnesium (mg)	20.6	20	16
Phosphorus (mg)	252	216	252
Iron (mg)	1.4	1.92	2.4
Copper (mg)	0.26	0.08	0.11
Zinc (mg)	1.25	1.32	1.68
Selenium (µg)	10.3	11	14
Vitamin A (µg)	231	368	246
Vitamin D (µg)	1.14	1.86	2.26
Vitamin E (mg)	1.16	1.48	1.43
Vitamin B_1 (mg)	0.13	0.08	0.08
Vitamin B_2 (mg)	0.3	0.4	0.56
Niacin (mg)	1.4	0.08	0.1
Vitamin B_6 (mg)	0.13	0.11	0.16
Vitamin B_{12} (µg)	0.1	2.5	1.4
Folate (µg)	19.1	34	53
Pantothenate (mg)	0.94	1.55	1.32
Biotin (µg)	9.87	19.8	19.2
Vitamin C (mg)	trace	trace	nil

Scotch egg	Soufflé cheese	Soufflé plain	FOOD
one	average portion	average portion	PORTION SIZE
			NUTRIENTS
301	278	221	Energy (kcals)
14.4	12.5	8.4	Protein (g)
20.5	21.1	16.2	Total fat (g)
5.2	9.1	5.5	Saturated fat (g)
7.9	7.5	6.3	Mono-unsat. fat (g)
4.0	3.0	3.1	Poly-unsat. fat (g)
15.7	10.2	11.4	Carbohydrate (g)
trace	2.6	3.0	Sugar (g)
unknown	0.3	0.3	Fibre (g)
804	484	264	Sodium (mg)
156	154	154	Potassium (mg)
60	231	105	Calcium (mg)
18	19	14	Magnesium (mg)
204	231	154	Phosphorus (mg)
2.16	1.1	1.1	Iron (mg)
0.28	0.05	0.05	Copper (mg)
1.44	1.21	0.88	Zinc (mg)
unknown	8	6	Selenium (µg)
36	267	213	Vitamin A (µg)
0.88	1.53	1.67	Vitamin D (µg)
unknown	1.4	1.34	Vitamin E (mg)
0.1	0.08	0.08	Vitamin B_1 (mg)
0.25	0.29	0.24	Vitamin B_2 (mg)
1.2	0.22	0.22	Niacin (mg)
0.16	0.09	0.09	Vitamin B_6 (mg)
0.6	1.3	1.2	Vitamin B_{12} (µg)
50	21	19	Folate (µg)
1.32	0.79	0.82	Pantothenate (mg)
10.4	9.5	10.0	Biotin (µg)
unknown	trace	trace	Vitamin C (mg)

FOOD	Baked beans	Baked beans low salt low sugar	Bean and vegetable casserole	Bean salad
PORTION SIZE	medium portion	medium portion	medium average portion	one tablespoon
NUTRIENTS				
Energy (kcals)	113	99	120	44
Protein (g)	7.0	7.3	7.8	1.3
Total fat (g)	0.8	0.8	1.6	2.8
Saturated fat (g)	0.1	0.1	0.3	0.3
Mono-unsat. fat (g)	0.1	0.1	0.3	1.0
Poly-unsat. fat (g)	0.4	0.4	0.5	1.3
Carbohydrate (g)	20.7	16.9	20.3	3.8
Sugar (g)	8.0	3.8	7.5	0.8
Fibre (g)	5.0	5.1	5.2	0.9
Sodium (mg)	716	446	242	84
Potassium (mg)	419	365	702	57
Calcium (mg)	72	61	60	11
Magnesium (mg)	42	39	44	7
Phosphorus (mg)	135	122	161	22
Iron (mg)	1.89	1.62	1.82	0.45
Copper (mg)	0.04	0.14	0.21	0.02
Zinc (mg)	0.68	0.68	0.78	0.15
Selenium (µg)	3	3	3	1
Vitamin A (µg)	16	17	333	12.5
Vitamin D (µg)	nil	nil	nil	nil
Vitamin E (mg)	0.5	0.53	1.46	0.08
Vitamin B_1 (mg)	0.12	0.12	0.26	0.03
Vitamin B_2 (mg)	0.08	0.08	0.21	0.01
Niacin (mg)	0.68	0.68	2.08	0.15
Vitamin B_6 (mg)	0.19	0.19	0.34	0.03
Vitamin B_{12} (µg)	nil	nil	nil	nil
Folate (µg)	30	31	44	13
Pantothenate (mg)	0.24	0.26	0.42	0.04
Biotin (µg)	3.4	3.5	6.2	unknown
Vitamin C (mg)	trace	trace	10	2

Broad beans frozen	**Butter beans** canned	**Chick peas** canned	**Dhal**	**FOOD**
two tablespoons	two tablespoons	two tablespoons	one tablespoon	**PORTION SIZE**
				NUTRIENTS
97	92	80	64	Energy (kcals)
9.5	7.1	25.0	3.0	Protein (g)
0.7	0.6	2.0	2.6	Total fat (g)
0.1	0.1	0.2	0.4	Saturated fat (g)
0.1	trace	0.4	0.9	Mono-unsat. fat (g)
0.4	0.2	1.0	2.2	Poly-unsat. fat (g)
14	15.6	11.2	7.6	Carbohydrate (g)
1.6	1.3	0.2	0.8	Sugar (g)
7.8	5.5	2.8	0.7	Fibre (g)
10	504	154	132	Sodium (mg)
336	348	78	112	Potassium (mg)
67	18	30	9.6	Calcium (mg)
43	32	16	12	Magnesium (mg)
180	82	56	44	Phosphorus (mg)
1.92	1.8	1.04	1.04	Iron (mg)
0.38	0.17	0.04	0.07	Copper (mg)
1.2	0.72	0.56	0.4	Zinc (mg)
unknown	unknown	trace	0.8	Selenium (µg)
45	trace	2	30	Vitamin A (µg)
nil	nil	nil	0.04	Vitamin D (µg)
0.73	0.4	1.08	unknown	Vitamin E (mg)
0.04	0.06	0.04	0.06	Vitamin B_1 (mg)
0.07	0.04	0.02	0.02	Vitamin B_2 (mg)
3.6	0.24	0.14	0.28	Niacin (mg)
0.1	0.06	0.02	0.07	Vitamin B_6 (mg)
nil	nil	nil	trace	Vitamin B_{12} (µg)
38	14	8	2.8	Folate (µg)
4.56	unknown	unknown	0.14	Pantothenate (mg)
2.5	unknown	unknown	unknown	Biotin (µg)
10	trace	trace	0.4	Vitamin C (mg)

FOOD	Kidney beans red	Lentils red split, boiled	Mushy peas canned	Peas frozen
PORTION SIZE	two tablespoons	one tablespoon	average portion	medium average
NUTRIENTS				
Energy (kcals)	70	40	65	48
Protein (g)	4.8	3.0	4.6	4.2
Total fat (g)	0.4	0.2	0.6	0.6
Saturated fat (g)	trace	trace	0.1	0.1
Mono-unsat. fat (g)	trace	trace	0.1	0.1
Poly-unsat. fat (g)	0.2	0.1	0.2	0.3
Carbohydrate (g)	12.4	7.0	11	6.8
Sugar (g)	2.6	0.3	1.4	1.9
Fibre (g)	4.4	0.8	1.4	3.6
Sodium (mg)	274	5	272	1
Potassium (mg)	196	88	136	105
Calcium (mg)	50	6	11	25
Magnesium (mg)	22	10	18	15
Phosphorus (mg)	92	40	80	69
Iron (mg)	1.4	0.96	1.04	1.12
Copper (mg)	trace	0.08	0.09	0.02
Zinc (mg)	0.48	0.4	0.56	0.49
Selenium (μg)	4	1	unknown	1
Vitamin A (μg)	trace	1	unknown	47
Vitamin D (μg)	nil	nil	nil	nil
Vitamin E (mg)	0.14	unknown	0.24	0.13
Vitamin B_1 (mg)	0.14	0.04	unknown	0.18
Vitamin B_2 (mg)	0.04	0.02	unknown	0.06
Niacin (mg)	0.42	0.16	unknown	1.12
Vitamin B_6 (mg)	0.08	0.04	unknown	0.06
Vitamin B_{12} (μg)	nil	nil	nil	nil
Folate (μg)	6	2	unknown	33
Pantothenate (mg)	0.1	0.12	unknown	0.1
Biotin (μg)	unknown	unknown	trace	0.3
Vitamin C (mg)	trace	trace	trace	8

Tofu steamed	**FOOD**
small cube (2-inch square)	**PORTION SIZE**
	NUTRIENTS
102	Energy (kcals)
11.3	Protein (g)
5.9	Total fat (g)
0.7	Saturated fat (g)
1.1	Mono-unsat. fat (g)
2.8	Poly-unsat. fat (g)
1.0	Carbohydrate (g)
0.4	Sugar (g)
unknown	Fibre (g)
6	Sodium (mg)
88	Potassium (mg)
714	Calcium (mg)
32	Magnesium (mg)
133	Phosphorus (mg)
1.68	Iron (mg)
0.28	Copper (mg)
0.98	Zinc (mg)
unknown	Selenium (μg)
0.5	Vitamin A (μg)
nil	Vitamin D (μg)
1.33	Vitamin E (mg)
0.08	Vitamin B_1 (mg)
0.03	Vitamin B_2 (mg)
0.14	Niacin (mg)
0.1	Vitamin B_6 (mg)
nil	Vitamin B_{12} (μg)
21	Folate (μg)
0.07	Pantothenate (mg)
unknown	Biotin (μg)
nil	Vitamin C (mg)

FOOD	Almonds	Brazil nuts	Cashew nuts	Chestnuts
PORTION SIZE	6 whole	3 whole	small bag	5 whole
NUTRIENTS				
Energy (kcals)	80	68	153	85
Protein (g)	2.7	1.4	5.1	1.0
Total fat (g)	7.3	6.8	12.7	1.4
Saturated fat (g)	0.6	1.6	2.5	0.3
Mono-unsat. fat (g)	4.5	2.6	7.3	0.5
Poly-unsat. fat (g)	1.8	2.3	2.3	0.6
Carbohydrate (g)	0.9	0.3	4.7	18.3
Sugar (g)	0.5	0.2	1.4	3.5
Fibre (g)	1.0	0.4	0.8	2.0
Sodium (mg)	2	trace	73	6
Potassium (mg)	101	66	183	250
Calcium (mg)	31	17	9	23
Magnesium (mg)	35	41	63	17
Phosphorus (mg)	72	59	128	37
Iron (mg)	0.39	0.25	1.55	0.45
Copper (mg)	0.13	0.18	0.51	0.12
Zinc (mg)	0.42	0.42	1.42	0.25
Selenium (μg)	1	153	9	trace
Vitamin A (μg)	nil	nil	trace	nil
Vitamin D (μg)	nil	nil	nil	nil
Vitamin E (mg)	3.11	0.72	0.32	0.6
Vitamin B_1 (mg)	0.03	0.07	0.1	0.07
Vitamin B_2 (mg)	0.1	trace	0.04	0.01
Niacin (mg)	0.4	0.03	0.32	0.25
Vitamin B_6 (mg)	0.02	0.03	0.11	0.17
Vitamin B_{12} (μg)	nil	nil	nil	nil
Folate (μg)	6	2	17	unknown
Pantothenate (mg)	0.06	0.04	0.27	0.25
Biotin (μg)	8.3	1.1	3.3	0.7
Vitamin C (mg)	nil	nil	nil	trace

Hazelnuts	Mixed nuts and raisins	Peanuts roasted	Peanuts dry roasted	FOOD
10 whole	medium bag	medium bag	medium bag	**PORTION SIZE**
				NUTRIENTS
65	241	301	295	Energy (kcals)
1.4	7.1	12.3	12.8	Protein (g)
6.3	17	26.5	24.9	Total fat (g)
0.5	2.8	4.8	4.4	Saturated fat (g)
5.0	8.9	12.1	11.4	Mono-unsat. fat (g)
0.6	4.4	8.3	7.8	Poly-unsat. fat (g)
0.6	15.8	3.5	5.2	Carbohydrate (g)
0.4	14.4	1.9	1.9	Sugar (g)
0.6	2.3	3.0	3.2	Fibre (g)
1	12	200	395	Sodium (mg)
73	410	405	365	Potassium (mg)
14	42	19	26	Calcium (mg)
16	80	90	95	Magnesium (mg)
30	155	205	210	Phosphorus (mg)
0.32	1.15	0.65	1.05	Iron (mg)
0.12	0.41	0.27	0.32	Copper (mg)
0.21	1.2	1.45	1.65	Zinc (mg)
trace	85	2	2	Selenium (μg)
nil	trace	nil	nil	Vitamin A (μg)
nil	nil	nil	nil	Vitamin D (μg)
2.5	unknown	0.33	0.56	Vitamin E (mg)
0.04	0.29	0.09	0.09	Vitamin B_1 (mg)
0.02	0.05	0.05	0.06	Vitamin B_2 (mg)
0.11	2.75	6.8	6.55	Niacin (mg)
0.06	0.21	0.31	0.27	Vitamin B_6 (mg)
nil	nil	nil	nil	Vitamin B_{12} (μg)
7	28	26	33	Folate (μg)
0.15	0.63	0.85	0.8	Pantothenate (mg)
7.6	19.8	51	65	Biotin (μg)
nil	trace	nil	nil	Vitamin C (mg)

FOOD	Pecan nuts	Pistachio nuts	Sunflower seeds	Walnuts
PORTION SIZE	3 whole	10 kernels	tablespoon	6 halves
NUTRIENTS				
Energy (kcals)	123	60	93	138
Protein (g)	1.8	1.8	3.2	2.9
Total fat (g)	12.6	5.5	7.6	13.7
Saturated fat (g)	0.9	0.7	0.7	1.1
Mono-unsat. fat (g)	7.5	2.8	1.6	2.5
Poly-unsat. fat (g)	3.3	1.8	5.0	9.5
Carbohydrate (g)	0.9	0.8	3.0	0.7
Sugar (g)	0.9	0.6	0.3	0.5
Fibre (g)	0.9	0.6	1.0	0.7
Sodium (mg)	trace	53	trace	1
Potassium (mg)	93	104	114	90
Calcium (mg)	12	11	18	19
Magnesium (mg)	24	13	62	32
Phosphorus (mg)	57	42	102	76
Iron (mg)	0.39	0.3	1.02	0.58
Copper (mg)	0.18	0.08	0.36	0.27
Zinc (mg)	0.96	0.22	0.82	0.54
Selenium (μg)	3	1	8	4
Vitamin A (μg)	1.5	2	trace	nil
Vitamin D (μg)	nil	nil	nil	nil
Vitamin E (mg)	0.78	0.42	6.04	0.77
Vitamin B_1 (mg)	0.12	0.07	0.26	0.08
Vitamin B_2 (mg)	0.03	0.02	0.03	0.03
Niacin (mg)	0.24	0.17	0.66	0.24
Vitamin B_6 (mg)	0.03	unknown	unknown	0.13
Vitamin B_{12} (μg)	nil	nil	nil	nil
Folate (μg)	6	6	unknown	13
Pantothenate (mg)	0.3	unknown	unknown	0.32
Biotin (μg)	unknown	unknown	unknown	3.8
Vitamin C (mg)	nil	nil	nil	nil

Segment Four

Dairy foods

About one sixth of the food we eat should come from this food group. All dairy foods are derived from milk, but some soya milk products have also been included in this section. Dairy foods are excellent sources of protein and calcium, but they can also contain a lot of fat. Having semi-skimmed or skimmed milk and low-fat cheeses and yoghurts reduces the fat but these products still contain plenty of protein and the same amount of calcium as the standard varieties. In this section, all standard cheese portions weigh 40 grams unless otherwise stated.

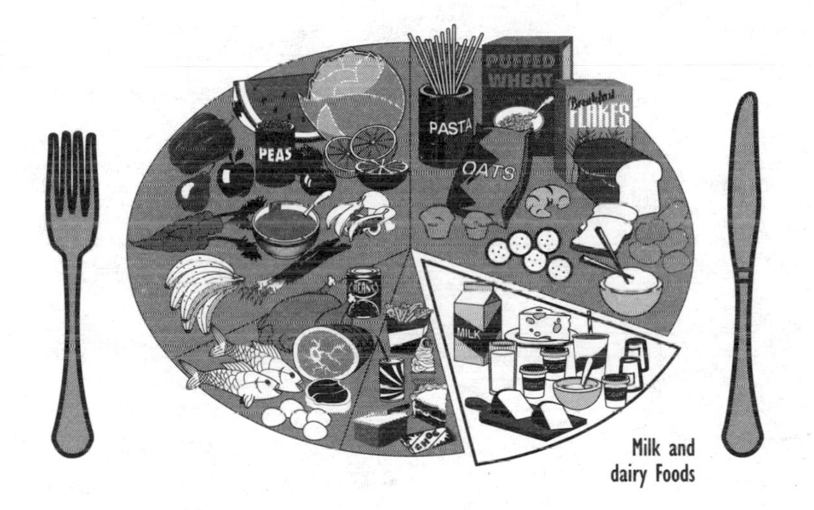

FOOD	Brie cheese	Camembert cheese	Cheddar cheese average	Cheddar cheese low fat
PORTION SIZE	standard	standard	standard	standard
NUTRIENTS				
Energy (kcals)	128	119	165	104
Protein (g)	7.7	8.4	10.2	12.6
Total fat (g)	10.8	9.5	13.8	6.0
Saturated fat (g)	6.7	5.9	8.7	3.8
Mono-unsat. fat (g)	3.1	2.8	3.8	1.8
Poly-unsat. fat (g)	0.3	0.3	0.6	0.2
Carbohydrate (g)	trace	trace	trace	trace
Sugar (g)	trace	trace	trace	trace
Fibre (g)	nil	nil	nil	nil
Sodium (mg)	280	260	268	268
Potassium (mg)	40	40	31	44
Calcium (mg)	216	140	288	336
Magnesium (mg)	11	8	10	16
Phosphorus (mg)	156	124	196	248
Iron (mg)	0.32	0.08	0.12	0.08
Copper (mg)	trace	0.03	0.01	0.02
Zinc (mg)	0.88	1.08	0.92	1.12
Selenium (µg)	unknown	unknown	5	6
Vitamin A (µg)	128	113	145	72
Vitamin D (µg)	0.08	0.07	0.1	0.04
Vitamin E (mg)	0.34	0.26	0.21	0.16
Vitamin B_1 (mg)	0.02	0.02	0.01	0.01
Vitamin B_2 (mg)	0.17	0.21	0.16	0.21
Niacin (mg)	0.17	0.38	0.03	0.04
Vitamin B_6 (mg)	0.06	0.09	0.04	0.05
Vitamin B_{12} (µg)	0.5	0.4	0.4	0.5
Folate (µg)	23	41	13	22
Pantothenate (mg)	0.14	0.14	0.14	0.2
Biotin (µg)	2.2	3.0	1.2	1.5
Vitamin C (mg)	trace	trace	trace	trace

Cheddar cheese vegetarian	Cheshire cheese	Cream cheese	Cottage cheese plain	FOOD
standard	standard	portion in a sandwich	one small tub	**PORTION SIZE**
				NUTRIENTS
170	152	132	110	Energy (kcals)
10.3	9.6	0.9	15.5	Protein (g)
14.3	12.6	14.2	4.4	Total fat (g)
9.0	7.8	8.9	2.7	Saturated fat (g)
3.9	3.6	4.1	1.2	Mono-unsat. fat (g)
0.6	0.4	0.4	0.1	Poly-unsat. fat (g)
trace	trace	trace	2.4	Carbohydrate (g)
trace	trace	trace	2.4	Sugar (g)
nil	nil	nil	nil	Fibre (g)
268	220	90	426	Sodium (mg)
27	35	48	100	Potassium (mg)
276	224	29	82	Calcium (mg)
12	8	3	10	Magnesium (mg)
196	160	30	179	Phosphorus (mg)
0.08	0.12	0.03	0.11	Iron (mg)
trace	0.05	0.01	0.04	Copper (mg)
0.76	1.32	0.15	0.67	Zinc (mg)
5	4	trace	4	Selenium (µg)
184	154	127	51	Vitamin A (µg)
0.11	0.1	0.08	0.03	Vitamin D (µg)
0.32	0.28	0.3	0.09	Vitamin E (mg)
0.01	0.01	0.01	0.03	Vitamin B_1 (mg)
0.18	0.19	0.04	0.29	Vitamin B_2 (mg)
0.02	0.04	0.03	0.11	Niacin (mg)
0.04	0.04	0.01	0.09	Vitamin B_6 (mg)
0.5	0.4	0.1	0.8	Vitamin B_{12} (µg)
10	16	3	30	Folate (µg)
0.18	0.12	0.08	0.45	Pantothenate (mg)
1.0	1.6	0.5	3.4	Biotin (µg)
trace	trace	trace	trace	Vitamin C (mg)

FOOD	**Cottage cheese** reduced fat	**Cottage cheese** with additions	**Danish blue cheese**	**Derby cheese**
PORTION SIZE	one small tub	one small tub	average (30g)	standard
NUTRIENTS				
Energy (kcals)	87	106	104	161
Protein (g)	14.9	14.3	6	9.7
Total fat (g)	1.6	4.3	8.9	13.6
Saturated fat (g)	1.0	2.7	5.6	8.5
Mono-unsat. fat (g)	0.4	1.2	2.6	3.9
Poly-unsat. fat (g)	trace	0.1	0.3	0.4
Carbohydrate (g)	3.7	2.9	trace	trace
Sugar (g)	3.7	2.9	trace	trace
Fibre (g)	nil	trace	nil	nil
Sodium (mg)	426	403	378	232
Potassium (mg)	100	146	27	35
Calcium (mg)	82	123	150	272
Magnesium (mg)	10	13	8	10
Phosphorus (mg)	179	179	111	188
Iron (mg)	0.11	0.11	0.06	0.16
Copper (mg)	0.04	0.06	0.02	0.01
Zinc (mg)	0.67	0.56	0.6	0.72
Selenium (µg)	4	4	1	4
Vitamin A (µg)	18.6	50	96	150
Vitamin D (µg)	0.01	0.03	0.07	0.1
Vitamin E (mg)	0.03	0.09	0.23	0.18
Vitamin B_1 (mg)	0.03	0.07	0.01	0.01
Vitamin B_2 (mg)	0.29	0.24	0.12	0.16
Niacin (mg)	0.15	0.22	0.14	0.01
Vitamin B_6 (mg)	0.09	0.09	0.04	0.04
Vitamin B_{12} (µg)	0.8	0.7	0.3	0.6
Folate (µg)	30	15	15	10
Pantothenate (mg)	0.45	0.35	0.16	0.12
Biotin (µg)	3.4	3.4	0.8	1.2
Vitamin C (mg)	trace	1	trace	trace

Double Gloucester cheese	Edam cheese	Emmental cheese	Feta cheese	FOOD
standard	standard	standard	standard	**PORTION SIZE**
				NUTRIENTS
162	133	153	75	Energy (kcals)
9.8	10.4	11.5	4.7	Protein (g)
13.6	10.2	11.9	6.1	Total fat (g)
8.5	6.4	7.4	4.1	Saturated fat (g)
4.0	3.0	3.4	1.2	Mono-unsat. fat (g)
0.4	0.3	0.4	0.2	Poly-unsat. fat (g)
trace	trace	trace	0.4	Carbohydrate (g)
trace	trace	trace	0.4	Sugar (g)
nil	nil	nil	nil	Fibre (g)
236	408	180	32	Sodium (mg)
32	39	36	29	Potassium (mg)
264	308	388	108	Calcium (mg)
9	16	14	6	Magnesium (mg)
184	212	236	84	Phosphorus (mg)
0.16	0.16	0.12	0.06	Iron (mg)
0.01	0.02	0.52	0.02	Copper (mg)
0.72	0.88	1.76	0.27	Zinc (mg)
5	unknown	3	unknown	Selenium (µg)
151	80	137	67	Vitamin A (µg)
0.1	0.08	unknown	0.15	Vitamin D (µg)
0.26	0.19	0.18	0.11	Vitamin E (mg)
0.01	0.01	0.02	0.01	Vitamin B_1 (mg)
0.18	0.14	0.14	0.06	Vitamin B_2 (mg)
0.03	0.03	0.04	0.06	Niacin (mg)
0.04	0.04	0.04	0.02	Vitamin B_6 (mg)
0.5	0.8	0.8	0.3	Vitamin B_{12} (µg)
12	16	8	7	Folate (µg)
0.13	0.15	0.16	0.11	Pantothenate (mg)
1.2	0.7	1.2	0.7	Biotin (µg)
trace	trace	trace	trace	Vitamin C (mg)

FOOD	Goats' cheese	Gouda cheese	Gruyere cheese	Lancashire cheese
PORTION SIZE	one individual	standard	standard	standard
NUTRIENTS				
Energy (kcals)	198	150	164	149
Protein (g)	13.1	9.6	10.9	9.3
Total fat (g)	15.8	12.4	13.3	12.4
Saturated fat (g)	10.4	7.8	8.3	7.8
Mono-unsat. fat (g)	3.6	3.6	3.9	3.6
Poly-unsat. fat (g)	0.5	0.4	0.4	0.4
Carbohydrate (g)	1.0	trace	trace	trace
Sugar (g)	1.0	trace	trace	trace
Fibre (g)	nil	nil	nil	nil
Sodium (mg)	470	364	268	236
Potassium (mg)	130	36	40	34
Calcium (mg)	190	296	380	224
Magnesium (mg)	14	15	15	7
Phosphorus (mg)	210	196	244	160
Iron (mg)	0.1	0.04	0.12	0.08
Copper (mg)	trace	trace	0.05	0.04
Zinc (mg)	0.7	0.72	0.92	0.96
Selenium (μg)	unknown	unknown	unknown	4
Vitamin A (μg)	310	107	145	144
Vitamin D (μg)	0.5	0.1	0.1	0.1
Vitamin E (mg)	0.79	0.21	0.23	0.28
Vitamin B_1 (mg)	0.04	0.01	0.01	0.01
Vitamin B_2 (mg)	0.63	0.12	0.16	0.18
Niacin (mg)	0.65	0.04	0.02	0.04
Vitamin B_6 (mg)	0.12	0.03	0.04	0.03
Vitamin B_{12} (μg)	2.0	0.7	0.6	0.4
Folate (μg)	19	17	5	18
Pantothenate (mg)	unknown	0.13	0.14	0.11
Biotin (μg)	unknown	0.6	0.6	1.6
Vitamin C (mg)	trace	trace	trace	trace

Leicester cheese	Mozzarella cheese	Parmesan cheese	Parmesan cheese	FOOD
standard	standard	one tablespoon grated	standard	**PORTION SIZE**
				NUTRIENTS
160	116	23	181	Energy (kcals)
9.7	10	2.0	15.8	Protein (g)
13.5	8.4	1.6	13.1	Total fat (g)
8.4	5.2	1.0	8.2	Saturated fat (g)
3.9	2.4	0.5	3.8	Mono-unsat. fat (g)
0.4	0.2	trace	0.4	Poly-unsat. fat (g)
trace	trace	trace	trace	Carbohydrate (g)
trace	trace	trace	trace	Sugar (g)
nil	nil	nil	nil	Fibre (g)
252	244	55	436	Sodium (mg)
34	30	6	44	Potassium (mg)
264	236	60	480	Calcium (mg)
9	11	2	18	Magnesium (mg)
188	168	41	324	Phosphorus (mg)
0.2	0.12	0.05	0.44	Iron (mg)
0.02	trace	0.02	0.13	Copper (mg)
1.32	0.56	0.27	2.12	Zinc (mg)
4	unknown	1	4	Selenium (µg)
145	107	19	152	Vitamin A (µg)
0.1	0.06	0.01	0.1	Vitamin D (µg)
0.15	0.13	0.04	0.28	Vitamin E (mg)
0.01	0.01	trace	0.01	Vitamin B_1 (mg)
0.18	0.12	0.02	0.18	Vitamin B_2 (mg)
0.04	0.03	0.01	0.05	Niacin (mg)
0.04	0.04	0.01	0.05	Vitamin B_6 (mg)
0.5	0.8	0.1	0.8	Vitamin B_{12} (µg)
10	8	1	5	Folate (µg)
0.15	0.1	0.02	0.17	Pantothenate (mg)
1.2	0.9	0.2	1.3	Biotin (µg)
trace	trace	trace	trace	Vitamin C (mg)

FOOD	Processed cheese	Processed cheese smoked	Red Windsor cheese	Ricotta cheese
PORTION SIZE	one slice	one 'sausage'	standard	heaped tablespoon
NUTRIENTS				
Energy (kcals)	66	242	160	79
Protein (g)	4.2	16.4	9.8	5.2
Total fat (g)	5.4	19.6	13.5	6.1
Saturated fat (g)	3.3	12.1	8.4	3.8
Mono-unsat. fat (g)	1.5	5.6	3.9	1.5
Poly-unsat. fat (g)	0.2	0.9	0.4	0.3
Carbohydrate (g)	0.2	trace	trace	1.1
Sugar (g)	0.2	trace	trace	1.1
Fibre (g)	nil	nil	nil	nil
Sodium (mg)	264	1016	276	55
Potassium (mg)	26	70	35	61
Calcium (mg)	120	544	276	132
Magnesium (mg)	4	22	12	7
Phosphorus (mg)	160	824	180	94
Iron (mg)	0.1	0.24	0.08	0.22
Copper (mg)	0.03	0.16	0.01	unknown
Zinc (mg)	0.64	2.56	0.84	0.71
Selenium (µg)	2	8	4	unknown
Vitamin A (µg)	57	207	149	110
Vitamin D (µg)	0.04	0.15	0.1	unknown
Vitamin E (mg)	0.11	0.18	0.24	0.02
Vitamin B_1 (mg)	0.01	0.02	0.01	0.01
Vitamin B_2 (mg)	0.06	0.22	0.15	0.1
Niacin (mg)	0.02	0.05	0.04	0.05
Vitamin B_6 (mg)	0.02	0.06	0.04	0.02
Vitamin B_{12} (µg)	0.2	0.7	0.6	0.2
Folate (µg)	4	14	13	unknown
Pantothenate (mg)	0.06	0.18	0.16	unknown
Biotin (µg)	0.5	1.2	1.0	unknown
Vitamin C (mg)	trace	trace	trace	trace

Roquefort cheese	Sage Derby cheese	Soft cheese full fat	Soft cheese medium fat	FOOD
standard	standard	heaped tablespoon	heaped tablespoon	**PORTION SIZE**
				NUTRIENTS
150	161	172	98	Energy (kcals)
7.9	9.7	4.7	5.1	Protein (g)
13.2	13.6	17.0	8.0	Total fat (g)
8.3	8.5	10.7	5.0	Saturated fat (g)
3.2	3.9	4.9	2.3	Mono-unsat. fat (g)
0.6	0.4	0.5	0.2	Poly-unsat. fat (g)
trace	trace	trace	1.7	Carbohydrate (g)
trace	trace	trace	1.7	Sugar (g)
nil	nil	nil	nil	Fibre (g)
668	240	182	unknown	Sodium (mg)
36	26	83	unknown	Potassium (mg)
212	244	61	unknown	Calcium (mg)
13	9	5	unknown	Magnesium (mg)
160	192	72	unknown	Phosphorus (mg)
0.16	0.28	0.05	unknown	Iron (mg)
0.04	trace	0.05	unknown	Copper (mg)
0.48	0.48	0.38	unknown	Zinc (mg)
unknown	4	2	2	Selenium (µg)
118	152	unknown	123	Vitamin A (µg)
unknown	0.1	unknown	0.06	Vitamin D (µg)
0.22	0.21	unknown	0.43	Vitamin E (mg)
0.02	0.01	0.02	unknown	Vitamin B_1 (mg)
0.26	0.17	0.09	unknown	Vitamin B_2 (mg)
0.23	0.02	0.05	unknown	Niacin (mg)
0.04	0.04	0.03	unknown	Vitamin B_6 (mg)
0.2	0.6	0.2	unknown	Vitamin B_{12} (µg)
18	10	7	unknown	Folate (µg)
0.2	0.14	0.17	unknown	Pantothenate (mg)
0.9	1.3	1.1	unknown	Biotin (µg)
trace	trace	trace	trace	Vitamin C (mg)

FOOD	Soya cheese	Cheese spread	Stilton cheese blue	Stilton cheese white
PORTION SIZE	standard	one triangle	average (35g)	standard
NUTRIENTS				
Energy (kcals)	128	39	144	145
Protein (g)	7.3	1.9	7.9	8.0
Total fat (g)	10.9	3.2	12.4	12.5
Saturated fat (g)	unknown	2.0	7.8	7.8
Mono-unsat. fat (g)	unknown	0.9	3.6	3.6
Poly-unsat. fat (g)	unknown	0.1	0.3	0.4
Carbohydrate (g)	trace	0.6	trace	trace
Sugar (g)	trace	0.6	trace	trace
Fibre (g)	nil	nil	nil	nil
Sodium (mg)	240	148	326	308
Potassium (mg)	52	34	46	37
Calcium (mg)	180	59	112	100
Magnesium (mg)	12	4	7	6
Phosphorus (mg)	140	111	109	104
Iron (mg)	0.44	0.03	0.11	0.12
Copper (mg)	trace	0.02	0.06	trace
Zinc (mg)	0.72	0.29	0.88	0.4
Selenium (µg)	unknown	1	4	4
Vitamin A (µg)	nil	41	135	137
Vitamin D (µg)	nil	0.02	0.09	0.1
Vitamin E (mg)	unknown	0.03	0.21	0.22
Vitamin B_1 (mg)	0.1	0.01	0.01	0.01
Vitamin B_2 (mg)	0.25	0.05	0.15	0.15
Niacin (mg)	0.45	0.01	0.17	0.04
Vitamin B_6 (mg)	0.08	0.01	0.06	0.03
Vitamin B_{12} (µg)	1.0	0.1	0.3	0.5
Folate (µg)	14	3	27	21
Pantothenate (mg)	unknown	0.07	0.25	0.09
Biotin (µg)	unknown	0.5	1.3	1.2
Vitamin C (mg)	nil	trace	trace	trace

Wensleydale cheese	FOOD
standard	**PORTION SIZE**
	NUTRIENTS
151	Energy (kcals)
9.3	Protein (g)
12.6	Total fat (g)
7.9	Saturated fat (g)
3.6	Mono-unsat. fat (g)
0.4	Poly-unsat. fat (g)
trace	Carbohydrate (g)
trace	Sugar (g)
nil	Fibre (g)
208	Sodium (mg)
36	Potassium (mg)
224	Calcium (mg)
8	Magnesium (mg)
164	Phosphorus (mg)
0.12	Iron (mg)
0.04	Copper (mg)
1.36	Zinc (mg)
4	Selenium (µg)
127	Vitamin A (µg)
0.1	Vitamin D (µg)
0.16	Vitamin E (mg)
0.01	Vitamin B_1 (mg)
0.18	Vitamin B_2 (mg)
0.04	Niacin (mg)
0.04	Vitamin B_6 (mg)
0.4	Vitamin B_{12} (µg)
17	Folate (µg)
0.12	Pantothenate (mg)
1.6	Biotin (µg)
trace	Vitamin C (mg)

FOOD	Canned cream UHT spray	Clotted cream	Double cream	Half cream
PORTION SIZE	amount on cake or dessert	tablespoon	tablespoon	tablespoon
NUTRIENTS				
Energy (kcals)	53	176	135	22
Protein (g)	0.3	0.5	0.5	0.4
Total fat (g)	5.4	19.0	14.4	2.0
Saturated fat (g)	3.4	11.9	9.0	1.2
Mono-unsat. fat (g)	1.6	5.5	4.2	0.6
Poly-unsat. fat (g)	0.2	0.5	0.4	0.1
Carbohydrate (g)	0.6	0.7	0.8	0.6
Sugar (g)	0.6	0.7	0.8	0.6
Fibre (g)	nil	nil	nil	nil
Sodium (mg)	6	5	11	7
Potassium (mg)	16	17	20	18
Calcium (mg)	11	11	15	15
Magnesium (mg)	1	2	2	2
Phosphorus (mg)	10	12	15	12
Iron (mg)	0.17	0.03	0.06	0.02
Copper (mg)	trace	0.03	trace	trace
Zinc (mg)	0.07	0.06	0.06	0.05
Selenium (μg)	trace	trace	trace	trace
Vitamin A (μg)	72	246	196	30
Vitamin D (μg)	0.03	0.08	0.08	0.02
Vitamin E (mg)	0.13	0.44	0.33	0.04
Vitamin B_1 (mg)	0.01	0.01	0.01	trace
Vitamin B_2 (mg)	0.03	0.05	0.05	0.03
Niacin (mg)	0.01	0.01	0.01	0.02
Vitamin B_6 (mg)	0.01	0.01	0.01	0.01
Vitamin B_{12} (μg)	trace	trace	0.1	trace
Folate (μg)	trace	2	2	1
Pantothenate (mg)	0.03	0.04	0.06	0.04
Biotin (μg)	0.3	0.3	0.3	0.3
Vitamin C (mg)	nil	trace	trace	trace

Single cream	Soured cream	Whipping cream	FOOD
tablespoon	tablespoon	tablespoon	**PORTION SIZE**
			NUTRIENTS
30	31	56	Energy (kcals)
0.4	0.4	0.3	Protein (g)
2.9	3.0	5.9	Total fat (g)
1.8	1.9	3.7	Saturated fat (g)
0.8	0.9	1.7	Mono-unsat. fat (g)
0.1	0.1	0.2	Poly-unsat. fat (g)
0.6	0.6	0.5	Carbohydrate (g)
0.6	0.6	0.5	Sugar (g)
nil	nil	nil	Fibre (g)
7	6	6	Sodium (mg)
18	17	12	Potassium (mg)
14	14	9	Calcium (mg)
1	2	1	Magnesium (mg)
11	12	9	Phosphorus (mg)
0.02	0.06	trace	Iron (mg)
trace	trace	trace	Copper (mg)
0.08	0.08	0.05	Zinc (mg)
trace	trace	trace	Selenium (μg)
50	52	91	Vitamin A (μg)
0.02	0.02	0.03	Vitamin D (μg)
0.06	0.07	0.13	Vitamin E (mg)
0.01	trace	trace	Vitamin B_1 (mg)
0.03	0.03	0.03	Vitamin B_2 (mg)
0.02	0.01	0.01	Niacin (mg)
0.01	0.01	0.01	Vitamin B_6 (mg)
trace	trace	trace	Vitamin B_{12} (μg)
1	2	1	Folate (μg)
0.04	0.04	0.03	Pantothenate (mg)
0.3	0.2	0.2	Biotin (μg)
trace	trace	trace	Vitamin C (mg)

FOOD	**Condensed milk** skimmed sweetened	**Condensed milk** full fat sweetened	**Cows' milk** calcium fortified	**Cows' milk** Channel Island
PORTION SIZE	tablespoon	tablespoon	½ pint	½ pint
NUTRIENTS				
Energy (kcals)	67	83	129	229
Protein (g)	2.5	2.1	11.7	10.5
Total fat (g)	0.1	2.5	1.5	14.9
Saturated fat (g)	trace	1.6	0.9	9.7
Mono-unsat. fat (g)	trace	0.7	0.3	3.8
Poly-unsat. fat (g)	trace	0.1	trace	0.3
Carbohydrate (g)	15.0	13.9	18.2	14.1
Sugar (g)	15.0	13.9	18.2	14.1
Fibre (g)	nil	nil	nil	nil
Sodium (mg)	38	35	161	158
Potassium (mg)	113	90	557	410
Calcium (mg)	83	73	498	381
Magnesium (mg)	8	7	38	35
Phosphorus (mg)	68	60	322	293
Iron (mg)	0.08	0.06	0.15	0.15
Copper (mg)	trace	trace	trace	trace
Zinc (mg)	0.3	0.25	1.17	1.17
Selenium (µg)	1	1	3	3
Vitamin A (µg)	8	31	18	169
Vitamin D (µg)	0.21	1.35	0.56	0.09
Vitamin E (mg)	0.01	0.05	0.09	0.32
Vitamin B_1 (mg)	0.03	0.02	0.18	0.12
Vitamin B_2 (mg)	0.13	0.12	1.52	0.56
Niacin (mg)	0.08	0.07	0.09	0.29
Vitamin B_6 (mg)	0.02	0.02	0.15	0.18
Vitamin B_{12} (µg)	0.2	0.2	5.3	1.2
Folate (µg)	4	4	12	18
Pantothenate (mg)	0.26	0.21	unknown	1.05
Biotin (µg)	1.3	1.0	unknown	5.6
Vitamin C (mg)	1	1	unknown	3

Cows' milk full fat (silver top)	Cows' milk semi-skimmed	Cows' milk skimmed	Cows' milk sterilised full fat	FOOD
½ pint	½ pint	½ pint	½ pint	PORTION SIZE
				NUTRIENTS
193	135	97	193	Energy (kcals)
9.4	9.7	9.7	10.3	Protein (g)
11.4	4.7	0.3	11.4	Total fat (g)
7.0	2.9	0.3	7.0	Saturated fat (g)
3.2	1.5	trace	3.2	Mono-unsat. fat (g)
0.3	trace	trace	0.3	Poly-unsat. fat (g)
14.1	14.6	14.6	13.2	Carbohydrate (g)
14.1	14.6	14.6	13.2	Sugar (g)
nil	nil	nil	nil	Fibre (g)
161	161	158	167	Sodium (mg)
410	440	440	410	Potassium (mg)
337	352	352	352	Calcium (mg)
32	32	35	38	Magnesium (mg)
270	278	275	267	Phosphorus (mg)
0.18	0.15	0.18	0.53	Iron (mg)
trace	trace	trace	trace	Copper (mg)
1.17	1.17	1.17	0.88	Zinc (mg)
3	3	3	3	Selenium (µg)
162	66	3	162	Vitamin A (µg)
0.09	0.03	trace	0.09	Vitamin D (µg)
0.26	0.09	trace	0.26	Vitamin E (mg)
0.09	0.12	0.12	0.09	Vitamin B_1 (mg)
0.5	0.53	0.50	0.41	Vitamin B_2 (mg)
0.29	0.29	0.29	0.29	Niacin (mg)
0.18	0.18	0.18	0.12	Vitamin B_6 (mg)
1.2	1.2	1.2	0.3	Vitamin B_{12} (µg)
18	18	15	trace	Folate (µg)
1.03	0.94	0.94	0.82	Pantothenate (mg)
5.6	5.9	5.6	5.3	Biotin (µg)
3	3	3	trace	Vitamin C (mg)

FOOD	**Dried milk** skimmed	**Dried milk** with added vegetable fat	**Evaporated milk**	**Goats' milk**
PORTION SIZE	teaspoon	teaspoon	small can	½ pint
NUTRIENTS				
Energy (kcals)	10	15	257	176
Protein (g)	1.1	0.7	14.3	9.1
Total fat (g)	trace	0.8	16.0	10.3
Saturated fat (g)	trace	0.5	10.0	6.7
Mono-unsat. fat (g)	trace	0.2	4.6	2.3
Poly-unsat. fat (g)	trace	trace	0.5	0.3
Carbohydrate (g)	1.6	1.3	14.4	12.9
Sugar (g)	1.6	1.3	14.4	12.9
Fibre (g)	nil	nil	nil	nil
Sodium (mg)	17	13	306	123
Potassium (mg)	48	31	612	498
Calcium (mg)	38	25	493	293
Magnesium (mg)	4	2	49	38
Phosphorus (mg)	29	20	442	264
Iron (mg)	0.01	0.01	0.44	0.35
Copper (mg)	trace	trace	0.03	0.09
Zinc (mg)	0.12	0.02	1.53	1.47
Selenium (µg)	trace	trace	5	unknown
Vitamin A (µg)	11	12	207	129
Vitamin D (µg)	0.06	0.31	6.72	0.32
Vitamin E (mg)	0.01	0.04	0.32	0.09
Vitamin B_1 (mg)	0.01	0.01	0.12	0.12
Vitamin B_2 (mg)	0.05	0.04	0.71	0.38
Niacin (mg)	0.03	0.02	0.39	0.91
Vitamin B_6 (mg)	0.02	0.01	0.12	0.18
Vitamin B_{12} (µg)	0.1	0.1	0.2	0.3
Folate (µg)	2	1	19	3
Pantothenate (mg)	0.1	0.06	1.27	1.2
Biotin (µg)	0.6	0.4	6.8	8.8
Vitamin C (mg)	trace	trace	2	3

Sheep's milk	Soya milk unflavoured	FOOD
½ pint	½ pint	**PORTION SIZE**
		NUTRIENTS
278	94	Energy (kcals)
15.8	8.5	Protein (g)
17.6	5.6	Total fat (g)
11.1	0.9	Saturated fat (g)
4.4	1.2	Mono-unsat. fat (g)
0.9	3.2	Poly-unsat. fat (g)
14.9	2.3	Carbohydrate (g)
14.9	2.3	Sugar (g)
nil	trace	Fibre (g)
129	94	Sodium (mg)
352	352	Potassium (mg)
498	38	Calcium (mg)
53	44	Magnesium (mg)
440	138	Phosphorus (mg)
0.09	1.17	Iron (mg)
0.29	0.18	Copper (mg)
2.05	0.59	Zinc (mg)
unknown	unknown	Selenium (µg)
243	trace	Vitamin A (µg)
0.53	nil	Vitamin D (µg)
0.32	2.17	Vitamin E (mg)
0.23	0.18	Vitamin B_1 (mg)
0.94	0.79	Vitamin B_2 (mg)
1.17	0.32	Niacin (mg)
0.23	0.21	Vitamin B_6 (mg)
1.8	nil	Vitamin B_{12} (µg)
15	56	Folate (µg)
1.32	unknown	Pantothenate (mg)
7.3	unknown	Biotin (µg)
15	nil	Vitamin C (mg)

FOOD	Yoghurt drinking	Yoghurt Greek, cows'	Yoghurt Greek, sheep's	Yoghurt low calorie
PORTION SIZE	average pot	average pot	average pot	average pot
NUTRIENTS				
Energy (kcals)	124	230	212	51
Protein (g)	6.2	12.8	8.8	5.4
Total fat (g)	trace	18.2	15.0	0.3
Saturated fat (g)	trace	10.4	9.6	0.1
Mono-unsat. fat (g)	trace	5.4	3.8	0.1
Poly-unsat. fat (g)	trace	1.0	0.8	trace
Carbohydrate (g)	26.2	4.0	11.2	7.5
Sugar (g)	26.2	4.0	11.2	7.5
Fibre (g)	unknown	nil	nil	unknown
Sodium (mg)	94	142	300	91
Potassium (mg)	260	300	380	225
Calcium (mg)	200	300	300	163
Magnesium (mg)	22	24	32	16
Phosphorus (mg)	162	260	280	138
Iron (mg)	0.2	0.6	trace	0.13
Copper (mg)	0.02	trace	trace	trace
Zinc (mg)	0.6	1.0	1.0	0.5
Selenium (µg)	2	4	2	1
Vitamin A (µg)	trace	242	175	trace
Vitamin D (µg)	trace	0.1	0.48	trace
Vitamin E (mg)	trace	0.76	1.46	0.04
Vitamin B_1 (mg)	0.06	0.06	0.1	0.05
Vitamin B_2 (mg)	0.32	0.72	0.66	0.36
Niacin (mg)	0.18	0.12	0.46	0.16
Vitamin B_6 (mg)	0.1	0.1	0.16	0.09
Vitamin B_{12} (µg)	0.4	0.4	0.4	0.3
Folate (µg)	24	12	6	10
Pantothenate (mg)	0.38	unknown	unknown	unknown
Biotin (µg)	1.8	unknown	unknown	unknown
Vitamin C (mg)	nil	trace	trace	1

Yoghurt full fat, fruit	**Yoghurt** full fat, plain	**Yoghurt** low fat, fruit	**Yoghurt** low fat, plain	**FOOD**
average pot	average pot	average pot	average pot	**PORTION SIZE**
				NUTRIENTS
131	99	113	70	Energy (kcals)
6.4	7.1	5.1	6.4	Protein (g)
3.5	3.8	0.9	1.0	Total fat (g)
1.9	2.1	0.5	0.6	Saturated fat (g)
1.0	1.1	0.3	0.3	Mono-unsat. fat (g)
0.3	0.3	trace	trace	Poly-unsat. fat (g)
19.6	9.8	22.4	9.4	Carbohydrate (g)
19.6	9.8	22.4	9.4	Sugar (g)
unknown	unknown	unknown	trace	Fibre (g)
103	100	80	104	Sodium (mg)
263	350	263	313	Potassium (mg)
200	250	188	238	Calcium (mg)
20	24	19	24	Magnesium (mg)
163	213	150	200	Phosphorus (mg)
trace	0.13	0.13	0.13	Iron (mg)
trace	trace	trace	trace	Copper (mg)
0.63	0.88	0.63	0.75	Zinc (mg)
1	3	1	1	Selenium (μg)
52	39	14	11	Vitamin A (μg)
0.05	0.05	0.01	0.01	Vitamin D (μg)
0.06	0.06	0.01	0.01	Vitamin E (mg)
0.07	0.07	0.06	0.06	Vitamin B_1 (mg)
0.38	0.34	0.26	0.31	Vitamin B_2 (mg)
0.16	0.25	0.17	0.19	Niacin (mg)
0.09	0.13	0.1	0.11	Vitamin B_6 (mg)
0.1	0.3	0.3	0.3	Vitamin B_{12} (μg)
13	23	20	21	Folate (μg)
0.38	0.63	0.41	0.56	Pantothenate (mg)
2.5	3.3	2.9	3.6	Biotin (μg)
1	1	1	1	Vitamin C (mg)

FOOD	Yoghurt soya
PORTION SIZE	average pot
NUTRIENTS	
Energy (kcals)	86
Protein (g)	6.0
Total fat (g)	5.0
Saturated fat (g)	0.7
Mono-unsat. fat (g)	1.1
Poly-unsat. fat (g)	2.9
Carbohydrate (g)	4.7
Sugar (g)	4.7
Fibre (g)	unknown
Sodium (mg)	unknown
Potassium (mg)	unknown
Calcium (mg)	unknown
Magnesium (mg)	unknown
Phosphorus (mg)	unknown
Iron (mg)	unknown
Copper (mg)	unknown
Zinc (mg)	unknown
Selenium (μg)	unknown
Vitamin A (μg)	28
Vitamin D (μg)	nil
Vitamin E (mg)	1.79
Vitamin B_1 (mg)	unknown
Vitamin B_2 (mg)	unknown
Niacin (mg)	unknown
Vitamin B_6 (mg)	unknown
Vitamin B_{12} (μg)	nil
Folate (μg)	unknown
Pantothenate (mg)	unknown
Biotin (μg)	unknown
Vitamin C (mg)	nil

Segment Five

Foods high in fat and sugar

This section is very large and probably contains a lot of what most of us would describe as convenience, or more unkindly, junk food. Although these foods are high in sugar and fat, they often contain a surprising number of nutrients. Foods from this section should make up only a very small part of our regular food intake, but a healthy diet can still contain them. Drinks have been included in this section, because most of the non-alcoholic ones are high in sugar, and the alcoholic ones should only be taken in moderation.

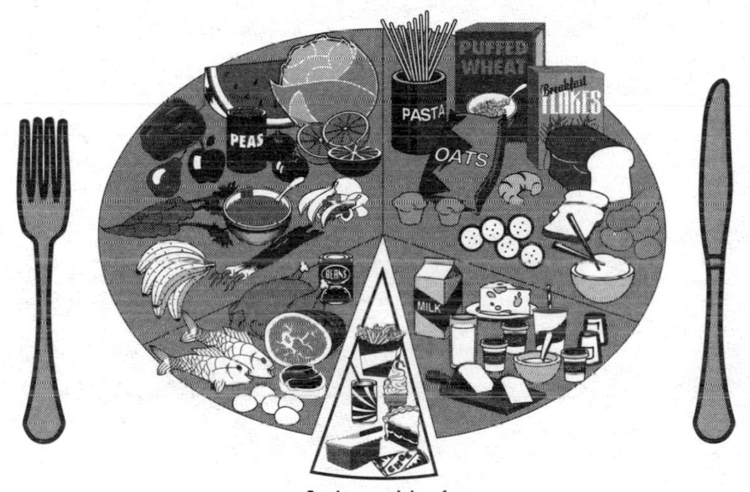

Foods containing fat
Foods containing sugar

For ease of use, the section is split into sub-sections as follows:

- Cakes, biscuits and puddings
- Confectionery
- Spreads, sugar and syrups
- Ice cream
- Snacks
- Fats and oils
- Sauces, soups and savoury spreads
- Beverages

Cakes, biscuits and puddings

I think most of us would agree that life without these sweet delights would be dull indeed, but such foods can be high in both sugar and fat. The best daily dessert to eat on a healthy diet is fruit; save those puds for an occasional treat and keep the cakes for that special occasion. Biscuits can be deceptively high in fat so if you feel a cup of tea is too wet without one, a low-fat, plain biscuit is best.

Trying to pick the right dessert when eating out is difficult, there really is no healthy pudding, and in any case they do not taste the same if made with low-fat or low-sugar ingredients. If you only eat out occasionally, then enjoy the dessert of your choice. If you can do without cream, so much the better. Anyone eating out a lot should try to stick to fruit of the fresh variety, and remember that cheese and biscuits might not contain the sugar, but are in a different league when it comes to fat.

There was insufficient data for this section from The Composition of Foods and therefore in order to enhance it, some manufacturer's data has been used.

[4] – Waitrose
[6] – Marks & Spencer

FOOD	Apple Strudel	Battenburg cake	Bourbon biscuits[4]	Brandy snaps
PORTION SIZE	average	average slice	one	one
NUTRIENTS				
Energy (kcals)	265	118	64	66
Protein (g)	3.7	1.9	0.6	0.4
Total fat (g)	13.9	5.6	2.6	3.0
Saturated fat (g)	4.6	1.5	0.9	unknown
Mono-unsat. fat (g)	unknown	2.5	1.4	unknown
Poly-unsat. fat (g)	1.7	1.4	0.2	unknown
Carbohydrate (g)	33	16	9.6	9.6
Sugar (g)	16.7	10.9	4.1	6.8
Fibre (g)	unknown	unknown	0.2	0.1
Sodium (mg)	unknown	141	25	38
Potassium (mg)	unknown	45	14.4	17
Calcium (mg)	unknown	28	unknown	7
Magnesium (mg)	unknown	8	unknown	1
Phosphorus (mg)	unknown	61	unknown	6
Iron (mg)	unknown	0.35	unknown	0.15
Copper (mg)	unknown	0.03	unknown	0.01
Zinc (mg)	unknown	0.22	unknown	0.05
Selenium (µg)	unknown	1	unknown	trace
Vitamin A (µg)	unknown	15	unknown	unknown
Vitamin D (µg)	unknown	0.13	unknown	0.03
Vitamin E (mg)	unknown	0.86	unknown	0.08
Vitamin B_1 (mg)	unknown	0.03	unknown	0.01
Vitamin B_2 (mg)	unknown	0.05	unknown	trace
Niacin (mg)	unknown	0.16	unknown	0.06
Vitamin B_6 (mg)	unknown	0.02	unknown	trace
Vitamin B_{12} (µg)	unknown	0.3	unknown	nil
Folate (µg)	unknown	4	unknown	trace
Pantothenate (mg)	unknown	0.13	unknown	0.02
Biotin (µg)	unknown	2.6	unknown	trace
Vitamin C (mg)	unknown	nil	unknown	nil

Carrot and orange cake[4]	Chelsea bun	Cherry cake	Chocolate biscuits full coated	FOOD
average slice	one	average slice	one	**PORTION SIZE**
				NUTRIENTS
227	285	165	63	Energy (kcals)
3.4	6.1	2.1	0.7	Protein (g)
10.2	10.8	6.6	3.3	Total fat (g)
1.82	3.3	unknown	unknown	Saturated fat (g)
4.5	4.1	unknown	unknown	Mono-unsat. fat (g)
2.4	2.9	unknown	unknown	Poly-unsat. fat (g)
30.4	43.8	25.9	8.1	Carbohydrate (g)
22.7	16.7	16.8	5.2	Sugar (g)
1.1	257	0.5	0.3	Fibre (g)
429	172	130	19	Sodium (mg)
91	86	31	28	Potassium (mg)
unknown	20	30	13	Calcium (mg)
unknown	94	4	5	Magnesium (mg)
unknown	1.17	46	16	Phosphorus (mg)
unknown	0.2	0.55	0.2	Iron (mg)
unknown	0.62	0.04	0.03	Copper (mg)
unknown	0.31	0.21	0.1	Zinc (mg)
unknown	unknown	unknown	unknown	Selenium (µg)
unknown	13	unknown	unknown	Vitamin A (µg)
unknown	0.08	0.66	nil	Vitamin D (µg)
unknown	1.16	0.72	0.17	Vitamin E (mg)
unknown	0.12	0.03	trace	Vitamin B_1 (mg)
unknown	0.1	0.04	0.02	Vitamin B_2 (mg)
unknown	1.09	0.17	0.06	Niacin (mg)
unknown	0.09	0.02	trace	Vitamin B_6 (mg)
unknown	trace	0.4	nil	Vitamin B_{12} (µg)
unknown	25	3	unknown	Folate (µg)
unknown	0.31	0.13	unknown	Pantothenate (mg)
unknown	4.7	2.1	unknown	Biotin (µg)
unknown	trace	nil	nil	Vitamin C (mg)

FOOD	Chocolate cake with butter icing	Chocolate chip cookies[4]	Chocolate Swiss roll individual	Choux buns
PORTION SIZE	average slice	one	one	one
NUTRIENTS				
Energy (kcals)	313	45	84	427
Protein (g)	3.7	0.5	1.1	6
Total fat (g)	19.3	2.2	2.8	36.4
Saturated fat (g)	unknown	1.2	unknown	unknown
Mono-unsat. fat (g)	unknown	0.7	unknown	unknown
Poly-unsat. fat (g)	unknown	0.2	unknown	unknown
Carbohydrate (g)	33.1	5.6	14.5	19.7
Sugar (g)	22.3	2.7	10.4	1.7
Fibre (g)	unknown	0.2	unknown	0.8
Sodium (mg)	273	59	88	235
Potassium (mg)	91	18.9	53	99
Calcium (mg)	38	unknown	19	73
Magnesium (mg)	23	unknown	5	11
Phosphorus (mg)	104	unknown	50	100
Iron (mg)	0.98	unknown	0.28	1.12
Copper (mg)	0.2	unknown	0.06	0.06
Zinc (mg)	0.58	unknown	0.13	0.56
Selenium (µg)	3	unknown	unknown	unknown
Vitamin A (µg)	unknown	unknown	unknown	unknown
Vitamin D (µg)	1.8	unknown	unknown	0.43
Vitamin E (mg)	1.9	unknown	unknown	1.95
Vitamin B_1 (mg)	0.05	unknown	0.03	0.08
Vitamin B_2 (mg)	0.06	unknown	0.05	0.18
Niacin (mg)	0.26	unknown	0.08	0.45
Vitamin B_6 (mg)	0.03	unknown	0.01	0.06
Vitamin B_{12} (µg)	0.6	unknown	trace	1.1
Folate (µg)	6	unknown	3	12
Pantothenate (mg)	0.26	unknown	unknown	0.45
Biotin (µg)	3.9	unknown	unknown	6.7
Vitamin C (mg)	nil	unknown	nil	trace

Coconut cake	Cream horn	Rice Krispie cake	Currant bun	FOOD
average slice	one	one	one	**PORTION SIZE**
				NUTRIENTS
174	261	116	178	Energy (kcals)
2.7	2.3	1.4	4.6	Protein (g)
9.5	21.5	4.7	4.5	Total fat (g)
unknown	10.0	2.7	unknown	Saturated fat (g)
unknown	8.0	1.5	unknown	Mono-unsat. fat (g)
unknown	2.5	0.2	unknown	Poly-unsat. fat (g)
20.5	15.5	18.3	31.6	Carbohydrate (g)
8.6	3.7	10.2	9.1	Sugar (g)
1.0	0.5	0.1	unknown	Fibre (g)
184	120	113	138	Sodium (mg)
68	43	58	126	Potassium (mg)
40	37	7	66	Calcium (mg)
8	7	19	16	Magnesium (mg)
100	34	30	60	Phosphorus (mg)
0.6	0.42	1.0	1.14	Iron (mg)
0.07	0.04	0.12	0.11	Copper (mg)
0.28	0.24	0.1	0.36	Zinc (mg)
unknown	unknown	unknown	unknown	Selenium (µg)
unknown	139	1	unknown	Vitamin A (µg)
0.68	0.06	0.2	nil	Vitamin D (µg)
0.82	1.3	0.19	unknown	Vitamin E (mg)
0.04	0.04	0.1	0.22	Vitamin B_1 (mg)
0.04	0.04	0.13	0.1	Vitamin B_2 (mg)
0.28	0.3	1.45	0.9	Niacin (mg)
0.06	0.02	0.17	0.07	Vitamin B_6 (mg)
trace	trace	0.2	trace	Vitamin B_{12} (µg)
4	4	25	24	Folate (µg)
0.16	0.06	0.15	unknown	Pantothenate (mg)
2	0.6	0.8	unknown	Biotin (µg)
nil	1	nil	nil	Vitamin C (mg)

FOOD	Custard tart individual	Custard Creams[4]	Danish pastry	Digestive biscuit plain
PORTION SIZE	one	one	one	one
NUTRIENTS				
Energy (kcals)	260	56	411	61
Protein (g)	5.9	0.6	6.4	0.8
Total fat (g)	13.6	2.6	19.4	2.7
Saturated fat (g)	5.3	1.6	6.2	unknown
Mono-unsat. fat (g)	5.8	0.6	8.5	unknown
Poly-unsat. fat (g)	1.6	0.1	3.5	unknown
Carbohydrate (g)	30.5	7.6	56.4	8.9
Sugar (g)	12.0	3.3	31.4	1.8
Fibre (g)	1.1	0.1	1.8	0.3
Sodium (mg)	122	20.6	209	78
Potassium (mg)	103	12.1	187	22
Calcium (mg)	89	unknown	101	12
Magnesium (mg)	13	unknown	26	3
Phosphorus (mg)	92	unknown	108	11
Iron (mg)	0.75	unknown	1.43	0.42
Copper (mg)	0.07	unknown	0.07	0.04
Zinc (mg)	0.47	unknown	0.55	0.06
Selenium (μg)	0.19	unknown	unknown	unknown
Vitamin A (μg)	30	unknown	unknown	unknown
Vitamin D (μg)	unknown	unknown	unknown	nil
Vitamin E (mg)	unknown	unknown	trace	unknown
Vitamin B_1 (mg)	0.13	unknown	0.14	0.02
Vitamin B_2 (mg)	0.15	unknown	0.08	0.01
Niacin (mg)	0.47	unknown	0.99	0.14
Vitamin B_6 (mg)	0.03	unknown	0.08	0.01
Vitamin B_{12} (μg)	trace	unknown	trace	nil
Folate (μg)	12	unknown	22	2
Pantothenate (mg)	unknown	unknown	0.55	unknown
Biotin (μg)	unknown	unknown	7.7	unknown
Vitamin C (mg)	nil	unknown	nil	nil

Digestive biscuit chocolate	Doughnut custard filled	Doughnut jam filled	Doughnut ring	FOOD
one	one	one	one	**PORTION SIZE**
				NUTRIENTS
99	269	252	238	Energy (kcals)
1.4	4.6	4.3	3.7	Protein (g)
4.8	14.3	10.9	13.0	Total fat (g)
unknown	unknown	3.2	3.8	Saturated fat (g)
unknown	unknown	4.1	5.0	Mono-unsat. fat (g)
unknown	unknown	2.7	3.3	Poly-unsat. fat (g)
13.3	32.5	36.6	28.3	Carbohydrate (g)
5.7	11.9	14.1	9.2	Sugar (g)
0.4	unknown	unknown	unknown	Fibre (g)
90	150	135	138	Sodium (mg)
42	74	83	52	Potassium (mg)
17	62	54	46	Calcium (mg)
8	15	14	13	Magnesium (mg)
26	68	53	49	Phosphorus (mg)
0.42	0.83	0.9	0.72	Iron (mg)
0.05	0.09	0.07	0.08	Copper (mg)
0.2	0.45	0.38	0.36	Zinc (mg)
unknown	unknown	unknown	unknown	Selenium (µg)
unknown	unknown	unknown	unknown	Vitamin A (µg)
nil	unknown	unknown	unknown	Vitamin D (µg)
0.22	0.07	trace	trace	Vitamin E (mg)
0.02	0.15	0.16	0.13	Vitamin B_1 (mg)
0.02	0.08	0.05	0.04	Vitamin B_2 (mg)
0.26	0.75	0.97	0.72	Niacin (mg)
0.02	0.02	0.02	0.01	Vitamin B_6 (mg)
nil	trace	trace	trace	Vitamin B_{12} (µg)
unknown	14	16	11	Folate (µg)
unknown	unknown	unknown	unknown	Pantothenate (mg)
unknown	unknown	unknown	unknown	Biotin (µg)
nil	unknown	unknown	nil	Vitamin C (mg)

FOOD	Doughnut ring iced	Eccles cake	Eclair fresh	Eclair frozen
PORTION SIZE	one	one	one (90g)	one (35g)
NUTRIENTS				
Energy (kcals)	287	214	336	139
Protein (g)	3.6	1.8	3.7	2.0
Total fat (g)	13.1	11.9	21.4	10.7
Saturated fat (g)	unknown	4.5	unknown	5.6
Mono-unsat. fat (g)	unknown	4.2	unknown	3.6
Poly-unsat. fat (g)	unknown	2.6	unknown	0.7
Carbohydrate (g)	41.3	26.7	34.1	9.1
Sugar (g)	23.0	18.5	23.8	2.3
Fibre (g)	unknown	0.7	0.4	0.3
Sodium (mg)	128	108	135	26
Potassium (mg)	57	162	79	56
Calcium (mg)	44	36	42	30
Magnesium (mg)	14	10	14	7
Phosphorus (mg)	50	30	66	42
Iron (mg)	0.75	0.54	0.81	0.39
Copper (mg)	0.1	0.19	0.1	0.08
Zinc (mg)	0.38	0.22	0.36	0.28
Selenium (µg)	unknown	unknown	unknown	unknown
Vitamin A (µg)	unknown	27	unknown	84
Vitamin D (µg)	unknown	0.05	0.22	nil
Vitamin E (mg)	0.02	0.9	1.13	0.44
Vitamin B_1 (mg)	0.13	0.05	0.05	0.04
Vitamin B_2 (mg)	0.04	0.01	0.1	0.07
Niacin (mg)	0.67	0.41	0.27	0.11
Vitamin B_6 (mg)	0.01	0.05	0.03	0.01
Vitamin B_{12} (µg)	trace	nil	trace	0.3
Folate (µg)	11	2	7	4
Pantothenate (mg)	unknown	0.05	0.27	0.11
Biotin (µg)	unknown	0.9	4.5	1.8
Vitamin C (mg)	nil	nil	trace	trace

Fancy iced cakes	Flapjacks	Fruit cake retail	Fruit cake rich iced	FOOD
one	one	one slice	one slice	**PORTION SIZE**
				NUTRIENTS
114	290	212	249	Energy (kcals)
1.1	2.7	3.1	2.9	Protein (g)
4.2	16.0	7.7	8.0	Total fat (g)
2.6	4.6	3.5	unknown	Saturated fat (g)
1.1	6.2	3.1	unknown	Mono-unsat. fat (g)
0.2	4.4	0.7	unknown	Poly-unsat. fat (g)
19.3	36.2	34.7	43.9	Carbohydrate (g)
15.1	21.3	25.9	38.6	Sugar (g)
unknown	1.6	unknown	1.2	Fibre (g)
70	168	150	98	Sodium (mg)
48	120	234	231	Potassium (mg)
12	22	36	53	Calcium (mg)
8	29	15	23	Magnesium (mg)
34	96	66	59	Phosphorus (mg)
0.39	1.26	1.02	1.12	Iron (mg)
0.07	0.14	0.15	0.13	Copper (mg)
0.2	0.9	0.30	0.42	Zinc (mg)
unknown	1	unknown	1	Selenium (μg)
nil	153	unknown	unknown	Vitamin A (μg)
nil	1.38	unknown	0.51	Vitamin D (μg)
unknown	1.71	unknown	1.64	Vitamin E (mg)
trace	0.16	0.05	0.05	Vitamin B_1 (mg)
0.01	0.02	0.04	0.09	Vitamin B_2 (mg)
0.06	0.18	0.36	0.35	Niacin (mg)
unknown	0.05	0.07	0.06	Vitamin B_6 (mg)
nil	nil	nil	trace	Vitamin B_{12} (μg)
unknown	7	5	9	Folate (μg)
unknown	0.18	0.12	0.14	Pantothenate (mg)
unknown	4.8	3.0	2.8	Biotin (μg)
nil	nil	nil	nil	Vitamin C (mg)

FOOD	Fruit shortcake[4]	Garibaldi biscuits[4]	Gateau	Gingerbread
PORTION SIZE	one	one	average slice	average slice
NUTRIENTS				
Energy (kcals)	48	38	303	190
Protein (g)	0.6	0.5	5.1	2.8
Total fat (g)	2.0	1.0	15.1	6.3
Saturated fat (g)	0.9	0.5	8.6	unknown
Mono-unsat. fat (g)	0.7	0.4	4.8	unknown
Poly-unsat. fat (g)	0.2	0.1	0.7	unknown
Carbohydrate (g)	7	6.7	39.1	32.3
Sugar (g)	2.5	3.6	29.1	17.5
Fibre (g)	0.2	0.1	0.4	0.6
Sodium (mg)	42	unknown	50	100
Potassium (mg)	unknown	unknown	79	80
Calcium (mg)	unknown	unknown	54	41
Magnesium (mg)	unknown	unknown	7	7
Phosphorus (mg)	unknown	unknown	85	43
Iron (mg)	unknown	unknown	0.81	0.8
Copper (mg)	unknown	unknown	0.05	0.05
Zinc (mg)	unknown	unknown	0.54	0.3
Selenium (µg)	unknown	unknown	unknown	unknown
Vitamin A (µg)	unknown	unknown	238	unknown
Vitamin D (µg)	unknown	unknown	0.45	0.59
Vitamin E (mg)	unknown	unknown	0.69	0.68
Vitamin B_1 (mg)	unknown	unknown	0.06	0.05
Vitamin B_2 (mg)	unknown	unknown	0.16	0.04
Niacin (mg)	unknown	unknown	0.27	0.3
Vitamin B_6 (mg)	unknown	unknown	0.05	0.03
Vitamin B_{12} (µg)	unknown	unknown	0.9	trace
Folate (µg)	unknown	unknown	10	4
Pantothenate (mg)	unknown	unknown	0.45	0.15
Biotin (µg)	unknown	unknown	7.2	2.0
Vitamin C (mg)	unknown	unknown	nil	nil

Ginger nut biscuits	Greek pastries	Hot cross buns	Jaffa cakes	FOOD
one	one	one	one	**PORTION SIZE**
				NUTRIENTS
46	322	155	47	Energy (kcals)
0.6	4.7	3.7	0.5	Protein (g)
1.5	17.0	3.4	1.4	Total fat (g)
unknown	unknown	1.0	unknown	Saturated fat (g)
unknown	unknown	1.1	unknown	Mono-unsat. fat (g)
unknown	unknown	0.8	unknown	Poly-unsat. fat (g)
7.9	40	29.3	8.8	Carbohydrate (g)
3.6	18.4	11.7	7.4	Sugar (g)
0.1	unknown	0.9	unknown	Fibre (g)
33	310	60	17	Sodium (mg)
22	90	100	22	Potassium (mg)
13	44	55	7	Calcium (mg)
3	22	12	4	Magnesium (mg)
9	70	55	17	Phosphorus (mg)
0.4	0.9	0.8	0.19	Iron (mg)
0.02	0.14	0.12	0.04	Copper (mg)
0.05	0.4	0.35	0.04	Zinc (mg)
unknown	unknown	unknown	unknown	Selenium (µg)
unknown	unknown	36	unknown	Vitamin A (µg)
nil	unknown	0.3	0.02	Vitamin D (µg)
0.15	unknown	0.35	0.11	Vitamin E (mg)
0.01	0.09	0.08	0.01	Vitamin B_1 (mg)
trace	0.04	0.05	0.01	Vitamin B_2 (mg)
0.09	1.0	0.65	0.04	Niacin (mg)
0.01	unknown	0.05	trace	Vitamin B_6 (mg)
nil	unknown	trace	nil	Vitamin B_{12} (µg)
trace	unknown	14	1	Folate (µg)
0.01	unknown	0.15	0.03	Pantothenate (mg)
0.1	unknown	2.5	0.4	Biotin (µg)
nil	unknown	nil	trace	Vitamin C (mg)

FOOD	Jam tart	Macaroon	Malt bread	Malted milk biscuits[4]
PORTION SIZE	one	one	one slice	one
NUTRIENTS				
Energy (kcals)	129	124	94	42
Protein (g)	1.1	2.4	2.9	0.6
Total fat (g)	5.1	5.5	0.8	1.9
Saturated fat (g)	1.7	0.4	0.1	0.9
Mono-unsat. fat (g)	2.2	3.8	0.1	0.7
Poly-unsat. fat (g)	1.0	1.0	0.3	0.1
Carbohydrate (g)	21.1	17.5	19.9	5.4
Sugar (g)	12.8	16.5	9.1	1.5
Fibre (g)	0.5	0.8	unknown	0.19
Sodium (mg)	78	13	98	45
Potassium (mg)	37	98	98	12.9
Calcium (mg)	19	26	39	unknown
Magnesium (mg)	4	27	16	unknown
Phosphorus (mg)	16	48	56	unknown
Iron (mg)	0.48	0.45	0.98	unknown
Copper (mg)	0.05	0.02	0.09	unknown
Zinc (mg)	0.1	0.36	0.39	unknown
Selenium (μg)	trace	1	unknown	unknown
Vitamin A (μg)	25	nil	nil	unknown
Vitamin D (μg)	0.2	nil	nil	unknown
Vitamin E (mg)	0.25	2.05	unknown	unknown
Vitamin B_1 (mg)	0.02	0.02	0.16	unknown
Vitamin B_2 (mg)	trace	0.1	0.05	unknown
Niacin (mg)	0.17	0.22	0.98	unknown
Vitamin B_6 (mg)	0.01	0.01	0.04	unknown
Vitamin B_{12} (μg)	nil	trace	nil	unknown
Folate (μg)	1	5	11	unknown
Pantothenate (mg)	0.03	0.06	unknown	unknown
Biotin (μg)	trace	0.5	unknown	unknown
Vitamin C (mg)	1	nil	nil	unknown

Morning Coffee biscuits[4]	Nice biscuits[4]	Rich Tea biscuits[4]	Rock cakes	FOOD
one	one	one	one	PORTION SIZE
				NUTRIENTS
23	22	31	178	Energy (kcals)
0.3	0.3	0.4	2.4	Protein (g)
0.7	0.8	1.0	7.4	Total fat (g)
0.3	0.5	0.4	unknown	Saturated fat (g)
0.2	0.2	0.4	unknown	Mono-unsat. fat (g)
0.08	0.06	0.1	unknown	Poly-unsat. fat (g)
3.8	3.3	5	27.2	Carbohydrate (g)
0.9	1.2	1.6	14.5	Sugar (g)
0.1	0.2	0.1	0.7	Fibre (g)
246	14	35	176	Sodium (mg)
5	7	12	95	Potassium (mg)
unknown	unknown	unknown	50	Calcium (mg)
unknown	unknown	unknown	7	Magnesium (mg)
unknown	unknown	unknown	108	Phosphorus (mg)
unknown	unknown	unknown	0.54	Iron (mg)
unknown	unknown	unknown	0.12	Copper (mg)
unknown	unknown	unknown	0.27	Zinc (mg)
unknown	unknown	unknown	1	Selenium (µg)
unknown	unknown	unknown	unknown	Vitamin A (µg)
unknown	unknown	unknown	0.7	Vitamin D (µg)
unknown	unknown	unknown	0.77	Vitamin E (mg)
unknown	unknown	unknown	0.05	Vitamin B_1 (mg)
unknown	unknown	unknown	0.03	Vitamin B_2 (mg)
unknown	unknown	unknown	0.31	Niacin (mg)
unknown	unknown	unknown	0.04	Vitamin B_6 (mg)
unknown	unknown	unknown	trace	Vitamin B_{12} (µg)
unknown	unknown	unknown	3	Folate (µg)
unknown	unknown	unknown	0.09	Pantothenate (mg)
unknown	unknown	unknown	1.8	Biotin (µg)
unknown	unknown	unknown	nil	Vitamin C (mg)

FOOD	Scones cheese	Scones fruit	Scones plain	Shortbread
PORTION SIZE	one	one	one	one
NUTRIENTS				
Energy (kcals)	174	152	174	65
Protein (g)	4.8	3.5	3.5	0.8
Total fat (g)	8.5	4.7	7.0	3.4
Saturated fat (g)	unknown	1.6	2.4	unknown
Mono-unsat. fat (g)	unknown	1.8	2.6	unknown
Poly-unsat. fat (g)	unknown	1.2	1.7	unknown
Carbohydrate (g)	20.7	25.4	25.8	8.3
Sugar (g)	1.1	8.1	2.8	2.2
Fibre (g)	0.8	unknown	0.9	0.2
Sodium (mg)	365	341	370	30
Potassium (mg)	67	106	72	13
Calcium (mg)	120	72	86	12
Magnesium (mg)	9	12	9	2
Phosphorus (mg)	226	173	221	10
Iron (mg)	0.53	0.72	0.62	0.17
Copper (mg)	0.09	0.11	0.09	0.01
Zinc (mg)	0.48	0.38	0.34	0.05
Selenium (µg)	2	unknown	1	trace
Vitamin A (µg)	unknown	unknown	77	unknown
Vitamin D (µg)	0.52	unknown	0.58	0.03
Vitamin E (mg)	0.62	unknown	0.69	0.1
Vitamin B_1 (mg)	0.07	0.12	0.08	0.02
Vitamin B_2 (mg)	0.06	0.05	0.03	trace
Niacin (mg)	0.43	0.58	0.48	0.13
Vitamin B_6 (mg)	0.04	0.02	0.04	0.01
Vitamin B_{12} (µg)	trace	trace	trace	nil
Folate (µg)	4	3	4	1
Pantothenate (mg)	0.1	unknown	0.1	0.01
Biotin (µg)	1.0	unknown	0.5	0.1
Vitamin C (mg)	trace	trace	trace	nil

Shortcake	Sponge cake	Sponge cake with butter icing	Sponge cake jam filled	FOOD
one	average slice	average slice	average slice	**PORTION SIZE**
				NUTRIENTS
51	266	294	181	Energy (kcals)
0.6	3.7	2.7	2.5	Protein (g)
2.4	15.3	18.4	2.9	Total fat (g)
0.9	4.6	5.6	1.0	Saturated fat (g)
1.0	6.1	7.4	1.0	Mono-unsat. fat (g)
0.3	3.8	4.6	0.4	Poly-unsat. fat (g)
6.8	30.4	31.4	38.5	Carbohydrate (g)
2.0	17.6	22.3	28.6	Sugar (g)
0.1	0.5	0.4	1.1	Fibre (g)
25	203	216	252	Sodium (mg)
unknown	48	35	84	Potassium (mg)
unknown	38	28	26	Calcium (mg)
unknown	5	4	8	Magnesium (mg)
unknown	87	66	132	Phosphorus (mg)
unknown	0.7	0.54	0.96	Iron (mg)
unknown	0.06	0.05	0.12	Copper (mg)
unknown	0.41	0.36	0.3	Zinc (mg)
unknown	3	2	6	Selenium (µg)
unknown	180	209	unknown	Vitamin A (µg)
unknown	1.62	1.86	unknown	Vitamin D (µg)
unknown	1.64	1.91	trace	Vitamin E (mg)
unknown	0.05	0.04	0.02	Vitamin B_1 (mg)
unknown	0.07	0.05	0.04	Vitamin B_2 (mg)
unknown	0.29	0.18	0.24	Niacin (mg)
unknown	0.03	0.02	unknown	Vitamin B_6 (mg)
unknown	0.6	0.6	0.6	Vitamin B_{12} (µg)
unknown	6	4	unknown	Folate (µg)
unknown	0.29	0.18	unknown	Pantothenate (mg)
unknown	4.1	3.0	unknown	Biotin (µg)
unknown	nil	nil	nil	Vitamin C (mg)

FOOD	Sponge cake frozen	Swiss roll	Teacakes	Vanilla slice
PORTION SIZE	average slice	one slice	one	one
NUTRIENTS				
Energy (kcals)	123	83	178	373
Protein (g)	1.3	2.2	4.8	5.1
Total fat (g)	6.5	1.3	4.5	20.2
Saturated fat (g)	Unknown	unknown	unknown	unknown
Mono-unsat. fat (g)	Unknown	unknown	unknown	unknown
Poly-unsat. fat (g)	Unknown	unknown	unknown	unknown
Carbohydrate (g)	15.9	16.6	31.5	45.4
Sugar (g)	10.8	12.3	8.9	22.4
Fibre (g)	unknown	0.2	unknown	0.9
Sodium (mg)	117	39	162	260
Potassium (mg)	47	33	132	113
Calcium (mg)	17	29	53	88
Magnesium (mg)	4	3	17	12
Phosphorus (mg)	70	54	60	86
Iron (mg)	0.27	0.45	1.56	0.9
Copper (mg)	0.05	0.03	0.14	0.08
Zinc (mg)	0.16	0.21	0.42	0.45
Selenium (μg)	unknown	2	unknown	unknown
Vitamin A (μg)	unknown	unknown	unknown	unknown
Vitamin D (μg)	0.16	0.15	nil	0.11
Vitamin E (mg)	trace	0.22	unknown	1.07
Vitamin B_1 (mg)	0.04	0.02	0.13	0.09
Vitamin B_2 (mg)	0.04	0.05	0.09	0.1
Niacin (mg)	0.12	0.09	1.08	0.45
Vitamin B_6 (mg)	0.02	0.02	0.03	0.06
Vitamin B_{12} (μg)	trace	0.3	trace	trace
Folate (μg)	2	4	22	8
Pantothenate (mg)	unknown	0.18	unknown	0.34
Biotin (μg)	unknown	3.3	unknown	3.4
Vitamin C (mg)	nil	trace	trace	1

Viennese fingers filled[4]	Wafer biscuits	Welsh cakes	FOOD
one	one	one	PORTION SIZE
			NUTRIENTS
110	37	121	Energy (kcals)
1.1	0.3	1.6	Protein (g)
6	2.1	5.5	Total fat (g)
2.3	unknown	unknown	Saturated fat (g)
2.5	unknown	unknown	Mono-unsat. fat (g)
0.8	unknown	unknown	Poly-unsat. fat (g)
12.8	4.6	17.3	Carbohydrate (g)
4.2	3.1	8.8	Sugar (g)
0.2	unknown	0.4	Fibre (g)
45	5	56	Sodium (mg)
19	11	53	Potassium (mg)
unknown	5	27	Calcium (mg)
unknown	2	4	Magnesium (mg)
unknown	6	36	Phosphorus (mg)
unknown	0.11	0.34	Iron (mg)
unknown	0.01	0.06	Copper (mg)
unknown	0.04	0.14	Zinc (mg)
unknown	unknown	unknown??	Selenium (µg)
unknown	unknown	unknown	Vitamin A (µg)
unknown	nil	0.05	Vitamin D (µg)
unknown	0.13	0.13	Vitamin E (mg)
unknown	0.01	0.03	Vitamin B_1 (mg)
unknown	0.01	0.02	Vitamin B_2 (mg)
unknown	0.04	0.22	Niacin (mg)
unknown	trace	0.02	Vitamin B_6 (mg)
unknown	nil	trace	Vitamin B_{12} (µg)
unknown	unknown	2	Folate (µg)
unknown	unknown	0.06	Pantothenate (mg)
unknown	unknown	1.1	Biotin (µg)
unknown	nil	trace	Vitamin C (mg)

FOOD	Apple pie pastry top and bottom	Arctic roll	Bakewell tart individual	Blancmange
PORTION SIZE	average	average slice	one	average
NUTRIENTS				
Energy (kcals)	293	100	196	171
Protein (g)	3.2	2.0	2.7	4.6
Total fat (g)	14.6	3.3	12.8	5.6
Saturated fat (g)	unknown	1.5	unknown	3.4
Mono-unsat. fat (g)	unknown	1.3	unknown	1.7
Poly-unsat. fat (g)	unknown	0.4	unknown	0.2
Carbohydrate (g)	39.4	16.6	18.7	27.2
Sugar (g)	15.1	12.6	9.8	17.7
Fibre (g)	1.9	unknown	0.8	trace
Sodium (mg)	220	75	125	83
Potassium (mg)	110	70	77	210
Calcium (mg)	47	45	34	165
Magnesium (mg)	9	6	18	15
Phosphorus (mg)	44	60	47	134
Iron (mg)	0.77	0.35	0.64	0.15
Copper (mg)	0.11	0.06	0.04	0.01
Zinc (mg)	0.33	0.2	0.34	0.6
Selenium (μg)	1	unknown	1	2
Vitamin A (μg)	unknown	unknown	unknown	79
Vitamin D (μg)	0.63	unknown	0.71	0.04
Vitamin E (mg)	0.84	unknown	1.84	0.11
Vitamin B_1 (mg)	0.09	0.04	0.04	0.04
Vitamin B_2 (mg)	0.02	0.05	0.06	0.21
Niacin (mg)	0.55	0.12	0.3	0.15
Vitamin B_6 (mg)	0.04	0.03	0.02	0.08
Vitamin B_{12} (μg)	nil	0.2	trace	0.6
Folate (μg)	4	6	5	6
Pantothenate (mg)	0.11	unknown	0.13	0.45
Biotin (μg)	trace	unknown	1.3	2.7
Vitamin C (mg)	6	nil	trace	trace

Bread pudding	Bread and butter pudding	Cheesecake	Christmas pudding	FOOD
average slice	average	average slice	average	**PORTION SIZE**
				NUTRIENTS
564	272	511	291	Energy (kcals)
11.2	10.5	4.4	4.6	Protein (g)
18.2	13.3	42.6	9.7	Total fat (g)
unknown	unknown	22.6	unknown	Saturated fat (g)
unknown	unknown	13.7	unknown	Mono-unsat. fat (g)
unknown	unknown	3.4	unknown	Poly-unsat. fat (g)
94.4	29.8	29.5	49.5	Carbohydrate (g)
62.9	21.1	16.3	34.3	Sugar (g)
2.3	0.5	0.5	1.3	Fibre (g)
589	255	348	200	Sodium (mg)
589	340	144	350	Potassium (mg)
228	221	78	79	Calcium (mg)
46	27	12	27	Magnesium (mg)
209	221	97	76	Phosphorus (mg)
3.04	1.19	0.96	1.5	Iron (mg)
0.38	0.14	0.1	0.22	Copper (mg)
1.14	1.19	0.48	0.5	Zinc (mg)
21	10	unknown	7	Selenium (µg)
unknown	unknown	416	unknown	Vitamin A (µg)
0.3	0.46	1.13	0.12	Vitamin D (µg)
0.72	0.75	unknown	0.64	Vitamin E (mg)
0.19	0.12	0.05	0.08	Vitamin B_1 (mg)
0.23	0.36	0.14	0.08	Vitamin B_2 (mg)
1.52	0.51	0.24	0.7	Niacin (mg)
0.17	0.12	0.05	0.08	Vitamin B_6 (mg)
trace	1.7	0.6	trace	Vitamin B_{12} (µg)
15	15	7	8	Folate (µg)
0.57	0.85	unknown	0.2	Pantothenate (mg)
7.6	11.9	3.5	4.0	Biotin (µg)
trace	2	1	nil	Vitamin C (mg)

FOOD	Crème Caramel individual	Crumble fruit	Custard made with milk	Custard canned
PORTION SIZE	one	average	average	half a can
NUTRIENTS				
Energy (kcals)	98	337	140	200
Protein (g)	2.7	3.4	4.4	5.5
Total fat (g)	2.0	11.7	5.4	6.3
Saturated fat (g)	unknown	unknown	3.4	3.6
Mono-unsat. fat (g)	unknown	unknown	1.6	1.9
Poly-unsat. fat (g)	unknown	unknown	0.2	0.2
Carbohydrate (g)	18.5	57.8	19.9	32.3
Sugar (g)	16.2	36.2	13.7	25.8
Fibre (g)	unknown	2.9	trace	trace
Sodium (mg)	63	116	97	141
Potassium (mg)	135	323	192	273
Calcium (mg)	85	83	156	210
Magnesium (mg)	8	15	16	17
Phosphorus (mg)	69	56	132	183
Iron (mg)	trace	1.02	0.12	0.42
Copper (mg)	trace	0.17	trace	0.04
Zinc (mg)	0.27	0.34	0.48	0.63
Selenium (µg)	unknown	2	unknown	unknown
Vitamin A (µg)	34	unknown	75.8	unknown
Vitamin D (µg)	0.06	1.12	0.04	unknown
Vitamin E (mg)	0.14	1.67	0.12	unknown
Vitamin B_1 (mg)	0.03	0.09	0.05	0.08
Vitamin B_2 (mg)	0.18	0.03	0.22	0.21
Niacin (mg)	0.09	0.85	0.12	trace
Vitamin B_6 (mg)	0.03	0.05	0.07	0.06
Vitamin B_{12} (µg)	0.3	nil	0.6	trace
Folate (µg)	7	5	6	4
Pantothenate (mg)	unknown	0.17	0.43	unknown
Biotin (µg)	unknown	trace	2.6	unknown
Vitamin C (mg)	nil	5	1	nil

Egg custard	Frozen ice cream dessert	Fruit fool	Ice cream dairy, vanilla	FOOD
average	average	average	average	PORTION SIZE
				NUTRIENTS
130	127	196	146	Energy (kcals)
6.3	1.8	1.2	2.7	Protein (g)
6.6	8.0	11.2	7.4	Total fat (g)
3.4	6.3	7.0	4.8	Saturated fat (g)
2.3	1.0	3.2	1.8	Mono-unsat. fat (g)
0.4	0.2	0.4	0.2	Poly-unsat. fat (g)
12.1	12.8	24.2	18.3	Carbohydrate (g)
12.1	12.8	19.3	16.6	Sugar (g)
nil	unknown	1.4	nil	Fibre (g)
90	47	16	52	Sodium (mg)
187	112	192	120	Potassium (mg)
143	62	46	98	Calcium (mg)
14	11	10	10	Magnesium (mg)
143	55	37	83	Phosphorus (mg)
0.44	0.28	0.48	0.08	Iron (mg)
0.02	0.02	0.07	0.01	Copper (mg)
0.66	0.22	0.24	0.23	Zinc (mg)
3	unknown	unknown	unknown	Selenium (µg)
101	1.5	180	110	Vitamin A (µg)
0.41	trace	0.06	0.09	Vitamin D (µg)
0.26	0.29	0.54	0.16	Vitamin E (mg)
0.05	0.02	0.02	0.03	Vitamin B_1 (mg)
0.26	0.17	0.07	0.19	Vitamin B_2 (mg)
0.11	0.1	0.24	0.1	Niacin (mg)
0.09	0.03	0.04	0.06	Vitamin B_6 (mg)
0.9	0.3	trace	0.3	Vitamin B_{12} (µg)
13	2	unknown	5	Folate (µg)
0.69	unknown	0.17	0.33	Pantothenate (mg)
6.4	unknown	1.1	1.9	Biotin (µg)
trace	nil	20	1	Vitamin C (mg)

FOOD	Instant dessert powder made with milk	Jelly	Kulfi Indian ice cream	Lemon meringue pie
PORTION SIZE	average	average	average	average
NUTRIENTS				
Energy (kcals)	133	70	339	303
Protein (g)	3.7	1.4	4.3	4.3
Total fat (g)	7.6	nil	31.9	13.7
Saturated fat (g)	5.9	nil	18.2	unknown
Mono-unsat. fat (g)	1.2	nil	10.5	unknown
Poly-unsat. fat (g)	0.1	nil	1.4	unknown
Carbohydrate (g)	17.8	17.4	9.4	43.6
Sugar (g)	13.6	17.4	9.4	23.6
Fibre (g)	unknown	nil	0.5	0.7
Sodium (mg)	288	6	61	190
Potassium (mg)	156	6	192	78
Calcium (mg)	116	8	128	43
Magnesium (mg)	12	trace	26	9
Phosphorus (mg)	228	1	120	63
Iron (mg)	0.12	0.46	0.4	0.85
Copper (mg)	0.05	0.01	0.01	0.08
Zinc (mg)	0.48	unknown	0.56	0.47
Selenium (µg)	unknown	unknown	1	4
Vitamin A (µg)	unknown	nil	392	unknown
Vitamin D (µg)	unknown	nil	0.17	0.84
Vitamin E (mg)	unknown	nil	unknown	0.98
Vitamin B_1 (mg)	0.04	nil	nil	0.07
Vitamin B_2 (mg)	0.17	nil	unknown	0.08
Niacin (mg)	0.12	nil	unknown	0.38
Vitamin B_6 (mg)	0.06	nil	unknown	0.05
Vitamin B_{12} (µg)	0.4	nil	unknown	trace
Folate (µg)	5	nil	unknown	8
Pantothenate (mg)	unknown	nil	unknown	0.29
Biotin (µg)	unknown	nil	unknown	4.8
Vitamin C (mg)	1	nil	nil	3

Milk pudding	**Mince pie** individual	**Mousse** chocolate	**Mousse** fruit	**FOOD**
average	one	average pot	average pot	**PORTION SIZE**
				NUTRIENTS
258	233	86	82	Energy (kcals)
7.8	2.4	2.5	2.7	Protein (g)
8.6	11.2	3.3	3.4	Total fat (g)
5.4	4.1	unknown	unknown	Saturated fat (g)
2.4	4.6	unknown	unknown	Mono-unsat. fat (g)
0.4	2.0	unknown	unknown	Poly-unsat. fat (g)
39.8	32.5	12.3	10.8	Carbohydrate (g)
21.4	15.5	10.9	10.8	Sugar (g)
0.2	1.2	trace	unknown	Fibre (g)
118	171	42	37	Sodium (mg)
320	99	136	90	Potassium (mg)
260	41	60	72	Calcium (mg)
26	8	17	7	Magnesium (mg)
220	32	62	58	Phosphorus (mg)
0.2	0.82	0.99	trace	Iron (mg)
0.02	0.08	0.07	trace	Copper (mg)
1.0	0.17	0.37	0.24	Zinc (mg)
unknown	unknown	unknown	unknown	Selenium (µg)
unknown	50	30	23	Vitamin A (µg)
0.06	0.44	trace	0.04	Vitamin D (µg)
0.2	0.51	0.36	0.47	Vitamin E (mg)
0.08	0.06	0.02	0.02	Vitamin B_1 (mg)
0.32	0.01	0.13	0.14	Vitamin B_2 (mg)
0.2	0.44	0.12	0.12	Niacin (mg)
0.12	0.04	0.02	0.03	Vitamin B_6 (mg)
0.8	nil	0.1	0.1	Vitamin B_{12} (µg)
6	3	4	4	Folate (µg)
0.6	0.05	unknown	unknown	Pantothenate (mg)
4.4	trace	unknown	unknown	Biotin (µg)
2	nil	nil	trace	Vitamin C (mg)

FOOD	**Pancakes** sweet	**Rice pudding** canned	**Sponge pudding** with jam or syrup	**Sponge pudding** with dried fruit
PORTION SIZE	one	one small can	average	average
NUTRIENTS				
Energy (kcals)	331	190	366	364
Protein (g)	6.5	7.2	5.6	5.9
Total fat (g)	17.8	5.3	15.8	15.7
Saturated fat (g)	7.8	3.4	unknown	unknown
Mono-unsat. fat (g)	7.5	1.5	unknown	unknown
Poly-unsat. fat (g)	1.6	0.2	unknown	unknown
Carbohydrate (g)	38.5	29.8	53.6	52.9
Sugar (g)	17.8	17.5	28	27.4
Fibre (g)	0.9	0.4	1.1	1.3
Sodium (mg)	58	107	319	297
Potassium (mg)	165	298	109	198
Calcium (mg)	121	198	84	90
Magnesium (mg)	15	23	11	14
Phosphorus (mg)	121	170	176	187
Iron (mg)	0.88	0.43	1.21	1.21
Copper (mg)	0.05	0.06	0.11	0.17
Zinc (mg)	0.66	0.85	0.55	0.55
Selenium (μg)	3	unknown	3	3
Vitamin A (μg)	64	unknown	unknown	unknown
Vitamin D (μg)	0.22	unknown	1.51	1.51
Vitamin E (mg)	0.36	unknown	1.69	1.73
Vitamin B_1 (mg)	0.11	0.06	0.09	0.1
Vitamin B_2 (mg)	0.19	0.3	0.09	0.09
Niacin (mg)	0.55	0.43	0.55	0.66
Vitamin B_6 (mg)	0.1	0.04	0.05	0.08
Vitamin B_{12} (μg)	1.1	trace	trace	trace
Folate (μg)	9	unknown	8	9
Pantothenate (mg)	0.55	unknown	0.33	0.33
Biotin (μg)	5.5	unknown	4.4	5.5
Vitamin C (mg)	1	nil	trace	trace

Strawberry tartlets	Treacle tart individual	Trifle homemade	Trifle frozen	FOOD
one	one	average	one individual	**PORTION SIZE**
				NUTRIENTS
196	129	272	156	Energy (kcals)
2.4	1.3	6.1	2.5	Protein (g)
10.3	4.9	10.7	6.6	Total fat (g)
unknown	1.8	5.3	3.6	Saturated fat (g)
unknown	2.0	3.4	2.1	Mono-unsat. fat (g)
unknown	0.9	1.2	0.3	Poly-unsat. fat (g)
24.9	21.1	37.9	23.3	Carbohydrate (g)
6.9	11.8	28.6	20.2	Sugar (g)
1.1	0.4	0.9	0.6	Fibre (g)
152	126	90	90	Sodium (mg)
88	53	238	33	Potassium (mg)
37	22	134	55	Calcium (mg)
9	5	26	6	Magnesium (mg)
33	18	145	59	Phosphorus (mg)
0.66	0.49	0.85	0.23	Iron (mg)
0.07	0.04	0.07	0.05	Copper (mg)
0.19	0.11	0.68	0.23	Zinc (mg)
1	1	unknown	unknown	Selenium (µg)
unknown	23	128	85	Vitamin A (µg)
nil	0.21	0.29	0.19	Vitamin D (µg)
0.57	0.24	0.68	0.45	Vitamin E (mg)
0.06	0.03	0.1	trace	Vitamin B_1 (mg)
0.02	trace	0.22	0.08	Vitamin B_2 (mg)
0.57	0.21	0.51	0.11	Niacin (mg)
0.05	0.01	0.1	0.02	Vitamin B_6 (mg)
nil	nil	0.7	0.2	Vitamin B_{12} (µg)
3	1	14	5	Folate (µg)
0.19	0.04	0.58	0.38	Pantothenate (mg)
0.9	trace	5.3	3.5	Biotin (µg)
25	nil	7	5	Vitamin C (mg)

FOOD	**Sorbet** lemon	**Sticky toffee pudding**[6]	**Suet pudding**
PORTION SIZE	average	individual	average
NUTRIENTS			
Energy (kcals)	124	305	302
Protein (g)	0.9	3.9	4.0
Total fat (g)	trace	12.4	16.5
Saturated fat (g)	trace	6.7	unknown
Mono-unsat. fat (g)	trace	unknown	unknown
Poly-unsat. fat (g)	trace	unknown	unknown
Carbohydrate (g)	32.5	50.3	36.5
Sugar (g)	32.5	42.2	12.8
Fibre (g)	nil	1.1	0.8
Sodium (mg)	17	unknown	378
Potassium (mg)	40	unknown	84
Calcium (mg)	2	unknown	86
Magnesium (mg)	2	unknown	12
Phosphorus (mg)	5	unknown	162
Iron (mg)	trace	unknown	0.63
Copper (mg)	0.03	unknown	0.09
Zinc (mg)	0.95	unknown	0.36
Selenium (µg)	1	unknown	5
Vitamin A (µg)	nil	unknown	unknown
Vitamin D (µg)	nil	unknown	0.01
Vitamin E (mg)	trace	unknown	0.08
Vitamin B_1 (mg)	trace	unknown	0.08
Vitamin B_2 (mg)	0.04	unknown	0.05
Niacin (mg)	trace	unknown	0.54
Vitamin B_6 (mg)	0.01	unknown	0.04
Vitamin B_{12} (µg)	trace	unknown	trace
Folate (µg)	1	unknown	5
Pantothenate (mg)	0.04	unknown	0.18
Biotin (µg)	0.7	unknown	0.9
Vitamin C (mg)	trace	unknown	trace

Confectionery

Although as a nation we are all having less sugar, our sugar intake from sweets is certainly not on the decrease. Are they the archetypal 'junk food', or is it acceptable to have them occasionally? The main issue about so-called junk foods is that if you eat too many of the foods which fall into this category, your diet might contain enough calories and even enough protein, but it will be sadly lacking in vitamins and minerals. Most of us enjoy the occasional sweet, but they should not be eaten at the expense of other foods.

Sweets do the most damage to our teeth when eaten on their own between meals, so try to eat them immediately after your main meal, rather than during the evening. If you do not eat many other sugary or fatty foods, eating confectionery two or three times a week is acceptable, unless you have a weight problem.

Most of this section is derived from manufacturer's data, and the majority of that data is only for energy, protein, fat and carbohydrate. There is no mention of the sugar content of these sweets. It is easy to work out however, because most if not all of the carbohydrate in sweets and chocolates is sugar, rather than starch or fibre. Only items containing fruit, nuts or cereal will contain any starch or fibre; even so most of the carbohydrate is still sugar.

[7] – Cadbury's
[8] – Mars
[9] – Nestlé Rowntree

FOOD	**Aero** medium, milk[9]	**After Eight Mints**[9]	**Black Magic**[9]	**Boiled sweets**
PORTION SIZE	average bar	one	one	100g
NUTRIENTS				
Energy (kcals)	204	33	3_6	327
Protein (g)	3.9	0.2	0.3	trace
Total fat (g)	14.3	1.0	1.5	trace
Saturated fat (g)	unknown	unknown	unknown	nil
Mono-unsat. fat (g)	unknown	unknown	unknown	nil
Poly-unsat. fat (g)	unknown	unknown	unknown	nil
Carbohydrate (g)	26	5.7	5.0	87.1
Sugar (g)	unknown	unknown	unknown	86.7
Fibre (g)	unknown	unknown	unknown	nil
Sodium (mg)	57	1.9	5.0	25
Potassium (mg)	216	12	16.5	8
Calcium (mg)	110	1.2	unknown	5
Magnesium (mg)	unknown	unknown	unknown	2
Phosphorus (mg)	unknown	unknown	unknown	12
Iron (mg)	unknown	unknown	unknown	0.4
Copper (mg)	unknown	unknown	unknown	0.09
Zinc (mg)	unknown	unknown	unknown	unknown
Selenium (µg)	unknown	unknown	unknown	trace
Vitamin A (µg)	unknown	unknown	unknown	nil
Vitamin D (µg)	unknown	unknown	unknown	nil
Vitamin E (mg)	unknown	unknown	unknown	nil
Vitamin B_1 (mg)	unknown	unknown	unknown	nil
Vitamin B_2 (mg)	unknown	unknown	unknown	nil
Niacin (mg)	unknown	unknown	unknown	nil
Vitamin B_6 (mg)	unknown	unknown	unknown	nil
Vitamin B_{12} (µg)	unknown	unknown	unknown	nil
Folate (µg)	unknown	unknown	unknown	nil
Pantothenate (mg)	unknown	unknown	unknown	nil
Biotin (µg)	unknown	unknown	unknown	nil
Vitamin C (mg)	unknown	unknown	unknown	nil

Bounty bar milk[8]	**Boost**	**Cadbury's Caramel**[7]	**Cadbury's Chocolate** Bournville[7]	**FOOD**
twin	standard bar	standard bar	standard bar	**PORTION SIZE**
				NUTRIENTS
276	285	245	250	Energy (kcals)
2.6	4.0	2.7	2.3	Protein (g)
15.2	15.2	12.1	13.4	Total fat (g)
unknown	unknown	unknown	unknown	Saturated fat (g)
unknown	unknown	unknown	unknown	Mono-unsat. fat (g)
unknown	unknown	unknown	unknown	Poly-unsat. fat (g)
32.1	33.5	31.8	29.8	Carbohydrate (g)
unknown	unknown	unknown	unknown	Sugar (g)
unknown	unknown	unknown	unknown	Fibre (g)
unknown	unknown	unknown	unknown	Sodium (mg)
unknown	unknown	unknown	unknown	Potassium (mg)
unknown	unknown	unknown	unknown	Calcium (mg)
unknown	unknown	unknown	unknown	Magnesium (mg)
unknown	unknown	unknown	unknown	Phosphorus (mg)
unknown	unknown	unknown	unknown	Iron (mg)
unknown	unknown	unknown	unknown	Copper (mg)
unknown	unknown	unknown	unknown	Zinc (mg)
unknown	unknown	unknown	unknown	Selenium (μg)
unknown	unknown	unknown	unknown	Vitamin A (μg)
unknown	unknown	unknown	unknown	Vitamin D (μg)
unknown	unknown	unknown	unknown	Vitamin E (mg)
unknown	unknown	unknown	unknown	Vitamin B_1 (mg)
unknown	unknown	unknown	unknown	Vitamin B_2 (mg)
unknown	unknown	unknown	unknown	Niacin (mg)
unknown	unknown	unknown	unknown	Vitamin B_6 (mg)
unknown	unknown	unknown	unknown	Vitamin B_{12} (μg)
unknown	unknown	unknown	unknown	Folate (μg)
unknown	unknown	unknown	unknown	Pantothenate (mg)
unknown	unknown	unknown	unknown	Biotin (μg)
unknown	unknown	unknown	unknown	Vitamin C (mg)

FOOD	Cadbury's Chocolate buttons[7]	Cadbury's Chocolate white buttons[7]	Cadbury's Chocolate dairy milk[7]	Cadbury's Chocolate fruit & nut[7]
PORTION SIZE	standard bag	standard bag	standard bar	standard bar
NUTRIENTS				
Energy (kcals)	175	170	255	240
Protein (g)	2.6	2.8	3.8	3.9
Total fat (g)	9.7	9.7	14.4	12.5
Saturated fat (g)	unknown	unknown	unknown	unknown
Mono-unsat. fat (g)	unknown	unknown	unknown	unknown
Poly-unsat. fat (g)	unknown	unknown	unknown	unknown
Carbohydrate (g)	18.7	18.1	27.8	27.1
Sugar (g)	unknown	unknown	unknown	unknown
Fibre (g)	unknown	unknown	unknown	unknown
Sodium (mg)	unknown	unknown	unknown	unknown
Potassium (mg)	unknown	unknown	unknown	unknown
Calcium (mg)	unknown	unknown	unknown	unknown
Magnesium (mg)	unknown	unknown	unknown	unknown
Phosphorus (mg)	unknown	unknown	unknown	unknown
Iron (mg)	unknown	unknown	unknown	unknown
Copper (mg)	unknown	unknown	unknown	unknown
Zinc (mg)	unknown	unknown	unknown	unknown
Selenium (µg)	unknown	unknown	unknown	unknown
Vitamin A (µg)	unknown	unknown	unknown	unknown
Vitamin D (µg)	unknown	unknown	unknown	unknown
Vitamin E (mg)	unknown	unknown	unknown	unknown
Vitamin B_1 (mg)	unknown	unknown	unknown	unknown
Vitamin B_2 (mg)	unknown	unknown	unknown	unknown
Niacin (mg)	unknown	unknown	unknown	unknown
Vitamin B_6 (mg)	unknown	unknown	unknown	unknown
Vitamin B_{12} (µg)	unknown	unknown	unknown	unknown
Folate (µg)	unknown	unknown	unknown	unknown
Pantothenate (mg)	unknown	unknown	unknown	unknown
Biotin (µg)	unknown	unknown	unknown	unknown
Vitamin C (mg)	unknown	unknown	unknown	unknown

Cadbury's Chocolate Wholenut[7]	Cadbury's Chocolate Assortment[7]	Caramac[9]	Cereal bar chewy	FOOD
standard bar	one chocolate	standard bar	one	PORTION SIZE
				NUTRIENTS
265	47	169	126	Energy (kcals)
4.5	0.4	1.7	2.2	Protein (g)
16.9	7	10.8	4.9	Total fat (g)
unknown	unknown	unknown	unknown	Saturated fat (g)
unknown	unknown	unknown	unknown	Mono-unsat. fat (g)
unknown	unknown	unknown	unknown	Poly-unsat. fat (g)
23.7	6.2	16.3	19.4	Carbohydrate (g)
unknown	unknown	unknown	9.8	Sugar (g)
unknown	unknown	unknown	1.0	Fibre (g)
unknown	unknown	45	33	Sodium (mg)
unknown	unknown	111	96	Potassium (mg)
unknown	unknown	34	21	Calcium (mg)
unknown	unknown	unknown	17	Magnesium (mg)
unknown	unknown	unknown	57	Phosphorus (mg)
unknown	unknown	unknown	0.57	Iron (mg)
unknown	unknown	unknown	0.05	Copper (mg)
unknown	unknown	unknown	0.33	Zinc (mg)
unknown	unknown	unknown	unknown	Selenium (μg)
unknown	unknown	unknown	unknown	Vitamin A (μg)
unknown	unknown	unknown	nil	Vitamin D (μg)
unknown	unknown	unknown	unknown	Vitamin E (mg)
unknown	unknown	unknown	0.07	Vitamin B_1 (mg)
unknown	unknown	unknown	0.05	Vitamin B_2 (mg)
unknown	unknown	unknown	0.36	Niacin (mg)
unknown	unknown	unknown	0.04	Vitamin B_6 (mg)
unknown	unknown	unknown	trace	Vitamin B_{12} (μg)
unknown	unknown	unknown	3	Folate (μg)
unknown	unknown	unknown	unknown	Pantothenate (mg)
unknown	unknown	unknown	unknown	Biotin (μg)
unknown	unknown	unknown	trace	Vitamin C (mg)

*composite of Milk Tray, Roses and Bournville selection

FOOD	Cereal bar crunchy	Coconut Ice	Creme Egg	Crunchie[7]
PORTION SIZE	one	standard bar	one	standard bar
NUTRIENTS				
Energy (kcals)	140	464	163	195
Protein (g)	3.1	2.1	1.6	1.8
Total fat (g)	6.7	15.9	5.7	7.7
Saturated fat (g)	1.4	13.4	1.8	unknown
Mono-unsat. fat (g)	3.4	1.1	1.8	unknown
Poly-unsat. fat (g)	1.6	0.4	0.2	unknown
Carbohydrate (g)	18.1	83.4	27.7	29.8
Sugar (g)	8.4	83.4	22.6	unknown
Fibre (g)	1.4	3.3	unknown	unknown
Sodium (mg)	22	20	21	unknown
Potassium (mg)	108	200	82	unknown
Calcium (mg)	23	35	47	unknown
Magnesium (mg)	26	24	11	unknown
Phosphorus (mg)	87	60	51	unknown
Iron (mg)	0.78	0.88	0.31	unknown
Copper (mg)	0.09	0.15	0.04	unknown
Zinc (mg)	0.51	0.5	0.23	unknown
Selenium (µg)	unknown	1	trace	unknown
Vitamin A (µg)	trace	14	21	unknown
Vitamin D (µg)	nil	nil	0.23	unknown
Vitamin E (mg)	1.15	0.26	0.42	unknown
Vitamin B_1 (mg)	0.07	0.01	0.02	unknown
Vitamin B_2 (mg)	0.04	0.05	0.13	unknown
Niacin (mg)	0.69	0.25	0.08	unknown
Vitamin B_6 (mg)	0.04	0.04	0.01	unknown
Vitamin B_{12} (µg)	nil	trace	0.4	unknown
Folate (µg)	5	3	5	unknown
Pantothenate (mg)	unknown	0.19	0.23	unknown
Biotin (µg)	unknown	unknown	1.2	unknown
Vitamin C (mg)	trace	trace	nil	unknown

Double Decker[7]	Drifter[9]	Flake[7]	Fox's Glacier Mints	FOOD
standard bar	standard bar	standard	tube	**PORTION SIZE**
				NUTRIENTS
210	267	180	146	Energy (kcals)
2.4	4.1	2.8	nil	Protein (g)
8.8	12.0	10.4	nil	Total fat (g)
unknown	unknown	unknown	nil	Saturated fat (g)
unknown	unknown	unknown	nil	Mono-unsat. fat (g)
unknown	unknown	unknown	nil	Poly-unsat. fat (g)
29.5	37.0	18.9	36.6	Carbohydrate (g)
unknown	unknown	unknown	unknown	Sugar (g)
unknown	unknown	unknown	unknown	Fibre (g)
unknown	75	unknown	22	Sodium (mg)
unknown	74	unknown	0.2	Potassium (mg)
unknown	67	unknown	0.19	Calcium (mg)
unknown	unknown	unknown	unknown	Magnesium (mg)
unknown	unknown	unknown	unknown	Phosphorus (mg)
unknown	unknown	unknown	unknown	Iron (mg)
unknown	unknown	unknown	unknown	Copper (mg)
unknown	unknown	unknown	unknown	Zinc (mg)
unknown	unknown	unknown	unknown	Selenium (µg)
unknown	unknown	unknown	unknown	Vitamin A (µg)
unknown	unknown	unknown	unknown	Vitamin D (µg)
unknown	unknown	unknown	unknown	Vitamin E (mg)
unknown	unknown	unknown	unknown	Vitamin B_1 (mg)
unknown	unknown	unknown	unknown	Vitamin B_2 (mg)
unknown	unknown	unknown	unknown	Niacin (mg)
unknown	unknown	unknown	unknown	Vitamin B_6 (mg)
unknown	unknown	unknown	unknown	Vitamin B_{12} (µg)
unknown	unknown	unknown	unknown	Folate (µg)
unknown	unknown	unknown	unknown	Pantothenate (mg)
unknown	unknown	unknown	unknown	Biotin (µg)
unknown	unknown	unknown	unknown	Vitamin C (mg)

FOOD	Fruit Gums[9]	Fruit Pastilles[9]	Fudge	Cadbury's Fudge[7]
PORTION SIZE	tube	tube	one square	standard bar
NUTRIENTS				
Energy (kcals)	134	146	49	135
Protein (g)	1.84	1.8	0.4	1.1
Total fat (g)	nil	nil	1.5	4.9
Saturated fat (g)	nil	nil	1.0	unknown
Mono-unsat. fat (g)	nil	nil	0.4	unknown
Poly-unsat. fat (g)	nil	nil	trace	unknown
Carbohydrate (g)	40	34.8	8.9	21.6
Sugar (g)	unknown	unknown	8.9	unknown
Fibre (g)	unknown	unknown	nil	unknown
Sodium (mg)	80	27	18	unknown
Potassium (mg)	64	37	15	unknown
Calcium (mg)	20	42	13	unknown
Magnesium (mg)	unknown	unknown	1	unknown
Phosphorus (mg)	unknown	unknown	11	unknown
Iron (mg)	unknown	unknown	0.03	unknown
Copper (mg)	unknown	unknown	0.01	unknown
Zinc (mg)	unknown	unknown	0.04	unknown
Selenium (µg)	unknown	unknown	trace	unknown
Vitamin A (µg)	unknown	unknown	17	unknown
Vitamin D (µg)	unknown	unknown	0.13	unknown
Vitamin E (mg)	unknown	unknown	0.03	unknown
Vitamin B_1 (mg)	unknown	unknown	trace	unknown
Vitamin B_2 (mg)	unknown	unknown	0.02	unknown
Niacin (mg)	unknown	unknown	0.01	unknown
Vitamin B_6 (mg)	unknown	unknown	trace	unknown
Vitamin B_{12} (µg)	unknown	unknown	nil	unknown
Folate (µg)	unknown	unknown	trace	unknown
Pantotheate (mg)	unknown	unknown	0.03	unknown
Biotin (µg)	unknown	unknown	0.2	unknown
Vitamin C (mg)	unknown	unknown	nil	unknown

Galaxy Chocolate block[8]	Galaxy Chocolate Double nut/raisin[8]	Galaxy Chocolate Hazelnut[8]	Galaxy Caramel[8]	FOOD
small bar (47g)	small bar (46g)	small bar (46g)	standard bar	PORTION SIZE
				NUTRIENTS
250	245	263	239	Energy (kcals)
4.2	3.8	3.5	2.5	Protein (g)
14.1	14.1	17.7	12.2	Total fat (g)
unknown	unknown	unknown	unknown	Saturated fat (g)
unknown	unknown	unknown	unknown	Mono-unsat. fat (g)
unknown	unknown	unknown	unknown	Poly-unsat. fat (g)
26.6	25.6	22.3	29.4	Carbohydrate (g)
unknown	unknown	unknown	unknown	Sugar (g)
unknown	unknown	unknown	unknown	Fibre (g)
unknown	unknown	unknown	unknown	Sodium (mg)
unknown	unknown	unknown	unknown	Potassium (mg)
unknown	unknown	unknown	unknown	Calcium (mg)
unknown	unknown	unknown	unknown	Magnesium (mg)
unknown	unknown	unknown	unknown	Phosphorus (mg)
unknown	unknown	unknown	unknown	Iron (mg)
unknown	unknown	unknown	unknown	Copper (mg)
unknown	unknown	unknown	unknown	Zinc (mg)
unknown	unknown	unknown	unknown	Selenium (µg)
unknown	unknown	unknown	unknown	Vitamin A (µg)
unknown	unknown	unknown	unknown	Vitamin D (µg)
unknown	unknown	unknown	unknown	Vitamin E (mg)
unknown	unknown	unknown	unknown	Vitamin B_1 (mg)
unknown	unknown	unknown	unknown	Vitamin B_2 (mg)
unknown	unknown	unknown	unknown	Niacin (mg)
unknown	unknown	unknown	unknown	Vitamin B_6 (mg)
unknown	unknown	unknown	unknown	Vitamin B_{12} (µg)
unknown	unknown	unknown	unknown	Folate (µg)
unknown	unknown	unknown	unknown	Pantothenate (mg)
unknown	unknown	unknown	unknown	Biotin (µg)
unknown	unknown	unknown	unknown	Vitamin C (mg)

FOODS HIGH IN FAT AND SUGAR

FOOD	Halva carrot	Halva semolina	Jellytots[9]	Kit Kat[9]
PORTION SIZE	one ounce	one ounce	packet	four- finger
NUTRIENTS				
Energy (kcals)	106	103	149	245
Protein (g)	1.4	0.7	0.04	3.6
Total fat (g)	5.7	5.0	nil	12.7
Saturated fat (g)	3.4	2.9	nil	unknown
Mono-unsat. fat (g)	1.5	1.4	nil	unknown
Poly-unsat. fat (g)	0.4	0.3	nil	unknown
Carbohydrate (g)	13.3	14.7	37	29
Sugar (g)	13.1	11.3	unknown	unknown
Fibre (g)	0.9	0.2	unknown	unknown
Sodium (mg)	30	4	34	78
Potassium (mg)	111	17	4.3	227
Calcium (mg)	45	4	2.1	94
Magnesium (mg)	6	4	unknown	unknown
Phosphorus (mg)	39	10	unknown	unknown
Iron (mg)	0.18	0.09	unknown	unknown
Copper (mg)	0.02	0.03	unknown	unknown
Zinc (mg)	0.18	0.06	unknown	unknown
Selenium (µg)	1	trace	unknown	unknown
Vitamin A (µg)	513	33	unknown	unknown
Vitamin D (µg)	0.09	0.09	unknown	unknown
Vitamin E (mg)	0.39	0.28	unknown	unknown
Vitamin B_1 (mg)	0.03	0.01	unknown	unknown
Vitamin B_2 (mg)	0.05	trace	unknown	unknown
Niacin (mg)	0.09	0.03	unknown	unknown
Vitamin B_6 (mg)	0.04	trace	unknown	unknown
Vitamin B_{12} (µg)	nil	trace	unknown	unknown
Folate (µg)	4	1	unknown	unknown
Pantothenate (mg)	0.19	0.01	unknown	unknown
Biotin (µg)	0.9	0.3	unknown	unknown
Vitamin C (mg)	trace	nil	unknown	unknown

Lion Bar[9]	Liquorice Allsorts	M&M's peanut[8]	M&M's chocolate[8]	FOOD
standard bar	small bag	small pack (45g)	small pack (45g)	PORTION SIZE
				NUTRIENTS
253	195	231	219	Energy (kcals)
2.7	2.1	4.59	2.1	Protein (g)
11.8	2.9	12.1	9.4	Total fat (g)
unknown	2.0	unknown	unknown	Saturated fat (g)
unknown	0.7	unknown	unknown	Mono-unsat. fat (g)
unknown	0.1	unknown	unknown	Poly-unsat. fat (g)
34	43.0	25.7	2.7	Carbohydrate (g)
unknown	34.9	unknown	unknown	Sugar (g)
unknown	1.1	unknown	unknown	Fibre (g)
82	32	unknown	unknown	Sodium (mg)
103	336	unknown	unknown	Potassium (mg)
76	95	unknown	unknown	Calcium (mg)
unknown	43	unknown	unknown	Magnesium (mg)
unknown	25	unknown	unknown	Phosphorus (mg)
unknown	4.09	unknown	unknown	Iron (mg)
unknown	0.19	unknown	unknown	Copper (mg)
unknown	0.28	unknown	unknown	Zinc (mg)
unknown	unknown	unknown	unknown	Selenium (µg)
unknown	nil	unknown	unknown	Vitamin A (µg)
unknown	nil	unknown	unknown	Vitamin D (µg)
unknown	nil	unknown	unknown	Vitamin E (mg)
unknown	nil	unknown	unknown	Vitamin B_1 (mg)
unknown	nil	unknown	unknown	Vitamin B_2 (mg)
unknown	nil	unknown	unknown	Niacin (mg)
unknown	nil	unknown	unknown	Vitamin B_6 (mg)
unknown	nil	unknown	unknown	Vitamin B_{12} (µg)
unknown	nil	unknown	unknown	Folate (µg)
unknown	nil	unknown	unknown	Pantothenate (mg)
unknown	nil	unknown	unknown	Biotin (µg)
unknown	nil	unknown	unknown	Vitamin C (mg)

FOOD	Mars[8]	Marshmallows	Maltesers[8]	Matchmakers[9]
PORTION SIZE	small bar (45g)	one	small pack (37g)	10 sticks
NUTRIENTS				
Energy (kcals)	203	16	182	95
Protein (g)	1.8	0.2	3.7	1.0
Total fat (g)	7.8	nil	8.5	4.1
Saturated fat (g)	unknown	nil	unknown	unknown
Mono-unsat. fat (g)	unknown	nil	unknown	unknown
Poly-unsat. fat (g)	unknown	nil	unknown	unknown
Carbohydrate (g)	31.2	4.2	22.7	13.5
Sugar (g)	unknown	3.2	unknown	unknown
Fibre (g)	unknown	nil	unknown	unknown
Sodium (mg)	unknown	1	unknown	9
Potassium (mg)	unknown	trace	unknown	51
Calcium (mg)	unknown	trace	unknown	20
Magnesium (mg)	unknown	trace	unknown	unknown
Phosphorus (mg)	unknown	trace	unknown	unknown
Iron (mg)	unknown	0.02	unknown	unknown
Copper (mg)	unknown	trace	unknown	unknown
Zinc (mg)	unknown	trace	unknown	unknown
Selenium (µg)	unknown	unknown	unknown	unknown
Vitamin A (µg)	unknown	nil	unknown	unknown
Vitamin D (µg)	unknown	nil	unknown	unknown
Vitamin E (mg)	unknown	nil	unknown	unknown
Vitamin B_1 (mg)	unknown	nil	unknown	unknown
Vitamin B_2 (mg)	unknown	nil	unknown	unknown
Niacin (mg)	unknown	trace	unknown	unknown
Vitamin B_6 (mg)	unknown	nil	unknown	unknown
Vitamin B_{12} (µg)	unknown	nil	unknown	unknown
Folate (µg)	unknown	nil	unknown	unknown
Pantothenate (mg)	unknown	nil	unknown	unknown
Biotin (µg)	unknown	nil	unknown	unknown
Vitamin C (mg)	unknown	nil	unknown	unknown

Milky Bar[9]	Milky Way[8]	Minstrels Galaxy[8]	Munchies[9]	FOOD
medium bar (20g)	standard single bar (26g)	single bar (26g)	tube	PORTION SIZE
				NUTRIENTS
109	118	206	260	Energy (kcals)
1.6	1.09	2.5	2.6	Protein (g)
6.5	4.3	8.8	12.3	Total fat (g)
unknown	unknown	unknown	unknown	Saturated fat (g)
unknown	unknown	unknown	unknown	Mono-unsat. fat (g)
unknown	unknown	unknown	unknown	Poly-unsat. fat (g)
11.1	1.8	29.1	34.6	Carbohydrate (g)
unknown	unknown	unknown	unknown	Sugar (g)
unknown	unknown	unknown	unknown	Fibre (g)
20	unknown	unknown	89	Sodium (mg)
80	unknown	unknown	192	Potassium (mg)
64	unknown	unknown	45	Calcium (mg)
unknown	unknown	unknown	unknown	Magnesium (mg)
unknown	unknown	unknown	unknown	Phosphorus (mg)
unknown	unknown	unknown	unknown	Iron (mg)
unknown	unknown	unknown	unknown	Copper (mg)
unknown	unknown	unknown	unknown	Zinc (mg)
unknown	unknown	unknown	unknown	Selenium (µg)
unknown	unknown	unknown	unknown	Vitamin A (µg)
unknown	unknown	unknown	unknown	Vitamin D (µg)
unknown	unknown	unknown	unknown	Vitamin E (mg)
unknown	unknown	unknown	unknown	Vitamin B_1 (mg)
unknown	unknown	unknown	unknown	Vitamin B_2 (mg)
unknown	unknown	unknown	unknown	Niacin (mg)
unknown	unknown	unknown	unknown	Vitamin B_6 (mg)
unknown	unknown	unknown	unknown	Vitamin B_{12} (µg)
unknown	unknown	unknown	unknown	Folate (µg)
unknown	unknown	unknown	unknown	Pantothenate (mg)
unknown	unknown	unknown	unknown	Biotin (µg)
unknown	unknown	unknown	unknown	Vitamin C (mg)

FOOD	Nougat	Opal Fruits[8]	Peanut Brittle	Peppermints
PORTION SIZE	medium bar	tube	one bar	tube
NUTRIENTS				
Energy (kcals)	269	184	280	200
Protein (g)	3.1	0.13	5.0	0.3
Total fat (g)	5.9	3.4	11.0	0.3
Saturated fat (g)	0.8	unknown	3.1	unknown
Mono-unsat. fat (g)	2.9	unknown	4.6	unknown
Poly-unsat. fat (g)	1.9	unknown	2.8	unknown
Carbohydrate (g)	54.1	38	42.8	52.3
Sugar (g)	53.8	unknown	41.6	52.3
Fibre (g)	0.6	unknown	1.2	nil
Sodium (mg)	84	unknown	64	5
Potassium (mg)	168	unknown	139	trace
Calcium (mg)	18	unknown	19	3
Magnesium (mg)	16	unknown	42	1.7
Phosphorus (mg)	51	unknown	81	trace
Iron (mg)	0.49	unknown	0.64	0.1
Copper (mg)	0.15	unknown	0.24	0.01
Zinc (mg)	0.35	unknown	0.7	unknown
Selenium (μg)	1	unknown	1	trace
Vitamin A (μg)	2	unknown	24	nil
Vitamin D (μg)	nil	unknown	nil	nil
Vitamin E (mg)	0.45	unknown	1.98	nil
Vitamin B_1 (mg)	0.08	unknown	0.22	nil
Vitamin B_2 (mg)	0.08	unknown	0.02	nil
Niacin (mg)	0.21	unknown	2.61	nil
Vitamin B_6 (mg)	trace	unknown	0.11	nil
Vitamin B_{12} (μg)	nil	unknown	nil	nil
Folate (μg)	8	unknown	21	nil
Pantothenate (mg)	0.04	unknown	0.51	nil
Biotin (μg)	unknown	unknown	13.9	nil
Vitamin C (mg)	nil	unknown	nil	nil

Peppermint Creams	Cadbury's Peppermint Cream[7]	Picnic[7]	Quality Street[9]	FOOD
one	standard bar	standard bar	one	**PORTION SIZE**
				NUTRIENTS
26	215	230	37	Energy (kcals)
trace	1.4	3.8	0.3	Protein (g)
trace	7.4	11.3	1.5	Total fat (g)
nil	unknown	unknown	unknown	Saturated fat (g)
nil	unknown	unknown	unknown	Mono-unsat. fat (g)
nil	unknown	unknown	unknown	Poly-unsat. fat (g)
6.9	34.9	28.5	5.3	Carbohydrate (g)
6.8	unknown	unknown	unknown	Sugar (g)
trace	unknown	unknown	unknown	Fibre (g)
2	unknown	unknown	6.8	Sodium (mg)
1	unknown	unknown	10.8	Potassium (mg)
trace	unknown	unknown	unknown	Calcium (mg)
trace	unknown	unknown	unknown	Magnesium (mg)
trace	unknown	unknown	unknown	Phosphorus (mg)
0.04	unknown	unknown	unknown	Iron (mg)
trace	unknown	unknown	unknown	Copper (mg)
0.01	unknown	unknown	unknown	Zinc (mg)
trace	unknown	unknown	unknown	Selenium (µg)
trace	unknown	unknown	unknown	Vitamin A (µg)
nil	unknown	unknown	unknown	Vitamin D (µg)
trace	unknown	unknown	unknown	Vitamin E (mg)
trace	unknown	unknown	unknown	Vitamin B_1 (mg)
trace	unknown	unknown	unknown	Vitamin B_2 (mg)
trace	unknown	unknown	unknown	Niacin (mg)
trace	unknown	unknown	unknown	Vitamin B_6 (mg)
nil	unknown	unknown	unknown	Vitamin B_{12} (µg)
trace	unknown	unknown	unknown	Folate (µg)
trace	unknown	unknown	unknown	Pantothenate (mg)
trace	unknown	unknown	unknown	Biotin (µg)
nil	unknown	unknown	unknown	Vitamin C (mg)

FOOD	Revels[8]	Ripple Galaxy[8]	Rolo[9]	Sherbert Fountain
PORTION SIZE	small pack (35g)	standard bar	tube	one
NUTRIENTS				
Energy (kcals)	173	175	271	85
Protein (g)	2.17	2.9	2.5	0.1
Total fat (g)	8.0	9.9	11.8	nil
Saturated fat (g)	unknown	unknown	unknown	nil
Mono-unsat. fat (g)	unknown	unknown	unknown	nil
Poly-unsat. fat (g)	unknown	unknown	unknown	nil
Carbohydrate (g)	22.9	18.6	38	22.5
Sugar (g)	unknown	unknown	unknown	22.5
Fibre (g)	unknown	unknown	unknown	trace
Sodium (mg)	unknown	unknown	142	252
Potassium (mg)	unknown	unknown	116	4
Calcium (mg)	unknown	unknown	92	10
Magnesium (mg)	unknown	unknown	unknown	17
Phosphorus (mg)	unknown	unknown	unknown	trace
Iron (mg)	unknown	unknown	unknown	0.05
Copper (mg)	unknown	unknown	unknown	0.01
Zinc (mg)	unknown	unknown	unknown	unknown
Selenium (µg)	unknown	unknown	unknown	nil
Vitamin A (µg)	unknown	unknown	unknown	nil
Vitamin D (µg)	unknown	unknown	unknown	nil
Vitamin E (mg)	unknown	unknown	unknown	nil
Vitamin B_1 (mg)	unknown	unknown	unknown	nil
Vitamin B_2 (mg)	unknown	unknown	unknown	nil
Niacin (mg)	unknown	unknown	unknown	trace
Vitamin B_6 (mg)	unknown	unknown	unknown	nil
Vitamin B_{12} (µg)	unknown	unknown	unknown	nil
Folate (µg)	unknown	unknown	unknown	nil
Pantothenate (mg)	unknown	unknown	unknown	nil
Biotin (µg)	unknown	unknown	unknown	nil
Vitamin C (mg)	unknown	unknown	unknown	nil

Skittles[8]	Smarties[9]	Snickers[8]	Toffees mixed	FOOD
small pack (60g)	tube	small bar (38g)	one	**PORTION SIZE**
				NUTRIENTS
243	169	193	34	Energy (kcals)
0.1	1.9	3.8	0.2	Protein (g)
2.5	6.2	10.4	1.5	Total fat (g)
unknown	unknown	unknown	0.8	Saturated fat (g)
unknown	unknown	unknown	0.6	Mono-unsat. fat (g)
unknown	unknown	unknown	0.1	Poly-unsat. fat (g)
54.9	26.3	21	5.3	Carbohydrate (g)
unknown	unknown	unknown	3.6	Sugar (g)
unknown	unknown	unknown	nil	Fibre (g)
unknown	42	unknown	27	Sodium (mg)
unknown	111	unknown	9	Potassium (mg)
unknown	60	unknown	6	Calcium (mg)
unknown	unknown	unknown	1	Magnesium (mg)
unknown	unknown	unknown	5	Phosphorus (mg)
unknown	unknown	unknown	0.02	Iron (mg)
unknown	unknown	unknown	trace	Copper (mg)
unknown	unknown	unknown	0.02	Zinc (mg)
unknown	unknown	unknown	unknown	Selenium (μg)
unknown	unknown	unknown	nil	Vitamin A (μg)
unknown	unknown	unknown	nil	Vitamin D (μg)
unknown	unknown	unknown	nil	Vitamin E (mg)
unknown	unknown	unknown	nil	Vitamin B_1 (mg)
unknown	unknown	unknown	nil	Vitamin B_2 (mg)
unknown	unknown	unknown	nil	Niacin (mg)
unknown	unknown	unknown	nil	Vitamin B_6 (mg)
unknown	unknown	unknown	nil	Vitamin B_{12} (μg)
unknown	unknown	unknown	nil	Folate (μg)
unknown	unknown	unknown	nil	Pantothenate (mg)
unknown	unknown	unknown	nil	Biotin (μg)
unknown	unknown	unknown	nil	Vitamin C (mg)

FOOD	Toffee Crisp[9]	Toffo selection[9]	Tooty Frooties[9]	Topic[8]
PORTION SIZE	standard bar (48g)	tube	bag	standard bar
NUTRIENTS				
Energy (kcals)	238	208	164	233
Protein (g)	2.0	1.0	0.16	3.4
Total fat (g)	12.5	7.7	1.4	12.5
Saturated fat (g)	unknown	unknown	unknown	unknown
Mono-unsat. fat (g)	unknown	unknown	unknown	unknown
Poly-unsat. fat (g)	unknown	unknown	unknown	unknown
Carbohydrate (g)	29	33.4	37	26.6
Sugar (g)	unknown	unknown	unknown	unknown
Fibre (g)	unknown	unknown	unknown	unknown
Sodium (mg)	52	119	37	unknown
Potassium (mg)	127	47	4.1	unknown
Calcium (mg)	57	54	1.6	unknown
Magnesium (mg)	unknown	unknown	unknown	unknown
Phosphorus (mg)	unknown	unknown	unknown	unknown
Iron (mg)	unknown	unknown	unknown	unknown
Copper (mg)	unknown	unknown	unknown	unknown
Zinc (mg)	unknown	unknown	unknown	unknown
Selenium (µg)	unknown	unknown	unknown	unknown
Vitamin A (µg)	unknown	unknown	unknown	unknown
Vitamin D (µg)	unknown	unknown	unknown	unknown
Vitamin E (mg)	unknown	unknown	unknown	unknown
Vitamin B_1 (mg)	unknown	unknown	unknown	unknown
Vitamin B_2 (mg)	unknown	unknown	unknown	unknown
Niacin (mg)	unknown	unknown	unknown	unknown
Vitamin B_6 (mg)	unknown	unknown	unknown	unknown
Vitamin B_{12} (µg)	unknown	unknown	unknown	unknown
Folate (µg)	unknown	unknown	unknown	unknown
Pantotheate (mg)	unknown	unknown	unknown	unknown
Biotin (µg)	unknown	unknown	unknown	unknown
Vitamin C (mg)	unknown	unknown	unknown	unknown

Tracker choc chip[8]	**Tracker** roast nut[8]	**Turkish Delight** without nuts	**Turkish Delight** with nuts	**FOOD**
standard bar		one square	one square	**PORTION SIZE**
				NUTRIENTS
196	200	44	52	Energy (kcals)
2.9	3.4	0.1	0.6	Protein (g)
10.7	11.2	nil	0.4	Total fat (g)
unknown	unknown	nil	trace	Saturated fat (g)
unknown	unknown	nil	0.2	Mono-unsat. fat (g)
unknown	unknown	nil	0.1	Poly-unsat. fat (g)
22	21.2	11.7	12.2	Carbohydrate (g)
unknown	unknown	10.3	12.1	Sugar (g)
unknown	unknown	nil	trace	Fibre (g)
unknown	unknown	5	13	Sodium (mg)
unknown	unknown	1	8	Potassium (mg)
unknown	unknown	2	3	Calcium (mg)
unknown	unknown	trace	1	Magnesium (mg)
unknown	unknown	1	3	Phosphorus (mg)
unknown	unknown	0.03	0.06	Iron (mg)
unknown	unknown	0.02	0.02	Copper (mg)
unknown	unknown	0.1	0.03	Zinc (mg)
unknown	unknown	trace	trace	Selenium (µg)
unknown	unknown	nil	trace	Vitamin A (µg)
unknown	unknown	nil	nil	Vitamin D (µg)
unknown	unknown	nil	0.03	Vitamin E (mg)
unknown	unknown	0.02	trace	Vitamin B_1 (mg)
unknown	unknown	unknown	trace	Vitamin B_2 (mg)
unknown	unknown	unknown	0.02	Niacin (mg)
unknown	unknown	unknown	nil	Vitamin B_6 (mg)
unknown	unknown	unknown	nil	Vitamin B_{12} (µg)
unknown	unknown	unknown	trace	Folate (µg)
unknown	unknown	unknown	trace	Pantothenate (mg)
unknown	unknown	unknown	trace	Biotin (µg)
unknown	unknown	nil	nil	Vitamin C (mg)

FOOD	**Cadbury's Turkish Delight**[7]	**Twirl**[7]	**Twix**[8]	**Walnut Whip** vanilla and coffee[9]
PORTION SIZE	standard bar	per finger	Twin bar	one
NUTRIENTS				
Energy (kcals)	180	115	287	155
Protein (g)	1.1	1.8	3.36	1.8
Total fat (g)	3.8	6.6	16	7.8
Saturated fat (g)	unknown	unknown	unknown	unknown
Mono-unsat. fat (g)	unknown	unknown	unknown	unknown
Poly-unsat. fat (g)	unknown	unknown	unknown	unknown
Carbohydrate (g)	35.2	12.3	36.8	19.2
Sugar (g)	unknown	unknown	unknown	unknown
Fibre (g)	unknown	unknown	unknown	unknown
Sodium (mg)	unknown	unknown	unknown	20
Potassium (mg)	unknown	unknown	unknown	52
Calcium (mg)	unknown	unknown	unknown	54
Magnesium (mg)	unknown	unknown	unknown	unknown
Phosphorus (mg)	unknown	unknown	unknown	unknown
Iron (mg)	unknown	unknown	unknown	unknown
Copper (mg)	unknown	unknown	unknown	unknown
Zinc (mg)	unknown	unknown	unknown	unknown
Selenium (µg)	unknown	unknown	unknown	unknown
Vitamin A (µg)	unknown	unknown	unknown	unknown
Vitamin D (µg)	unknown	unknown	unknown	unknown
Vitamin E (mg)	unknown	unknown	unknown	unknown
Vitamin B_1 (mg)	unknown	unknown	unknown	unknown
Vitamin B_2 (mg)	unknown	unknown	unknown	unknown
Niacin (mg)	unknown	unknown	unknown	unknown
Vitamin B_6 (mg)	unknown	unknown	unknown	unknown
Vitamin B_{12} (µg)	unknown	unknown	unknown	unknown
Folate (µg)	unknown	unknown	unknown	unknown
Pantothenate (mg)	unknown	unknown	unknown	unknown
Biotin (µg)	unknown	unknown	unknown	unknown
Vitamin C (mg)	unknown	unknown	unknown	unknown

Wispa[7]	Cadbury's white chocolate buttons[7]	XXX mints[9]	Yorkie milk[9]	FOOD
standard bar	standard bag	tube	standard bar	**PORTION SIZE**
				NUTRIENTS
210	170	190	346	Energy (kcals)
2.7	2.8	0.3	4.6	Protein (g)
12.8	9.7	trace	19.4	Total fat (g)
unknown	unknown	unknown	unknown	Saturated fat (g)
unknown	unknown	unknown	unknown	Mono-unsat. fat (g)
unknown	unknown	unknown	unknown	Poly-unsat. fat (g)
20.7	18.1	47	38	Carbohydrate (g)
unknown	unknown	unknown	unknown	Sugar (g)
unknown	unknown	unknown	unknown	Fibre (g)
unknown	unknown	5	45	Sodium (mg)
unknown	unknown	5	254	Potassium (mg)
unknown	unknown	1	62	Calcium (mg)
unknown	unknown	unknown	unknown	Magnesium (mg)
unknown	unknown	unknown	unknown	Phosphorus (mg)
unknown	unknown	unknown	unknown	Iron (mg)
unknown	unknown	unknown	unknown	Copper (mg)
unknown	unknown	unknown	unknown	Zinc (mg)
unknown	unknown	unknown	unknown	Selenium (μg)
unknown	unknown	unknown	unknown	Vitamin A (μg)
unknown	unknown	unknown	unknown	Vitamin D (μg)
unknown	unknown	unknown	unknown	Vitamin E (mg)
unknown	unknown	unknown	unknown	Vitamin B_1 (mg)
unknown	unknown	unknown	unknown	Vitamin B_2 (mg)
unknown	unknown	unknown	unknown	Niacin (mg)
unknown	unknown	unknown	unknown	Vitamin B_6 (mg)
unknown	unknown	unknown	unknown	Vitamin B_{12} (μg)
unknown	unknown	unknown	unknown	Folate (μg)
unknown	unknown	unknown	unknown	Pantothenate (mg)
unknown	unknown	unknown	unknown	Biotin (μg)
unknown	unknown	unknown	unknown	Vitamin C (mg)

FOOD	Yorkie[9] peanut	Yorkie[9] raisin and biscuit
PORTION SIZE	standard bar	standard bar
NUTRIENTS		
Energy (kcals)	325	293
Protein (g)	6.9	3.8
Total fat (g)	20.1	14.5
Saturated fat (g)	unknown	unknown
Mono-unsat. fat (g)	unknown	unknown
Poly-unsat. fat (g)	unknown	unknown
Carbohydrate (g)	29	37
Sugar (g)	unknown	unknown
Fibre (g)	unknown	unknown
Sodium (mg)	unknown	38
Potassium (mg)	unknown	265
Calcium (mg)	unknown	53
Magnesium (mg)	unknown	unknown
Phosphorus (mg)	unknown	unknown
Iron (mg)	unknown	unknown
Copper (mg)	unknown	unknown
Zinc (mg)	unknown	unknown
Selenium (µg)	unknown	unknown
Vitamin A (µg)	unknown	unknown
Vitamin D (µg)	unknown	unknown
Vitamin E (mg)	unknown	unknown
Vitamin B_1 (mg)	unknown	unknown
Vitamin B_2 (mg)	unknown	unknown
Niacin (mg)	unknown	unknown
Vitamin B_6 (mg)	unknown	unknown
Vitamin B_{12} (µg)	unknown	unknown
Folate (µg)	unknown	unknown
Pantothenate (mg)	unknown	unknown
Biotin (µg)	unknown	unknown
Vitamin C (mg)	unknown	unknown

Spreads, sugar and syrups

This food group has much in common with sweets, in that all the products contain a great deal of sugar. However, unlike sweets, it has often been suggested that some of these foods have health-giving properties, which as you can see from the nutritional analysis, simply doesn't make sense. It is true that in its most natural state, sugar can contain some minerals, treacle being an especially good source of iron. However, there are other foods which are equally as good providers of those minerals, without having the drawback of being bad for your teeth.

Honey has been especially promoted as being better for your health than cane sugar, but the only difference between them, apart from the taste, is the minute amounts of minerals honey contains. Similarly, the difference between brown and white sugar are so small that the main factor becomes one of personal taste rather than which is better for your health.

Giving up sugar in beverages can be difficult; your taste buds will only begin to taste sweet food at a certain level of sweetness, and getting them used to a less sweet taste is often a long process. However, if you are serious about giving up sugar, then you should try to cut down on your sugar intake from all sources. The day when something suddenly tastes too sweet, is the day you have been successful.

FOOD	Chocolate nut spread	Chocolate spread	Honey	Jam average of two types
PORTION SIZE	average on a slice of bread	average on a slice of bread	average on a slice of bread	average on a slice of bread
NUTRIENTS				
Energy (kcals)	110	114	58	39
Protein (g)	1.2	0.8	0.1	0.1
Total fat (g)	6.6	7.5	nil	nil
Saturated fat (g)	2.0	unknown	nil	nil
Mono-unsat. fat (g)	3.4	unknown	nil	nil
Poly-unsat. fat (g)	0.9	unknown	nil	nil
Carbohydrate (g)	12.1	11.4	15.3	10.4
Sugar (g)	11.9	11.4	15.3	10.4
Fibre (g)	0.2	unknown	nil	unknown
Sodium (mg)	10	unknown	2	5
Potassium (mg)	78	unknown	10	8
Calcium (mg)	26	unknown	1	2
Magnesium (mg)	13	unknown	0	0.5
Phosphorus (mg)	36	unknown	3	1.5
Iron (mg)	0.44	unknown	0.08	0.03
Copper (mg)	0.1	unknown	0.01	trace
Zinc (mg)	0.2	unknown	0.18	0.01
Selenium (µg)	unknown	unknown	0	trace
Vitamin A (µg)	trace	trace	nil	nil
Vitamin D (µg)	trace	trace	nil	nil
Vitamin E (mg)	unknown	unknown	nil	nil
Vitamin B_1 (mg)	0.01	unknown	trace	trace
Vitamin B_2 (mg)	0.02	unknown	0.01	trace
Niacin (mg)	0.1	unknown	0.04	trace
Vitamin B_6 (mg)	0.02	unknown	unknown	trace
Vitamin B_{12} (µg)	trace	trace	nil	nil
Folate (µg)	unknown	unknown	unknown	trace
Pantotheate (mg)	unknown	unknown	unknown	trace
Biotin (µg)	unknown	unknown	unknown	trace
Vitamin C (mg)	trace	nil	nil	1

Lemon curd	Ice cream syrup	Maple syrup	Marmalade	FOOD
average on a slice of bread	average topping	serving on top of waffles	average on a slice of bread	PORTION SIZE
				NUTRIENTS
42	58	144	39	Energy (kcals)
0.1	0.2	nil	trace	Protein (g)
0.8	0.1	0.1	nil	Total fat (g)
0.2	trace	trace	nil	Saturated fat (g)
0.3	trace	trace	nil	Mono-unsat. fat (g)
0.2	trace	trace	nil	Poly-unsat. fat (g)
9.4	15.1	37	10.4	Carbohydrate (g)
6.1	14.3	33.4	10.4	Sugar (g)
trace	nil	nil	trace	Fibre (g)
10	39	5	10	Sodium (mg)
2	19	110	5	Potassium (mg)
1	3	37	4	Calcium (mg)
trace	4	8	trace	Magnesium (mg)
2	7	1	1	Phosphorus (mg)
0.08	0.22	0.66	0.03	Iron (mg)
0.05	0.03	0.04	trace	Copper (mg)
0.19	0.03	2.31	0.02	Zinc (mg)
unknown	unknown	trace	1	Selenium (µg)
2	trace	nil	1	Vitamin A (µg)
0.02	nil	nil	nil	Vitamin D (µg)
unknown	unknown	nil	trace	Vitamin E (mg)
trace	trace	0.01	trace	Vitamin B_1 (mg)
trace	trace	0.01	trace	Vitamin B_2 (mg)
trace	trace	trace	trace	Niacin (mg)
trace	trace	trace	trace	Vitamin B_6 (mg)
trace	nil	nil	nil	Vitamin B_{12} (µg)
trace	trace	nil	1	Folate (µg)
0.02	trace	0.02	trace	Pantothenate (mg)
0.2	trace	trace	trace	Biotin (µg)
trace	nil	nil	2	Vitamin C (mg)

FOOD	Sugar brown	Sugar white	Syrup golden	Treacle black
PORTION SIZE	heaped teaspoon/ individual packet	heaped teaspoon/ individual packet	tablespoon	tablespoon
NUTRIENTS				
Energy (kcals)	22	24	60	51
Protein (g)	trace	trace	0.1	0.2
Total fat (g)	nil	nil	nil	nil
Saturated fat (g)	nil	nil	nil	nil
Mono-unsat. fat (g)	nil	nil	nil	nil
Poly-unsat. fat (g)	nil	nil	nil	nil
Carbohydrate (g)	6.0	6.0	15.8	13.4
Sugar (g)	6.0	6.0	15.8	13.4
Fibre (g)	nil	nil	nil	trace
Sodium (mg)	2	trace	54	36
Potassium (mg)	8	trace	12	352
Calcium (mg)	3	1	3	110
Magnesium (mg)	1	trace	1	36
Phosphorus (mg)	trace	trace	trace	6
Iron (mg)	0.1	0.01	0.08	4.2
Copper (mg)	trace	0.01	0.01	0.16
Zinc (mg)	0.01	0.01	0.02	0.16
Selenium (µg)	trace	trace	trace	unknown
Vitamin A (µg)	nil	nil	nil	nil
Vitamin D (µg)	nil	nil	nil	nil
Vitamin E (mg)	nil	nil	nil	nil
Vitamin B_1 (mg)	trace	nil	trace	trace
Vitamin B_2 (mg)	trace	nil	trace	trace
Niacin (mg)	trace	nil	trace	trace
Vitamin B_6 (mg)	trace	nil	trace	trace
Vitamin B_{12} (µg)	nil	nil	nil	nil
Folate (µg)	trace	nil	trace	trace
Pantothenate (mg)	trace	nil	trace	trace
Biotin (µg)	trace	nil	trace	trace
Vitamin C (mg)	nil	nil	nil	nil

Ice Cream

In the old days, ice cream came in a cone or in a tub, but today we are increasingly eating it on a stick. It used to be reserved for the beach or during the intermission at the pictures, but now it is part of every day life, sold along side sweets and snacks in most local newsagents. Another change is the variety of ice cream available, no longer just Neapolitan or Cornish, but a huge variety of different tastes and flavours. The nineties saw a move back towards traditional ingredients for ice cream, including cream and eggs. This makes some types of ice cream particularly high in fat and calories, so check on the pack before you buy. Whatever your particular downfall, remember this, if it is in your freezer you will eat it. Always buy small amounts at a time and have it occasionally - how you eat it is entirely up to you!

This section concentrates on the ice cream and lollies you might buy from a shop or ice cream van. However, ice cream is also included in the puddings section earlier in this segment. Some manufacturer's data has been used in this section.

[7] – Cadbury's
[8] – Mars
[10] – Walls

FOOD	Blue Ribbon choc ice[10]	Bounty[8]	Calippo orange[10]	Cadbury's Caramel choc bar[7]
PORTION SIZE	one	one	one	one
NUTRIENTS				
Energy (kcals)	125	299	105	185
Protein (g)	1.5	3.7	0.1	2.5
Total fat (g)	8.0	20.9	trace	11.0
Saturated fat (g)	unknown	unknown	unknown	unknown
Mono-unsat. fat (g)	unknown	unknown	unknown	unknown
Poly-unsat. fat (g)	unknown	unknown	unknown	unknown
Carbohydrate (g)	12.0	24	26.0	20.0
Sugar (g)	unknown	unknown	unknown	unknown
Fibre (g)	0.15	unknown	unknown	0.2
Sodium (mg)	trace	unknown	trace	trace
Potassium (mg)	2.0	unknown	0.5	2.0
Calcium (mg)	50	unknown	4.5	74.0
Magnesium (mg)	10.5	unknown	9.5	16.0
Phosphorus (mg)	unknown	unknown	unknown	unknown
Iron (mg)	unknown	unknown	unknown	unknown
Copper (mg)	unknown	unknown	unknown	unknown
Zinc (mg)	unknown	unknown	unknown	unknown
Selenium (µg)	unknown	unknown	unknown	unknown
Vitamin A (µg)	unknown	unknown	unknown	unknown
Vitamin D (µg)	unknown	unknown	unknown	unknown
Vitamin E (mg)	unknown	unknown	unknown	unknown
Vitamin B_1 (mg)	unknown	unknown	unknown	unknown
Vitamin B_2 (mg)	unknown	unknown	unknown	unknown
Niacin (mg)	unknown	unknown	unknown	unknown
Vitamin B_6 (mg)	unknown	unknown	unknown	unknown
Vitamin B_{12} (µg)	unknown	unknown	unknown	unknown
Folate (µg)	unknown	unknown	unknown	unknown
Pantothenate (mg)	unknown	unknown	unknown	unknown
Biotin (µg)	unknown	unknown	unknown	unknown
Vitamin C (mg)	unknown	unknown	unknown	unknown

Cadbury's Crunchie choc bar[7]	Choc Ice	Chocolate-covered ice cream bar	Cornetto	FOOD
one	one	one	one	**PORTION SIZE**
				NUTRIENTS
200	139	182	195	Energy (kcals)
2.5	1.8	2.8	2.8	Protein (g)
10.5	8.8	13.3	9.7	Total fat (g)
unknown	5.4	8.6	5.0	Saturated fat (g)
unknown	2.4	3.8	3.1	Mono-unsat. fat (g)
unknown	0.6	0.9	1.0	Poly-unsat. fat (g)
22.0	14.1	13.7	25.9	Carbohydrate (g)
unknown	unknown	13.3	19.1	Sugar (g)
0.3	nil	unknown	unknown	Fibre (g)
0.1	46	52	68	Sodium (mg)
2.5	100	143	128	Potassium (mg)
81.0	65	80	90	Calcium (mg)
19.0	14	18	16	Magnesium (mg)
unknown	unknown	86	unknown	Phosphorus (mg)
unknown	0.05	0.4	unknown	Iron (mg)
unknown	trace	0.02	unknown	Copper (mg)
unknown	0.1	0.4	unknown	Zinc (mg)
unknown	unknown	unknown	unknown	Selenium (µg)
unknown	1.5	48	unknown	Vitamin A (µg)
unknown	trace	0.11	unknown	Vitamin D (µg)
unknown	unknown	unknown	unknown	Vitamin E (mg)
unknown	unknown	0.03	unknown	Vitamin B_1 (mg)
unknown	unknown	0.17	unknown	Vitamin B_2 (mg)
unknown	unknown	0.34	unknown	Niacin (mg)
unknown	unknown	0.02	unknown	Vitamin B_6 (mg)
unknown	unknown	nil	unknown	Vitamin B_{12} (µg)
unknown	unknown	7	unknown	Folate (µg)
unknown	unknown	0.28	unknown	Pantothenate (mg)
unknown	unknown	4.0	unknown	Biotin (µg)
unknown	unknown	nil	unknown	Vitamin C (mg)

FOOD	Dennis the Menace[10]	Feast[10]	Galaxy milk[8]	Ice cream
PORTION SIZE	one	one	one	one tub
NUTRIENTS				
Energy (kcals)	90	230	302	116
Protein (g)	0.5	3.5	3.8	2.2
Total fat (g)	3.5	13.0	19.5	5.9
Saturated fat (g)	unknown	unknown	unknown	3.8
Mono-unsat. fat (g)	unknown	unknown	unknown	1.4
Poly-unsat. fat (g)	unknown	unknown	unknown	0.2
Carbohydrate (g)	14.0	25.0	27.6	14.6
Sugar (g)	unknown	unknown	unknown	13.3
Fibre (g)	nil	0.3	unknown	nil
Sodium (mg)	0.1	0.1	unknown	41
Potassium (mg)	1.0	3.5	unknown	96
Calcium (mg)	23.0	90.0	unknown	78
Magnesium (mg)	5.0	17.0	unknown	8
Phosphorus (mg)	unknown	unknown	unknown	66
Iron (mg)	unknown	unknown	unknown	0.06
Copper (mg)	unknown	unknown	unknown	0.01
Zinc (mg)	unknown	unknown	unknown	0.18
Selenium (μg)	unknown	unknown	unknown	unknown
Vitamin A (μg)	unknown	unknown	unknown	88
Vitamin D (μg)	unknown	unknown	unknown	0.07
Vitamin E (mg)	unknown	unknown	unknown	0.13
Vitamin B_1 (mg)	unknown	unknown	unknown	0.02
Vitamin B_2 (mg)	unknown	unknown	unknown	0.15
Niacin (mg)	unknown	unknown	unknown	0.08
Vitamin B_6 (mg)	unknown	unknown	unknown	0.05
Vitamin B_{12} (μg)	unknown	unknown	unknown	0.2
Folate (μg)	unknown	unknown	unknown	4
Pantothenate (mg)	unknown	unknown	unknown	0.26
Biotin (μg)	unknown	unknown	unknown	1.5
Vitamin C (mg)	unknown	unknown	unknown	1

Ice cream in a cone	Whippy ice cream in a cone[10]	Magnum[10] dark chocolate	Magnum[10] white	FOOD
one	one	one	one	**PORTION SIZE**
				NUTRIENTS
117	85	295	300	Energy (kcals)
2.2	2.5	4.0	4.0	Protein (g)
5.4	3.5	20.0	20.0	Total fat (g)
unknown	unknown	unknown	unknown	Saturated fat (g)
unknown	unknown	unknown	unknown	Mono-unsat. fat (g)
unknown	unknown	unknown	unknown	Poly-unsat. fat (g)
16.1	12.0	26.0	27.0	Carbohydrate (g)
11.6	unknown	unknown	unknown	Sugar (g)
trace	0.1	unknown	unknown	Fibre (g)
48	trace	0.1	0.1	Sodium (mg)
107	2.5	4.5	4.5	Potassium (mg)
76	74.0	112	138	Calcium (mg)
9	8.0	27.0	13.0	Magnesium (mg)
63	unknown	unknown	unknown	Phosphorus (mg)
0.13	unknown	unknown	unknown	Iron (mg)
trace	unknown	unknown	unknown	Copper (mg)
0.19	unknown	unknown	unknown	Zinc (mg)
unknown	unknown	unknown	unknown	Selenium (µg)
0.5	unknown	unknown	unknown	Vitamin A (µg)
trace	unknown	unknown	unknown	Vitamin D (µg)
0.49	unknown	unknown	unknown	Vitamin E (mg)
0.03	unknown	unknown	unknown	Vitamin B_1 (mg)
0.14	unknown	unknown	unknown	Vitamin B_2 (mg)
0.13	unknown	unknown	unknown	Niacin (mg)
0.04	unknown	unknown	unknown	Vitamin B_6 (mg)
0.3	unknown	unknown	unknown	Vitamin B_{12} (µg)
5	unknown	unknown	unknown	Folate (µg)
unknown	unknown	unknown	unknown	Pantothenate (mg)
unknown	unknown	unknown	unknown	Biotin (µg)
1	unknown	unknown	unknown	Vitamin C (mg)

FOOD	Mars[8]	Mini juice[10]	Mini milk[10] vanilla	Opal Fruits[8] average
PORTION SIZE	one	one	one	one
NUTRIENTS				
Energy (kcals)	209	30	35	87
Protein (g)	2.8	trace	1.0	0.1
Total fat (g)	12.0	trace	1.0	0.1
Saturated fat (g)	unknown	unknown	unknown	unknown
Mono-unsat. fat (g)	unknown	unknown	unknown	unknown
Poly-unsat. fat (g)	unknown	unknown	unknown	unknown
Carbohydrate (g)	22.2	7.0	6.0	21.4
Sugar (g)	unknown	unknown	unknown	unknown
Fibre (g)	unknown	nil	nil	unknown
Sodium (mg)	unknown	trace	trace	unknown
Potassium (mg)	unknown	0.5	1.0	unknown
Calcium (mg)	unknown	1.0	34.0	unknown
Magnesium (mg)	unknown	1.0	4.5	unknown
Phosphorus (mg)	unknown	unknown	unknown	unknown
Iron (mg)	unknown	unknown	unknown	unknown
Copper (mg)	unknown	unknown	unknown	unknown
Zinc (mg)	unknown	unknown	unknown	unknown
Selenium (µg)	unknown	unknown	unknown	unknown
Vitamin A (µg)	unknown	unknown	unknown	unknown
Vitamin D (µg)	unknown	unknown	unknown	unknown
Vitamin E (mg)	unknown	unknown	unknown	unknown
Vitamin B_1 (mg)	unknown	unknown	unknown	unknown
Vitamin B_2 (mg)	unknown	unknown	unknown	unknown
Niacin (mg)	unknown	unknown	unknown	unknown
Vitamin B_6 (mg)	unknown	unknown	unknown	unknown
Vitamin B_{12} (µg)	unknown	unknown	unknown	unknown
Folate (µg)	unknown	unknown	unknown	unknown
Pantothenate (mg)	unknown	unknown	unknown	unknown
Biotin (µg)	unknown	unknown	unknown	unknown
Vitamin C (mg)	unknown	unknown	unknown	unknown

Skittles[8]	Snickers[8]	Solero[10]	Strawberry Split	FOOD
one	one	one	one	**PORTION SIZE**
				NUTRIENTS
52	230	130	105	Energy (kcals)
0.1	4.5	2.0	1.0	Protein (g)
trace	14.9	4.5	3.0	Total fat (g)
unknown	unknown	unknown	unknown	Saturated fat (g)
unknown	unknown	unknown	unknown	Mono-unsat. fat (g)
unknown	unknown	unknown	unknown	Poly-unsat. fat (g)
13.0	20	20.0	18.0	Carbohydrate (g)
unknown	unknown	unknown	unknown	Sugar (g)
unknown	unknown	0.2	0.3	Fibre (g)
unknown	unknown	trace	trace	Sodium (mg)
unknown	unknown	2.5	2.0	Potassium (mg)
unknown	unknown	66.0	45.0	Calcium (mg)
unknown	unknown	9.0	7.5	Magnesium (mg)
unknown	unknown	unknown	unknown	Phosphorus (mg)
unknown	unknown	unknown	unknown	Iron (mg)
unknown	unknown	unknown	unknown	Copper (mg)
unknown	unknown	unknown	unknown	Zinc (mg)
unknown	unknown	unknown	unknown	Selenium (µg)
unknown	unknown	unknown	unknown	Vitamin A (µg)
unknown	unknown	unknown	unknown	Vitamin D (µg)
unknown	unknown	unknown	unknown	Vitamin E (mg)
unknown	unknown	unknown	unknown	Vitamin B_1 (mg)
unknown	unknown	unknown	unknown	Vitamin B_2 (mg)
unknown	unknown	unknown	unknown	Niacin (mg)
unknown	unknown	unknown	unknown	Vitamin B_6 (mg)
unknown	unknown	unknown	unknown	Vitamin B_{12} (µg)
unknown	unknown	unknown	unknown	Folate (µg)
unknown	unknown	unknown	unknown	Pantothenate (mg)
unknown	unknown	unknown	unknown	Biotin (µg)
unknown	unknown	unknown	unknown	Vitamin C (mg)

FOOD	Super Mario[10]	Tangle Twister	Twix[8]
PORTION SIZE	one	one	one
NUTRIENTS			
Energy (kcals)	115	90	228
Protein (g)	2.5	1.0	3.1
Total fat (g)	5.5	2.0	13.6
Saturated fat (g)	unknown	unknown	unknown
Mono-unsat. fat (g)	unknown	unknown	unknown
Poly-unsat. fat (g)	unknown	unknown	unknown
Carbohydrate (g)	14.0	18.0	23.2
Sugar (g)	unknown	unknown	unknown
Fibre (g)	0.2	trace	unknown
Sodium (mg)	trace	trace	unknown
Potassium (mg)	3.0	1.0	unknown
Calcium (mg)	82.0	29.0	unknown
Magnesium (mg)	14.0	5.0	unknown
Phosphorus (mg)	unknown	unknown	unknown
Iron (mg)	unknown	unknown	unknown
Copper (mg)	unknown	unknown	unknown
Zinc (mg)	unknown	unknown	unknown
Selenium (μg)	unknown	unknown	unknown
Vitamin A (μg)	unknown	unknown	unknown
Vitamin D (μg)	unknown	unknown	unknown
Vitamin E (mg)	unknown	unknown	unknown
Vitamin B_1 (mg)	unknown	unknown	unknown
Vitamin B_2 (mg)	unknown	unknown	unknown
Niacin (mg)	unknown	unknown	unknown
Vitamin B_6 (mg)	unknown	unknown	unknown
Vitamin B_{12} (μg)	unknown	unknown	unknown
Folate (μg)	unknown	unknown	unknown
Pantothenate (mg)	unknown	unknown	unknown
Biotin (μg)	unknown	unknown	unknown
Vitamin C (mg)	unknown	unknown	unknown

Snacks

Bags of savoury snacks are another part of our everyday life which simply were not around twenty years ago. The only snack available were plain crisps with the blue screw of salt hidden inside the bag. Technology has ensured that today we have enough different types of savoury snack to satisfy even the most demanding five year old child. Are they all bad for us? Some are very high in fat, but others are probably not as high as you might think, it comes down to the same argument about junk diets rather than junk foods. If you eat only crisps and chocolate for lunch, then your diet is very unbalanced. If you eat a low fat sandwich and some fruit for lunch, then a bag of crisps will not push most people's daily fat intake into the danger zone.

It is usually when we are 'grazing' that savoury snack foods pose the most danger. How many parties or buffets have you been to and eaten the equivalent of three bags of savoury snacks, especially if there are dips to be had! Some people have compared a bag of crisps to an apple, pointing out that the crisps have more fibre and as much Vitamin C as the apple. What is forgotten is that an apple contains less energy, no fat and no salt, and its fibre is of the soluble variety. We must also remember that it is very time consuming and filling to eat more than one apple at a time!

Some manufacturer's data has been used in this section.

[11] – KP Foods

[12] – Walkers Snack Foods

FOOD	Bombay Mix	Brannigans thick cut crisps[11]	Chipsticks all flavours[12]	Corn Snacks
PORTION SIZE	small bag	one bag	one bag	average bag (50g)
NUTRIENTS				
Energy (kcals)	151	187	107	260
Protein (g)	5.6	2.6	1.5	3.5
Total fat (g)	9.9	5.5	5.3	15.9
Saturated fat (g)	1.2	unknown	unknown	5.9
Mono-unsat. fat (g)	4.9	unknown	unknown	6.4
Poly-unsat. fat (g)	3.4	unknown	unknown	2.9
Carbohydrate (g)	10.5	18.9	13.4	27.1
Sugar (g)	0.7	unknown	unknown	2.3
Fibre (g)	1.9	unknown	unknown	0.5
Sodium (mg)	231	unknown	unknown	565
Potassium (mg)	231	unknown	unknown	100
Calcium (mg)	17	unknown	unknown	34
Magnesium (mg)	30	unknown	unknown	9
Phosphorus (mg)	87	unknown	unknown	70
Iron (mg)	1.14	unknown	unknown	0.4
Copper (mg)	0.19	unknown	unknown	0.02
Zinc (mg)	0.75	unknown	unknown	0.25
Selenium (μg)	unknown	unknown	unknown	2
Vitamin A (μg)	trace	unknown	unknown	38
Vitamin D (μg)	nil	unknown	unknown	nil
Vitamin E (mg)	1.41	unknown	unknown	2.9
Vitamin B_1 (mg)	0.11	unknown	unknown	0.09
Vitamin B_2 (mg)	0.03	unknown	unknown	0.08
Niacin (mg)	1.29	unknown	unknown	0.45
Vitamin B_6 (mg)	0.16	unknown	unknown	0.06
Vitamin B_{12} (μg)	nil	unknown	unknown	nil
Folate (μg)	unknown	unknown	unknown	25
Pantothenate (mg)	0.36	unknown	unknown	unknown
Biotin (μg)	7.2	unknown	unknown	unknown
Vitamin C (mg)	trace	unknown	unknown	trace

Crisps standard	Crisps 'jacket'	Crisps low fat	Crisps thick cut	FOOD
average bag (30g)	average bag	average bag	average bag	**PORTION SIZE**
				NUTRIENTS
159	153	137	150	Energy (kcals)
1.7	1.9	2.0	2.2	Protein (g)
10.3	9.7	6.4	8.4	Total fat (g)
4.2	4.0	2.8	3.5	Saturated fat (g)
4.1	3.9	2.6	3.4	Mono-unsat. fat (g)
1.5	1.4	0.8	1.2	Poly-unsat. fat (g)
16.0	15.4	19.0	17.4	Carbohydrate (g)
0.2	0.2	0.4	0.4	Sugar (g)
1.6	1.4	1.8	unknown	Fibre (g)
252	156	219	159	Sodium (mg)
282	387	306	432	Potassium (mg)
9	14	11	11	Calcium (mg)
12	15	14	19	Magnesium (mg)
33	42	39	36	Phosphorus (mg)
0.45	0.6	0.54	0.57	Iron (mg)
0.05	0.06	0.11	0.07	Copper (mg)
0.15	0.27	0.27	0.3	Zinc (mg)
unknown	unknown	unknown	unknown	Selenium (µg)
trace	trace	trace	trace	Vitamin A (µg)
nil	nil	nil	nil	Vitamin D (µg)
1.75	1.65	1.04	1.44	Vitamin E (mg)
0.06	0.06	0.06	0.08	Vitamin B_1 (mg)
0.02	0.04	0.04	0.03	Vitamin B_2 (mg)
0.96	1.53	1.5	1.2	Niacin (mg)
0.24	0.15	0.14	0.31	Vitamin B_6 (mg)
nil	nil	nil	nil	Vitamin B_{12} (µg)
11	21	14	14	Folate (µg)
0.28	0.31	unknown	0.35	Pantothenate (mg)
unknown	unknown	unknown	unknown	Biotin (µg)
2	6	4	trace	Vitamin C (mg)

FOOD	Doritos all flavours[9]	Frazzles[12]	Hula Hoops[11] average	McCoys thick & crunchy potato chips[11] average
PORTION SIZE	one bag	one bag	one bag	one bag
NUTRIENTS				
Energy (kcals)	177	108	155	206
Protein (g)	2.5	1.8	1.2	2.4
Total fat (g)	8.8	5.2	9.1	12.6
Saturated fat (g)	unknown	unknown	unknown	unknown
Mono-unsat. fat (g)	unknown	unknown	unknown	unknown
Poly-unsat. fat (g)	unknown	unknown	unknown	unknown
Carbohydrate (g)	22.2	13.6	16.8	13.6
Sugar (g)	unknown	unknown	unknown	unknown
Fibre (g)	unknown	unknown	unknown	unknown
Sodium (mg)	unknown	unknown	unknown	unknown
Potassium (mg)	unknown	unknown	unknown	unknown
Calcium (mg)	unknown	unknown	unknown	unknown
Magnesium (mg)	unknown	unknown	unknown	unknown
Phosphorus (mg)	unknown	unknown	unknown	unknown
Iron (mg)	unknown	unknown	unknown	unknown
Copper (mg)	unknown	unknown	unknown	unknown
Zinc (mg)	unknown	unknown	unknown	unknown
Selenium (µg)	unknown	unknown	unknown	unknown
Vitamin A (µg)	unknown	unknown	unknown	unknown
Vitamin D (µg)	unknown	unknown	unknown	unknown
Vitamin E (mg)	unknown	unknown	unknown	unknown
Vitamin B_1 (mg)	unknown	unknown	unknown	unknown
Vitamin B_2 (mg)	unknown	unknown	unknown	unknown
Niacin (mg)	unknown	unknown	unknown	unknown
Vitamin B_6 (mg)	unknown	unknown	unknown	unknown
Vitamin B_{12} (µg)	unknown	unknown	unknown	unknown
Folate (µg)	unknown	unknown	unknown	unknown
Pantothenate (mg)	unknown	unknown	unknown	unknown
Biotin (µg)	unknown	unknown	unknown	unknown
Vitamin C (mg)	unknown	unknown	unknown	unknown

Monster Munch[12] all except flamin' hot flavour	Pretzels	Potato hoops	Popcorn plain	FOOD
one bag	small bag	average bag	average bag	**PORTION SIZE**
				NUTRIENTS
123	114	157	148	Energy (kcals)
1.6	2.7	1.2	1.5	Protein (g)
6.3	1.0	9.6	10.7	Total fat (g)
unknown	0.2	unknown	1.1	Saturated fat (g)
unknown	0.4	unknown	3.6	Mono-unsat. fat (g)
unknown	0.4	unknown	4.9	Poly-unsat. fat (g)
15.1	23.8	17.5	12.2	Carbohydrate (g)
unknown	unknown	0.2	0.3	Sugar (g)
unknown	unknown	0.8	unknown	Fibre (g)
unknown	516	321	1	Sodium (mg)
unknown	45	162	55	Potassium (mg)
unknown	11	7	3	Calcium (mg)
unknown	11	8	20	Magnesium (mg)
unknown	33	30	43	Phosphorus (mg)
unknown	1.29	0.3	0.28	Iron (mg)
unknown	0.08	0.05	unknown	Copper (mg)
unknown	0.27	0.21	0.43	Zinc (mg)
unknown	unknown	unknown	1	Selenium (µg)
unknown	nil	trace	9	Vitamin A (µg)
unknown	nil	nil	nil	Vitamin D (µg)
unknown	unknown	unknown	2.76	Vitamin E (mg)
unknown	0.14	unknown	0.05	Vitamin B_1 (mg)
unknown	0.19	unknown	0.03	Vitamin B_2 (mg)
unknown	1.59	unknown	0.25	Niacin (mg)
unknown	0.04	unknown	0.05	Vitamin B_6 (mg)
unknown	nil	nil	nil	Vitamin B_{12} (µg)
unknown	unknown	unknown	2	Folate (µg)
unknown	0.09	unknown	0.08	Pantothenate (mg)
unknown	unknown	unknown	1.0	Biotin (µg)
unknown	nil	1	nil	Vitamin C (mg)

FOOD	Popcorn candied	Quavers[12] all flavours	Roysters Idaho chips[11] all flavours	Scampi Fries[12]
PORTION SIZE	average bag	one bag	one bag	one bag
NUTRIENTS				
Energy (kcals)	120	96	144	134
Protein (g)	0.5	0.5	1.8	3.5
Total fat (g)	5.0	6.4	8.8	7.0
Saturated fat (g)	0.5	unknown	unknown	unknown
Mono-unsat. fat (g)	1.7	unknown	unknown	unknown
Poly-unsat. fat (g)	2.3	unknown	unknown	unknown
Carbohydrate (g)	19.4	9.0	14.4	14.2
Sugar (g)	15.5	unknown	unknown	unknown
Fibre (g)	unknown	unknown	unknown	unknown
Sodium (mg)	14	unknown	unknown	unknown
Potassium (mg)	19	unknown	unknown	unknown
Calcium (mg)	2	unknown	unknown	unknown
Magnesium (mg)	7	unknown	unknown	unknown
Phosphorus (mg)	15	unknown	unknown	unknown
Iron (mg)	0.1	unknown	unknown	unknown
Copper (mg)	unknown	unknown	unknown	unknown
Zinc (mg)	0.17	unknown	unknown	unknown
Selenium (µg)	unknown	unknown	unknown	unknown
Vitamin A (µg)	17	unknown	unknown	unknown
Vitamin D (µg)	0.03	unknown	unknown	unknown
Vitamin E (mg)	0.94	unknown	unknown	unknown
Vitamin B_1 (mg)	0.01	unknown	unknown	unknown
Vitamin B_2 (mg)	0.01	unknown	unknown	unknown
Niacin (mg)	0.08	unknown	unknown	unknown
Vitamin B_6 (mg)	0.02	unknown	unknown	unknown
Vitamin B_{12} (µg)	nil	unknown	unknown	unknown
Folate (µg)	1	unknown	unknown	unknown
Pantotheate (mg)	0.03	unknown	unknown	unknown
Biotin (µg)	0.3	unknown	unknown	unknown
Vitamin C (mg)	nil	unknown	unknown	unknown

Skips[11]	Solo's[11] all flavours	Space Raiders[11] average of all flavours except hot and spicy	Tortilla chips	FOOD
one bag	one bag	one bag	average bag	**PORTION SIZE**
				NUTRIENTS
87	108	84	230	Energy (kcals)
0.7	1.6	1.2	3.8	Protein (g)
4.8	5.3	3.8	11.3	Total fat (g)
unknown	unknown	unknown	2.0	Saturated fat (g)
unknown	unknown	unknown	5.3	Mono-unsat. fat (g)
unknown	unknown	unknown	3.3	Poly-unsat. fat (g)
10.1	13.5	11.0	30.0	Carbohydrate (g)
unknown	unknown	unknown	0.6	Sugar (g)
unknown	unknown	unknown	3.0	Fibre (g)
unknown	unknown	unknown	430	Sodium (mg)
unknown	unknown	unknown	110	Potassium (mg)
unknown	unknown	unknown	75	Calcium (mg)
unknown	unknown	unknown	45	Magnesium (mg)
unknown	unknown	unknown	120	Phosphorus (mg)
unknown	unknown	unknown	0.8	Iron (mg)
unknown	unknown	unknown	0.05	Copper (mg)
unknown	unknown	unknown	0.6	Zinc (mg)
unknown	unknown	unknown	unknown	Selenium (µg)
unknown	unknown	unknown	38	Vitamin A (µg)
unknown	unknown	unknown	nil	Vitamin D (µg)
unknown	unknown	unknown	0.97	Vitamin E (mg)
unknown	unknown	unknown	0.09	Vitamin B_1 (mg)
unknown	unknown	unknown	0.05	Vitamin B_2 (mg)
unknown	unknown	unknown	0.9	Niacin (mg)
unknown	unknown	unknown	0.16	Vitamin B_6 (mg)
unknown	unknown	unknown	nil	Vitamin B_{12} (µg)
unknown	unknown	unknown	10	Folate (µg)
unknown	unknown	unknown	unknown	Pantothenate (mg)
unknown	unknown	unknown	unknown	Biotin (µg)
unknown	unknown	unknown	trace	Vitamin C (mg)

FOOD	Twiglets	Walkers crisps[12] average of all flavours
PORTION SIZE	small bag (25g)	one bag
NUTRIENTS		
Energy (kcals)	96	165
Protein (g)	2.8	1.8
Total fat (g)	2.9	11.4
Saturated fat (g)	1.2	unknown
Mono-unsat. fat (g)	1.1	unknown
Poly-unsat. fat (g)	0.4	unknown
Carbohydrate (g)	15.5	13.8
Sugar (g)	0.3	unknown
Fibre (g)	unknown	unknown
Sodium (mg)	335	unknown
Potassium (mg)	115	unknown
Calcium (mg)	11	unknown
Magnesium (mg)	20	unknown
Phosphorus (mg)	93	unknown
Iron (mg)	0.73	unknown
Copper (mg)	0.08	unknown
Zinc (mg)	0.5	unknown
Selenium (μg)	unknown	unknown
Vitamin A (μg)	trace	unknown
Vitamin D (μg)	nil	unknown
Vitamin E (mg)	0.62	unknown
Vitamin B_1 (mg)	0.09	unknown
Vitamin B_2 (mg)	0.12	unknown
Niacin (mg)	1.95	unknown
Vitamin B_6 (mg)	0.09	unknown
Vitamin B_{12} (μg)	nil	unknown
Folate (μg)	20	unknown
Pantotheate (mg)	0.38	unknown
Biotin (μg)	3.8	unknown
Vitamin C (mg)	trace	unknown

Fats and oils

The message about the amount of fats and oils we can include in a healthy diet, has become very confusing in the last few years, thanks to the proliferation of margarines, low-fat spreads and vegetable oils. We knew where we were with butter and lard, they were bad for us and should be replaced. However, their replacements are not always as safe or healthy as we thought, and also they are still fat, something we should eat less of. That is why all fats and oils appear in this section, even olive oil, savour of the Mediterranean heart.

So what should you cook your chips in, and how different are margarine, butter and low-fat spreads? All margarine has the same fat content as butter, unless it is labelled as being a low-fat spread, or is a light version of a standard brand. Only margarines which say they are, will be high in poly-unsaturated or mono-unsaturated fat. Most oils are high in poly-unsaturated fat but only olive oil and rapeseed oil are high in mono-unsaturated fat. The most important message is that whatever you use, be sparing with it, so avoid deep fat frying, and thickly spread butter or margarine. Also think about other sources of fat in your diet. If you do not eat a lot of red meat, cheese, pastry, biscuits and cakes, or foods with cream in, then the chances are that your fat intake will already be quite low. In this case, a little butter or an occasional fry up are well deserved treats.

The standard portion size for all spreads, unless otherwise stated, is the amount spread on one slice of bread and weighs 7g.

FOOD	Butter	Butter	Coconut oil	Corn oil
PORTION SIZE	10g	standard	tablespoon	tablespoon
NUTRIENTS				
Energy (kcals)	74	52	99	99
Protein (g)	0.1	trace	trace	trace
Total fat (g)	8.2	5.7	11.0	11.0
Saturated fat (g)	5.4	3.8	9.5	1.6
Mono-unsat. fat (g)	2.0	1.4	0.7	3.3
Poly-unsat. fat (g)	0.3	0.2	0.2	5.6
Carbohydrate (g)	trace	trace	nil	nil
Sugar (g)	trace	trace	nil	nil
Fibre (g)	nil	nil	nil	nil
Sodium (mg)	75	53	trace	trace
Potassium (mg)	2	1	trace	trace
Calcium (mg)	2	1	trace	trace
Magnesium (mg)	trace	trace	trace	trace
Phosphorus (mg)	2	2	trace	trace
Iron (mg)	0.02	0.01	trace	0.01
Copper (mg)	trace	trace	trace	trace
Zinc (mg)	0.01	0.01	trace	trace
Selenium (µg)	trace	trace	trace	trace
Vitamin A (µg)	89	62	trace	trace
Vitamin D (µg)	0.08	0.06	nil	nil
Vitamin E (mg)	0.2	0.14	0.07	1.9
Vitamin B_1 (mg)	trace	trace	trace	trace
Vitamin B_2 (mg)	trace	trace	trace	trace
Niacin (mg)	trace	trace	trace	trace
Vitamin B_6 (mg)	trace	trace	trace	trace
Vitamin B_{12} (µg)	trace	trace	nil	nil
Folate (µg)	trace	trace	trace	trace
Pantothenate (mg)	trace	trace	trace	trace
Biotin (µg)	trace	trace	trace	trace
Vitamin C (mg)	trace	nil	nil	nil

Hazelnut oil	Low-fat spread	Margarine hard	Margarine soft	FOOD
tablespoon	standard	standard	standard	PORTION SIZE
				NUTRIENTS
99	27	50	52	Energy (kcals)
trace	0.4	trace	trace	Protein (g)
11.0	2.8	5.5	5.7	Total fat (g)
0.9	0.8	2.4	1.9	Saturated fat (g)
8.4	1.2	2.5	2.7	Mono-unsat. fat (g)
1.2	0.7	0.3	0.9	Poly-unsat. fat (g)
nil	trace	0.07	0.1	Carbohydrate (g)
nil	trace	0.07	0.1	Sugar (g)
nil	nil	nil	nil	Fibre (g)
trace	46	65	62	Sodium (mg)
trace	8	0.7	trace	Potassium (mg)
trace	3	trace	trace	Calcium (mg)
trace	trace	trace	trace	Magnesium (mg)
trace	6	0.7	1	Phosphorus (mg)
trace	trace	0.02	0.02	Iron (mg)
trace	0.01	trace	trace	Copper (mg)
trace	0.01	trace	trace	Zinc (mg)
trace	unknown	unknown	unknown	Selenium (µg)
trace	75	55	57	Vitamin A (µg)
nil	0.56	0.55	0.55	Vitamin D (µg)
1.9	0.44	0.3	0.86	Vitamin E (mg)
trace	trace	trace	trace	Vitamin B_1 (mg)
trace	trace	trace	trace	Vitamin B_2 (mg)
trace	trace	trace	trace	Niacin (mg)
trace	trace	trace	trace	Vitamin B_6 (mg)
nil	trace	trace	trace	Vitamin B_{12} (µg)
trace	trace	trace	trace	Folate (µg)
trace	trace	trace	trace	Pantothenate (mg)
trace	trace	trace	trace	Biotin (µg)
nil	nil	nil	nil	Vitamin C (mg)

FOOD	Margarine poly-unsaturated soft	Olive oil spread	Olive oil	Peanut oil (groundnut)
PORTION SIZE	standard	standard	tablespoon	tablespoon
Nutrients				
Energy (kcals)	52	40	99	99
Protein (g)	trace	trace	trace	trace
Total fat (g)	5.8	4.4	11.0	11.0
Saturated fat (g)	1.2	0.8	1.6	2.1
Mono-unsat. fat (g)	1.9	2.5	8.0	5.3
Poly-unsat. fat (g)	2.5	0.9	0.9	3.1
Carbohydrate (g)	trace	0.1	nil	nil
Sugar (g)	trace	0.1	nil	nil
Fibre (g)	nil	nil	nil	nil
Sodium (mg)	48	42	trace	trace
Potassium (mg)	trace	unknown	trace	trace
Calcium (mg)	trace	unknown	trace	trace
Magnesium (mg)	trace	unknown	trace	trace
Phosphorus (mg)	1	unknown	trace	trace
Iron (mg)	0.02	unknown	0.04	trace
Copper (mg)	trace	unknown	trace	trace
Zinc (mg)	trace	unknown	trace	trace
Selenium (μg)	unknown	unknown	trace	trace
Vitamin A (μg)	51	nil	trace	trace
Vitamin D (μg)	0.55	unknown	nil	nil
Vitamin E (mg)	2.28	nil	0.56	1.67
Vitamin B_1 (mg)	trace	trace	trace	trace
Vitamin B_2 (mg)	trace	trace	trace	trace
Niacin (mg)	trace	trace	trace	trace
Vitamin B_6 (mg)	trace	trace	trace	trace
Vitamin B_{12} (μg)	trace	nil	nil	nil
Folate (μg)	trace	trace	trace	trace
Pantothenate (mg)	trace	trace	trace	trace
Biotin (μg)	trace	trace	trace	trace
Vitamin C (mg)	nil	nil	nil	nil

Rapeseed oil	Safflower oil	Sesame oil	Soya oil	FOOD
tablespoon	tablespoon	tablespoon	tablespoon	**PORTION SIZE**
				NUTRIENTS
99	99	99	99	Energy (kcals)
trace	trace	trace	trace	Protein (g)
11.0	11.0	11.0	11.0	Total fat (g)
0.7	1.1	1.6	1.7	Saturated fat (g)
6.5	1.3	4.1	2.3	Mono-unsat. fat (g)
3.2	8.1	4.8	6.5	Poly-unsat. fat (g)
nil	nil	nil	nil	Carbohydrate (g)
nil	nil	nil	nil	Sugar (g)
nil	nil	nil	nil	Fibre (g)
trace	trace	trace	trace	Sodium (mg)
trace	trace	2	trace	Potassium (mg)
trace	trace	1	trace	Calcium (mg)
trace	trace	trace	trace	Magnesium (mg)
trace	trace	trace	trace	Phosphorus (mg)
0.01	trace	0.01	0.01	Iron (mg)
trace	trace	trace	trace	Copper (mg)
trace	trace	trace	trace	Zinc (mg)
trace	trace	trace	trace	Selenium (µg)
trace	trace	trace	trace	Vitamin A (µg)
nil	nil	nil	nil	Vitamin D (µg)
2.44	4.47	unknown	1.77	Vitamin E (mg)
trace	trace	trace	trace	Vitamin B_1 (mg)
trace	trace	0.01	trace	Vitamin B_2 (mg)
trace	trace	0.01	trace	Niacin (mg)
trace	trace	trace	trace	Vitamin B_6 (mg)
nil	nil	nil	nil	Vitamin B_{12} (µg)
trace	trace	trace	trace	Folate (µg)
trace	trace	trace	trace	Pantothenate (mg)
trace	trace	trace	trace	Biotin (µg)
nil	nil	nil	nil	Vitamin C (mg)

FOOD	Sunflower oil	Vegetable oil	Walnut oil	Wheatgerm oil
PORTION SIZE	tablespoon	tablespoon	tablespoon	tablespoon
NUTRIENTS				
Energy (kcals)	99	99	99	99
Protein (g)	trace	trace	trace	trace
Total fat (g)	11.0	11.0	11.0	11.0
Saturated fat (g)	1.3	1.1	1.0	2.0
Mono-unsat. fat (g)	2.3	3.9	1.8	1.8
Poly-unsat. fat (g)	7.0	5.3	7.7	6.6
Carbohydrate (g)	nil	nil	nil	nil
Sugar (g)	nil	nil	nil	nil
Fibre (g)	nil	nil	nil	nil
Sodium (mg)	trace	trace	trace	trace
Potassium (mg)	trace	trace	trace	trace
Calcium (mg)	trace	trace	trace	trace
Magnesium (mg)	trace	trace	trace	trace
Phosphorus (mg)	trace	trace	trace	trace
Iron (mg)	0.01	trace	trace	trace
Copper (mg)	trace	trace	trace	trace
Zinc (mg)	trace	trace	trace	trace
Selenium (μg)	trace	trace	trace	trace
Vitamin A (μg)	trace	trace	trace	trace
Vitamin D (μg)	nil	nil	nil	nil
Vitamin E (mg)	5.41	nil	unknown	15.03
Vitamin B_1 (mg)	trace	trace	trace	trace
Vitamin B_2 (mg)	trace	trace	trace	trace
Niacin (mg)	trace	trace	trace	trace
Vitamin B_6 (mg)	trace	trace	trace	trace
Vitamin B_{12} (μg)	nil	nil	nil	nil
Folate (μg)	trace	trace	trace	trace
Pantothenate (mg)	trace	trace	trace	trace
Biotin (μg)	trace	trace	trace	trace
Vitamin C (mg)	nil	nil	nil	nil

Soups, sauces and savoury spreads

The reason this section has been included in the last segment, is partly because these are foods which do not fit in easily elsewhere. However, many are high in fat, a few are also high in sugar, and most contain a great deal of salt. All good reasons for using them sparingly. However, they all add interest and taste to our food and life would be very dull without them.

If you are watching your weight or have been advised to cut down on your salt intake, you would be well advised to study this section carefully. It is often the case that we eat these foods almost without realising, and forget that a blob of sauce here and a drizzle of mayo there can all add up to a lot of calories and salt.

FOOD	Bovril	Bread sauce	Brown sauce bottled	Cheese sauce made with full fat milk
PORTION SIZE	thin scraping on bread	average	sachet	medium
NUTRIENTS				
Energy (kcals)	2	50	12	122
Protein (g)	0.4	1.9	0.1	5.0
Total fat (g)	trace	2.3	nil	9.1
Saturated fat (g)	unknown	1.2	nil	4.7
Mono-unsat. fat (g)	unknown	0.7	nil	2.9
Poly-unsat. fat (g)	unknown	0.3	nil	1.1
Carbohydrate (g)	trace	5.7	3.0	5.6
Sugar (g)	nil	2.1	2.8	2.7
Fibre (g)	nil	0.1	0.1	0.1
Sodium (mg)	48	216	118	279
Potassium (mg)	12	63	47	93
Calcium (mg)	trace	54	5	149
Magnesium (mg)	1	7	3	11
Phosphorus (mg)	6	43	4	112
Iron (mg)	0.14	0.14	0.37	0.12
Copper (mg)	trace	0.01	0.04	0.01
Zinc (mg)	0.02	0.18	0.02	0.5
Selenium (µg)	unknown	3	unknown	2
Vitamin A (µg)	nil	28	1	104
Vitamin D (µg)	nil	0.07	nil	0.34
Vitamin E (mg)	unknown	0.09	unknown	0.42
Vitamin B_1 (mg)	0.09	0.02	0.02	0.03
Vitamin B_2 (mg)	0.07	0.06	0.01	0.14
Niacin (mg)	0.82	0.14	0.01	0.1
Vitamin B_6 (mg)	0.01	0.02	0.01	0.04
Vitamin B_{12} (µg)	0.1	0.1	nil	0.3
Folate (µg)	10	2	1	4
Pantothenate (mg)	unknown	0.12	unknown	0.19
Biotin (µg)	unknown	0.8	unknown	1.4
Vitamin C (mg)	nil	trace	trace	1

Chicken soup canned	Chutney mixed fruit	Cranberry sauce	Curry sauce canned	FOOD
one small can	one teaspoon	average	average	PORTION SIZE
				NUTRIENTS
174	16	45	117	Energy (kcals)
5.1	0.1	0.1	2.3	Protein (g)
11.4	trace	trace	7.5	Total fat (g)
1.8	trace	trace	unknown	Saturated fat (g)
6.0	trace	trace	unknown	Mono-unsat. fat (g)
3.0	trace	trace	unknown	Poly-unsat. fat (g)
13.5	4.0	12.0	10.6	Carbohydrate (g)
3.3	3.7	11.8	5.6	Sugar (g)
trace	unknown	unknown	unknown	Fibre (g)
1200	80	trace	1470	Sodium (mg)
123	21	12	270	Potassium (mg)
81	3	2	45	Calcium (mg)
15	1	1	27	Magnesium (mg)
81	2	2	47	Phosphorus (mg)
1.2	0.09	0.03	1.65	Iron (mg)
0.06	0.01	0.03	0.08	Copper (mg)
0.9	trace	trace	0.3	Zinc (mg)
trace	trace	trace	unknown	Selenium (μg)
125	1	unknown	unknown	Vitamin A (μg)
trace	nil	nil	nil	Vitamin D (μg)
1.65	unknown	unknown	unknown	Vitamin E (mg)
0.03	trace	0.01	trace	Vitamin B_1 (mg)
0.09	nil	0.01	0.04	Vitamin B_2 (mg)
0.6	0.07	0.03	0.15	Niacin (mg)
0.03	trace	trace	0.03	Vitamin B_6 (mg)
trace	nil	nil	nil	Vitamin B_{12} (μg)
3	trace	unknown	unknown	Folate (μg)
0.12	trace	unknown	unknown	Pantothenate (mg)
nil	trace	unknown	unknown	Biotin (μg)
nil	trace	trace	trace	Vitamin C (mg)

FOOD	Dressing blue cheese	Dressing French	Dressing Thousand island	Dressing yoghurt-based
PORTION SIZE	tablespoon	tablespoon	tablespoon	tablespoon
NUTRIENTS				
Energy (kcals)	114	69	97	88
Protein (g)	0.5	trace	0.3	0.7
Total fat (g)	11.6	7.4	9.1	8.3
Saturated fat (g)	unknown	unknown	unknown	unknown
Mono-unsat. fat (g)	unknown	unknown	unknown	unknown
Poly-unsat. fat (g)	unknown	unknown	unknown	unknown
Carbohydrate (g)	2.2	0.7	3.8	2.9
Sugar (g)	1.9	0.7	3.2	2.2
Fibre (g)	nil	nil	0.1	unknown
Sodium (mg)	278	69	270	195
Potassium (mg)	13	unknown	39	36
Calcium (mg)	15	unknown	7	17
Magnesium (mg)	2	unknown	3	2
Phosphorus (mg)	15	unknown	10	18
Iron (mg)	0.15	unknown	0.09	0.03
Copper (mg)	trace	unknown	0.02	trace
Zinc (mg)	0.1	unknown	0.06	0.09
Selenium (µg)	trace	unknown	trace	unknown
Vitamin A (µg)	13	nil	12	unknown
Vitamin D (µg)	0.05	nil	0.03	unknown
Vitamin E (mg)	1.48	unknown	2.43	unknown
Vitamin B_1 (mg)	trace	nil	trace	unknown
Vitamin B_2 (mg)	0.01	nil	0.01	unknown
Niacin (mg)	nil	nil	0.03	unknown
Vitamin B_6 (mg)	trace	nil	0.01	unknown
Vitamin B_{12} (µg)	nil	nil	nil	unknown
Folate (µg)	1	nil	1	unknown
Pantothenate (mg)	0.03	nil	0.03	unknown
Biotin (µg)	0.3	nil	0.3	unknown
Vitamin C (mg)	nil	nil	trace	trace

Dip sour cream	Gravy instant granules	Horseradish sauce	Hummus	FOOD
tablespoon	medium average	sachet	average	**PORTION SIZE**
				NUTRIENTS
108	17	18	112	Energy (kcals)
0.87	0.2	0.3	4.6	Protein (g)
11.1	1.2	1.0	7.6	Total fat (g)
unknown	unknown	0.1	unknown	Saturated fat (g)
unknown	unknown	0.5	unknown	Mono-unsat. fat (g)
unknown	unknown	0.4	unknown	Poly-unsat. fat (g)
1.2	1.5	2.1	7.0	Carbohydrate (g)
0.6	0.1	1.8	1.1	Sugar (g)
unknown	trace	0.3	1.4	Fibre (g)
99	230	109	402	Sodium (mg)
39	5	26	114	Potassium (mg)
21.6	1	5	25	Calcium (mg)
3	1	2	37	Magnesium (mg)
23.7	3	5	96	Phosphorus (mg)
0.12	trace	0.07	1.14	Iron (mg)
0.29	0.01	0.01	0.18	Copper (mg)
0.27	trace	0.05	0.84	Zinc (mg)
trace	unknown	unknown	unknown	Selenium (µg)
unknown	unknown	trace	unknown	Vitamin A (µg)
unknown	nil	trace	nil	Vitamin D (µg)
unknown	unknown	unknown	unknown	Vitamin E (mg)
unknown	unknown	unknown	0.1	Vitamin B_1 (mg)
unknown	unknown	unknown	0.03	Vitamin B_2 (mg)
unknown	unknown	unknown	0.66	Niacin (mg)
unknown	unknown	unknown	unknown	Vitamin B_6 (mg)
trace	nil	trace	nil	Vitamin B_{12} (µg)
unknown	nil	unknown	unknown	Folate (µg)
unknown	unknown	unknown	unknown	Pantothenate (mg)
unknown	unknown	unknown	unknown	Biotin (µg)
unknown	nil	trace	1	Vitamin C (mg)

FOOD	**Mango chutney**	**Marmite**	**Mayonnaise**	**Mayonnaise** low calorie
PORTION SIZE	teaspoon	thin scrape on bread	tablespoon	tablespoon
NUTRIENTS				
Energy (kcals)	19	2	207	86
Protein (g)	0.1	0.4	0.3	0.3
Total fat (g)	trace	trace	22.7	8.4
Saturated fat (g)	trace	unknown	3.3	unknown
Mono-unsat. fat (g)	trace	unknown	5.2	unknown
Poly-unsat. fat (g)	trace	unknown	13.2	unknown
Carbohydrate (g)	4.8	trace	0.5	2.5
Sugar (g)	4.6	nil	0.4	1.4
Fibre (g)	unknown	nil	nil	nil
Sodium (mg)	130	45	135	282
Potassium (mg)	4	26	5	unknown
Calcium (mg)	1	1	2	unknown
Magnesium (mg)	2	2	trace	unknown
Phosphorus (mg)	1	17	8	unknown
Iron (mg)	0.11	0.04	0.09	unknown
Copper (mg)	trace	trace	0.01	unknown
Zinc (mg)	trace	0.02	0.03	unknown
Selenium (µg)	unknown	unknown	unknown	unknown
Vitamin A (µg)	unknown	nil	31	unknown
Vitamin D (µg)	nil	nil	0.1	unknown
Vitamin E (mg)	unknown	unknown	5.68	unknown
Vitamin B_1 (mg)	nil	0.03	0.01	unknown
Vitamin B_2 (mg)	trace	0.11	0.02	unknown
Niacin (mg)	0.02	0.58	trace	unknown
Vitamin B_6 (mg)	unknown	0.01	trace	unknown
Vitamin B_{12} (µg)	nil	trace	0.2	unknown
Folate (µg)	unknown	10	1	unknown
Pantothenate (mg)	unknown	unknown	unknown	unknown
Biotin (µg)	unknown	unknown	unknown	unknown
Vitamin C (mg)	trace	nil	unknown	unknown

Mint sauce	Mushroom soup tinned	Mustard	Oxo cubes	FOOD
average	one small tin	teaspoon	one	**PORTION SIZE**
				NUTRIENTS
10	138	11	16	Energy (kcals)
0.2	3.3	0.6	2.7	Protein (g)
trace	9.0	0.7	0.2	Total fat (g)
trace	1.5	trace	unknown	Saturated fat (g)
trace	4.8	0.5	unknown	Mono-unsat. fat (g)
trace	2.7	0.1	unknown	Poly-unsat. fat (g)
2.2	11.7	0.8	0.8	Carbohydrate (g)
2.2	2.4	0.6	nil	Sugar (g)
unknown	0.3	unknown	nil	Fibre (g)
69	1410	236	721	Sodium (mg)
21	165	16	51	Potassium (mg)
12	90	6	13	Calcium (mg)
5	12	7	4	Magnesium (mg)
3	90	15	25	Phosphorus (mg)
0.74	0.9	0.23	1.72	Iron (mg)
0.03	0.12	0.02	0.05	Copper (mg)
0.02	0.9	0.08	unknown	Zinc (mg)
trace	3	unknown	unknown	Selenium (µg)
trace	128	unknown	nil	Vitamin A (µg)
nil	nil	nil	nil	Vitamin D (µg)
trace	1.62	unknown	unknown	Vitamin E (mg)
trace	trace	unknown	unknown	Vitamin B_1 (mg)
trace	0.15	unknown	unknown	Vitamin B_2 (mg)
trace	0.9	unknown	unknown	Niacin (mg)
trace	0.03	unknown	unknown	Vitamin B_6 (mg)
nil	trace	nil	unknown	Vitamin B_{12} (µg)
trace	6	nil	unknown	Folate (µg)
trace	0.3	unknown	unknown	Pantothenate (mg)
trace	3.0	unknown	unknown	Biotin (µg)
trace	nil	nil	nil	Vitamin C (mg)

FOOD	Oxtail soup tinned	Peanut butter smooth	Pesto sauce	Piccalilli
PORTION SIZE	one small tin	thickly spread on bread	tablespoon	teaspoon
NUTRIENTS				
Energy (kcals)	132	125	134	17
Protein (g)	7.2	4.5	5.3	0.2
Total fat (g)	5.1	10.7	12.4	0.1
Saturated fat (g)	1.8	2.3	3.3	trace
Mono-unsat. fat (g)	1.8	4.3	5.8	trace
Poly-unsat. fat (g)	0.6	3.7	2.6	0.1
Carbohydrate (g)	15.3	2.6	0.5	3.5
Sugar (g)	2.7	1.3	0.4	3.0
Fibre (g)	0.3	1.1	unknown	0.2
Sodium (mg)	1320	70	125	268
Potassium (mg)	279	140	65	8
Calcium (mg)	120	7	146	3
Magnesium (mg)	18	36	18	1
Phosphorus (mg)	111	66	125	3
Iron (mg)	3	0.42	0.62	0.12
Copper (mg)	0.12	0.14	0.1	0.01
Zinc (mg)	1.2	0.6	0.94	0.02
Selenium (µg)	trace	1	unknown	unknown
Vitamin A (µg)	nil	nil	67	unknown
Vitamin D (µg)	nil	nil	0.03	nil
Vitamin E (mg)	0.6	1.0	0.98	unknown
Vitamin B_1 (mg)	0.06	0.03	0.04	trace
Vitamin B_2 (mg)	0.09	0.02	0.07	trace
Niacin (mg)	2.1	2.5	0.23	0.02
Vitamin B_6 (mg)	0.09	0.12	unknown	trace
Vitamin B_{12} (µg)	nil	nil	0.2	nil
Folate (µg)	3	11	unknown	unknown
Pantothenate (mg)	0.15	0.31	unknown	unknown
Biotin (µg)	nil	18.8	unknown	trace
Vitamin C (mg)	nil	nil	1	trace

Pickle sweet	**Relish** chilli/tomato	**Relish** corn/onion/ cucumber	**Salad cream**	**FOOD**
one pack portion	average in a burger	average in a burger	tablespoon	**PORTION SIZE**
				NUTRIENTS
28	17	18	105	Energy (kcals)
0.1	0.2	0.2	0.5	Protein (g)
trace	trace	trace	9.2	Total fat (g)
trace	trace	trace	1.2	Saturated fat (g)
trace	trace	trace	1.75	Mono-unsat. fat (g)
trace	trace	trace	5.75	Poly-unsat. fat (g)
7.2	4.1	4.4	5	Carbohydrate (g)
6.8	3.8	3.8	5	Sugar (g)
0.2	0.2	0.2	unknown	Fibre (g)
322	72	51	312	Sodium (mg)
19	44	17	12	Potassium (mg)
3	2	2	5	Calcium (mg)
1	2	1	2.5	Magnesium (mg)
2	4	4	15	Phosphorus (mg)
0.12	0.05	0.05	0.12	Iron (mg)
trace	0.01	0.01	trace	Copper (mg)
0.02	0.02	0.03	0.1	Zinc (mg)
unknown	unknown	unknown	unknown	Selenium (µg)
8	unknown	unknown	2.5	Vitamin A (µg)
nil	nil	nil	0.05	Vitamin D (µg)
unknown	unknown	unknown	3.15	Vitamin E (mg)
0.01	0.01	unknown	unknown	Vitamin B_1 (mg)
trace	0.01	unknown	unknown	Vitamin B_2 (mg)
0.02	0.03	unknown	unknown	Niacin (mg)
trace	unknown	unknown	trace	Vitamin B_6 (mg)
nil	nil	nil	0.25	Vitamin B_{12} (µg)
trace	unknown	unknown	trace	Folate (µg)
unknown	unknown	unknown	unknown	Pantothenate (mg)
trace	unknown	unknown	unknown	Biotin (µg)
trace	unknown	unknown	nil	Vitamin C (mg)

FOOD	Salad cream low calorie	Soy sauce	Stock cube chicken	Sweet and sour sauce
PORTION SIZE	tablespoon	teaspoon	one	average
NUTRIENTS				
Energy (kcals)	57	4	21	66
Protein (g)	0.25	0.3	1.4	0.6
Total fat (g)	5.25	trace	1.4	0.2
Saturated fat (g)	0.75	unknown	unknown	0.2
Mono-unsat. fat (g)	1.5	unknown	unknown	nil
Poly-unsat. fat (g)	2.75	unknown	unknown	nil
Carbohydrate (g)	2.75	0.7	0.9	15.9
Sugar (g)	2.75	unknown	0.2	11.0
Fibre (g)	unknown	unknown	nil	unknown
Sodium (mg)	unknown	unknown	1467	585
Potassium (mg)	unknown	14	36	140
Calcium (mg)	unknown	4	11	15
Magnesium (mg)	unknown	unknown	4	9
Phosphorus (mg)	unknown	unknown	18	15
Iron (mg)	unknown	0.22	0.44	0.75
Copper (mg)	unknown	unknown	0.01	0.03
Zinc (mg)	unknown	unknown	0.11	0.15
Selenium (µg)	unknown	unknown	unknown	unknown
Vitamin A (µg)	unknown	nil	unknown	unknown
Vitamin D (µg)	unknown	nil	nil	nil
Vitamin E (mg)	unknown	unknown	unknown	unknown
Vitamin B_1 (mg)	unknown	0.01	unknown	0.16
Vitamin B_2 (mg)	unknown	unknown	unknown	trace
Niacin (mg)	unknown	0.06	unknown	nil
Vitamin B_6 (mg)	unknown	unknown	unknown	unknown
Vitamin B_{12} (µg)	unknown	nil	unknown	nil
Folate (µg)	unknown	unknown	unknown	unknown
Pantothenate (mg)	unknown	unknown	unknown	unknown
Biotin (µg)	unknown	unknown	unknown	unknown
Vitamin C (mg)	nil	nil	nil	unknown

Tahini paste	Tartare sauce	Tomato ketchup	Tomato soup cream of, tinned	FOOD
heaped teaspoon	sachet	sachet	one small tin	PORTION SIZE
				NUTRIENTS
115	36	14	156	Energy (kcals)
3.5	0.2	0.2	2.4	Protein (g)
11.2	3.0	trace	9.0	Total fat (g)
1.6	unknown	trace	1.5	Saturated fat (g)
4.2	unknown	trace	4.8	Mono-unsat. fat (g)
4.9	unknown	trace	2.4	Poly-unsat. fat (g)
0.2	2.1	3.4	17.7	Carbohydrate (g)
0.1	1.9	3.3	7.8	Sugar (g)
1.5	trace	0.1	2.1	Fibre (g)
4	96	196	1200	Sodium (mg)
110	5	42	570	Potassium (mg)
129	2	2	51	Calcium (mg)
72	2	2	24	Magnesium (mg)
139	4	4	60	Phosphorus (mg)
2.01	0.06	0.04	1.2	Iron (mg)
0.28	trace	0.01	0.18	Copper (mg)
1.03	0.04	0.01	0.6	Zinc (mg)
unknown	trace	unknown	trace	Selenium (µg)
1	6	4	225	Vitamin A (µg)
nil	0.02	nil	nil	Vitamin D (µg)
0.49	1.21	unknown	4.2	Vitamin E (mg)
0.18	trace	0.12	0.09	Vitamin B_1 (mg)
0.03	trace	0.01	0.06	Vitamin B_2 (mg)
0.97	trace	0.25	1.5	Niacin (mg)
0.14	trace	trace	0.18	Vitamin B_6 (mg)
nil	nil	nil	trace	Vitamin B_{12} (µg)
19	trace	trace	36	Folate (µg)
0.41	0.01	unknown	0.36	Pantothenate (mg)
2.1	0.1	unknown	3.0	Biotin (µg)
nil	trace	trace	trace	Vitamin C (mg)

FOOD	**Vegetable soup** tinned	**Vinegar**
PORTION SIZE	one small tin	teaspoon
NUTRIENTS		
Energy (kcals)	144	1
Protein (g)	4.2	trace
Total fat (g)	1.8	nil
Saturated fat (g)	unknown	nil
Mono-unsat. fat (g)	unknown	nil
Poly-unsat. fat (g)	unknown	nil
Carbohydrate (g)	29.7	trace
Sugar (g)	15.3	trace
Fibre (g)	4.5	nil
Sodium (mg)	1290	trace
Potassium (mg)	330	2
Calcium (mg)	36	trace
Magnesium (mg)	24	trace
Phosphorus (mg)	87	1
Iron (mg)	1.2	trace
Copper (mg)	0.12	trace
Zinc (mg)	0.6	trace
Selenium (µg)	unknown	trace
Vitamin A (µg)	9	nil
Vitamin D (µg)	nil	nil
Vitamin E (mg)	unknown	nil
Vitamin B_1 (mg)	0.27	nil
Vitamin B_2 (mg)	0.06	nil
Niacin (mg)	7.5	nil
Vitamin B_6 (mg)	0.03	nil
Vitamin B_{12} (µg)	nil	nil
Folate (µg)	30	nil
Pantothenate (mg)	unknown	nil
Biotin (µg)	unknown	nil
Vitamin C (mg)	trace	nil

Beverages

This last section is difficult to place within the plate model, because that really applies to food. However, beverages can be just as high in fat and/or sugar, and so this seemed like an obvious place for them to go. The section is divided up into alcoholic beverages, cold beverages and hot beverages. Alcoholic beverages are a part of most people's social life, but it is important to remember that a healthy diet should be part of a healthy lifestyle, and this includes following the Health Education Authority guidelines on alcohol. The recommendation is no more than three or four alcoholic beverages daily for men and two to three for women. It is also better to have a small amount of alcohol regularly, than to abstain on most nights and have a binge on Friday or Saturday night. The alcoholic content of all appropriate beverages is listed where the fibre content normally appears.

With regard to other beverages, apart from tea, coffee and cocoa, to which you add your own sugar, many hot or cold non-alcoholic beverages contain substantial amounts of sugar. This sugar is not always of the added variety, but can be a natural part of the beverage, for example in fruit juice. However, it is still sugar and can have as much effect on children's teeth as squash, particularly as fruit juice is often highly acidic. Whatever you give your children to drink, make sure they clean their teeth regularly.

BEVERAGE	**Barley wine**	**Beer** bitter draught	**Beer** bitter premium	**Brown ale**
PORTION SIZE	one small bottle	one pint	one pint	one small bottle
NUTRIENTS				
Energy (kcals)	119	172	189	90
Protein (g)	1.3	1.7	1.7	0.9
Total fat (g)	trace	trace	trace	trace
Saturated fat (g)	trace	trace	trace	trace
Mono-unsat. fat (g)	trace	trace	trace	trace
Poly-unsat. fat (g)	trace	trace	trace	trace
Carbohydrate (g)	11.0	12.6	12.6	9.0
Sugar (g)	11.0	12.6	12.6	9.0
Alcohol (g)	10.3	16.6	19.5	7.5
Sodium (mg)	27	34	46	48
Potassium (mg)	198	184	264	99
Calcium (mg)	25	46	52	21
Magnesium (mg)	36	40	46	18
Phosphorus (mg)	72	80	92	33
Iron (mg)	nil	0.57	trace	nil
Copper (mg)	0.14	0.06	0.17	0.21
Zinc (mg)	trace	0.57	0.57	0.9
Selenium (µg)	trace	trace	trace	trace
Vitamin A (µg)	trace	trace	trace	trace
Vitamin D (µg)	nil	nil	nil	nil
Vitamin E (mg)	unknown	unknown	unknown	unknown
Vitamin B_1 (mg)	trace	trace	trace	trace
Vitamin B_2 (mg)	0.11	0.17	0.23	0.06
Niacin (mg)	1.44	1.15	4.59	0.9
Vitamin B_6 (mg)	0.07	0.4	0.52	0.03
Vitamin B_{12} (µg)	trace	trace	trace	trace
Folate (µg)	16	17	46	12
Pantothenate (mg)	unknown	57.4	0.4	0.3
Biotin (µg)	unknown	5.7	5.7	3.0
Vitamin C (mg)	nil	nil	nil	nil

Cider dry	Cider sweet	Cider vintage	Lager ordinary	BEVERAGE
one pint	one pint	one pint	one pint	PORTION SIZE
				NUTRIENTS
207	241	580	166	Energy (kcals)
trace	trace	trace	1.7	Protein (g)
nil	nil	nil	trace	Total fat (g)
nil	nil	nil	trace	Saturated fat (g)
nil	nil	nil	trace	Mono-unsat. fat (g)
nil	nil	nil	trace	Poly-unsat. fat (g)
14.9	24.7	41.9	trace	Carbohydrate (g)
14.9	24.7	41.9	trace	Sugar (g)
21.8	21.2	60.3	22.9	Alcohol (g)
40	40	11	40	Sodium (mg)
413	413	557	224	Potassium (mg)
46	46	29	29	Calcium (mg)
17	17	23	40	Magnesium (mg)
17	17	52	109	Phosphorus (mg)
2.87	2.87	1.72	trace	Iron (mg)
0.23	0.23	0.11	trace	Copper (mg)
trace	trace	trace	trace	Zinc (mg)
trace	trace	trace	trace	Selenium (µg)
trace	trace	trace	trace	Vitamin A (µg)
nil	nil	nil	nil	Vitamin D (µg)
unknown	unknown	unknown	unknown	Vitamin E (mg)
trace	trace	trace	trace	Vitamin B_1 (mg)
trace	trace	trace	0.23	Vitamin B_2 (mg)
nil	nil	nil	4.02	Niacin (mg)
0.06	0.06	0.06	0.34	Vitamin B_6 (mg)
trace	trace	trace	trace	Vitamin B_{12} (µg)
unknown	unknown	unknown	69	Folate (µg)
0.23	0.17	0.17	0.17	Pantothenate (mg)
5.7	5.7	5.7	5.7	Biotin (µg)
nil	nil	nil	nil	Vitamin C (mg)

BEVERAGE	Lager premium	Lager low alcohol	Liqueurs cream	Liqueurs low-medium strength
PORTION SIZE	one pint	one pint	one measure	one measure
NUTRIENTS				
Energy (kcals)	339	57	81	66
Protein (g)	1.7	1.1	trace	trace
Total fat (g)	trace	trace	4.0	nil
Saturated fat (g)	trace	trace	unknown	nil
Mono-unsaturated fat (g)	trace	trace	unknown	nil
Poly-unsaturated fat (g)	trace	trace	unknown	nil
Carbohydrate (g)	13.8	8.6	5.7	8.2
Sugar (g)	13.8	5.7	5.7	8.2
Alcohol (g)	39.6	2.8	3.3	4.9
Sodium (mg)	40	69	22	3
Potassium (mg)	224	321	5	9
Calcium (mg)	29	46	5	1
Magnesium (mg)	40	69	1	1
Phosphorus (mg)	109	57	10	2
Iron (mg)	trace	trace	0.03	0.03
Copper (mg)	trace	trace	trace	trace
Zinc (mg)	trace	trace	0.05	trace
Selenium (µg)	trace	trace	trace	unknown
Vitamin A (µg)	trace	trace	52	trace
Vitamin D (µg)	nil	nil	trace	nil
Vitamin E (mg)	unknown	unknown	0.14	nil
Vitamin B_1 (mg)	trace	trace	unknown	trace
Vitamin B_2 (mg)	0.23	0.11	unknown	trace
Niacin (mg)	4.02	2.87	unknown	trace
Vitamin B_6 (mg)	0.34	0.17	unknown	trace
Vitamin B_{12} (µg)	trace	trace	nil	trace
Folate (µg)	69	34	trace	trace
Pantothenate (mg)	0.17	0.4	unknown	trace
Biotin (µg)	5.7	trace	unknown	trace
Vitamin C (mg)	nil	nil	nil	nil

Liqueurs high strength	Port	Shandy half bitter, half lemonade	Sherry dry	BEVERAGE
one measure	small glass	one pint	small glass	PORTION SIZE
				NUTRIENTS
79	79	149	58	Energy (kcals)
trace	0.1	1.1	0.1	Protein (g)
nil	nil	nil	nil	Total fat (g)
nil	nil	nil	nil	Saturated fat (g)
nil	nil	nil	nil	Mono-unsat. fat (g)
nil	nil	nil	nil	Poly-unsat. fat (g)
6.1	6.0	16.6	0.7	Carbohydrate (g)
6.1	6.0	16.6	0.7	Sugar (g)
7.9	7.9	11.5	7.8	Alcohol (g)
2	2	40	5	Sodium (mg)
1	49	155	29	Potassium (mg)
trace	2	29	4	Calcium (mg)
trace	6	23	7	Magnesium (mg)
trace	6	6	6	Phosphorus (mg)
trace	0.2	trace	0.2	Iron (mg)
trace	0.05	trace	0.01	Copper (mg)
trace	unknown	trace	unknown	Zinc (mg)
trace	trace	trace	trace	Selenium (µg)
trace	trace	trace	trace	Vitamin A (µg)
nil	nil	nil	nil	Vitamin D (µg)
nil	nil	unknown	nil	Vitamin E (mg)
trace	trace	trace	trace	Vitamin B_1 (mg)
trace	trace	0.11	trace	Vitamin B_2 (mg)
trace	0.05	1.72	0.05	Niacin (mg)
trace	trace	0.17	trace	Vitamin B_6 (mg)
trace	trace	trace	trace	Vitamin B_{12} (µg)
trace	trace	34	trace	Folate (µg)
trace	unknown	0.11	unknown	Pantothenate (mg)
trace	unknown	trace	unknown	Biotin (µg)
nil	nil	nil	nil	Vitamin C (mg)

BEVERAGE	**Sherry** medium	**Sherry** sweet	**Spirits** 40%	**Spirits** 40%
PORTION SIZE	one measure	one measure	one measure (England) (23g)	one measure (Scotland) (27g)
NUTRIENTS				
Energy (kcals)	58	68	51	60
Protein (g)	0.1	0.2	trace	trace
Total fat (g)	nil	nil	nil	nil
Saturated fat (g)	nil	nil	nil	nil
Mono-unsat. fat (g)	nil	nil	nil	nil
Poly-unsat. fat (g)	nil	nil	nil	nil
Carbohydrate (g)	3.0	3.5	trace	trace
Sugar (g)	3.0	3.5	trace	trace
Alcohol (g)	6.6	7.8	7.3	8.5
Sodium (mg)	14	7	trace	trace
Potassium (mg)	228	55	trace	trace
Calcium (mg)	4	4	trace	trace
Magnesium (mg)	3	6	trace	trace
Phosphorus (mg)	12	5	trace	trace
Iron (mg)	0.2	0.2	trace	trace
Copper (mg)	0.02	0.05	trace	trace
Zinc (mg)	trace	unknown	trace	trace
Selenium (µg)	trace	trace	trace	trace
Vitamin A (µg)	trace	trace	nil	nil
Vitamin D (µg)	nil	nil	nil	nil
Vitamin E (mg)	nil	nil	nil	nil
Vitamin B_1 (mg)	trace	trace	nil	nil
Vitamin B_2 (mg)	trace	trace	nil	nil
Niacin (mg)	0.05	0.05	nil	nil
Vitamin B_6 (mg)	0.01	trace	nil	nil
Vitamin B_{12} (µg)	trace	trace	nil	nil
Folate (µg)	trace	trace	nil	nil
Pantothenate (mg)	0.01	unknown	nil	nil
Biotin (µg)	0.5	unknown	nil	nil
Vitamin C (mg)	nil	nil	nil	nil

Stout	Champagne	Wine, rosé medium	Wine, red	BEVERAGE
one pint	one wine glass	one wine glass	one wine glass	PORTION SIZE
				NUTRIENTS
172	95	89	85	Energy (kcals)
2.3	0.4	0.1	0.1	Protein (g)
trace	nil	nil	nil	Total fat (g)
trace	nil	nil	nil	Saturated fat (g)
trace	nil	nil	nil	Mono-unsat. fat (g)
trace	nil	nil	nil	Poly-unsat. fat (g)
8.6	1.8	3.1	0.3	Carbohydrate (g)
8.6	1.8	3.1	0.3	Sugar (g)
18.9	12.4	10.8	12	Alcohol (g)
34	5	5	9	Sodium (mg)
276	71	94	138	Potassium (mg)
23	4	15	9	Calcium (mg)
46	8	9	14	Magnesium (mg)
149	9	8	16	Phosphorus (mg)
1.15	0.63	1.25	1.13	Iron (mg)
trace	0.01	0.02	0.07	Copper (mg)
trace	trace	trace	0.13	Zinc (mg)
trace	trace	trace	trace	Selenium (µg)
trace	trace	trace	trace	Vitamin A (µg)
nil	nil	nil	nil	Vitamin D (µg)
unknown	unknown	unknown	unknown	Vitamin E (mg)
trace	trace	trace	trace	Vitamin B_1 (mg)
0.17	0.01	0.01	0.02	Vitamin B_2 (mg)
4.59	0.13	0.13	0.13	Niacin (mg)
0.46	0.02	0.02	0.04	Vitamin B_6 (mg)
trace	trace	trace	trace	Vitamin B_{12} (µg)
34	trace	trace	1	Folate (µg)
0.23	0.04	0.05	0.05	Pantothenate (mg)
5.7	unknown	unknown	2.5	Biotin (µg)
nil	nil	nil	nil	Vitamin C (mg)

BEVERAGE	**Wine, sparkling** white	**Wine, white** dry	**Wine, white** medium	**Wine, white** sweet
PORTION SIZE	one wine glass	one wine glass	one wine glass	one wine glass
NUTRIENTS				
Energy (kcals)	93	83	93	118
Protein (g)	0.4	0.1	0.1	0.3
Total fat (g)	nil	nil	nil	nil
Saturated fat (g)	nil	nil	nil	nil
Mono-unsat. fat (g)	nil	nil	nil	nil
Poly-unsat. fat (g)	nil	nil	nil	nil
Carbohydrate (g)	6.4	0.8	3.8	7.4
Sugar (g)	6.4	0.8	3.8	7.4
Alcohol (g)	9.5	11.3	11.1	12.7
Sodium (mg)	6	5	14	16
Potassium (mg)	73	76	101	138
Calcium (mg)	11	11	15	18
Magnesium (mg)	9	10	10	14
Phosphorus (mg)	11	8	10	16
Iron (mg)	0.63	0.63	1.0	0.75
Copper (mg)	0.01	0.01	trace	0.06
Zinc (mg)	trace	trace	trace	trace
Selenium (µg)	trace	trace	trace	trace
Vitamin A (µg)	trace	trace	trace	trace
Vitamin D (µg)	nil	nil	nil	nil
Vitamin E (mg)	unknown	unknown	unknown	unknown
Vitamin B_1 (mg)	trace	trace	trace	trace
Vitamin B_2 (mg)	0.01	0.01	trace	0.01
Niacin (mg)	0.13	0.13	0.13	0.13
Vitamin B_6 (mg)	0.02	0.02	0.01	0.01
Vitamin B_{12} (µg)	trace	trace	trace	trace
Folate (µg)	trace	trace	trace	trace
Pantothenate (mg)	0.05	0.04	0.07	0.04
Biotin (µg)	1.3	unknown	1.3	unknown
Vitamin C (mg)	nil	nil	nil	nil

Apple juice	Blackcurrant drink concentrate	Blackcurrant drink ready to drink	Coca-Cola	BEVERAGE
one small glass	one tumbler	one carton	one standard can	PORTION SIZE
				NUTRIENTS
61	90	79	129	Energy (kcals)
0.2	trace	trace	trace	Protein (g)
0.2	nil	nil	nil	Total fat (g)
trace	nil	nil	nil	Saturated fat (g)
trace	nil	nil	nil	Mono-unsat. fat (g)
0.2	nil	nil	nil	Poly-unsat. fat (g)
15.8	24	21.0	34.7	Carbohydrate (g)
15.8	23.4	20.5	34.7	Sugar (g)
trace	nil	nil	nil	Fibre (g)
3	6	5	26	Sodium (mg)
176	36	32	3	Potassium (mg)
11	3	3	13	Calcium (mg)
8	tracc	trace	3	Magnesium (mg)
10	trace	trace	50	Phosphorous (mg)
0.16	trace	trace	trace	Iron (mg)
trace	trace	trace	0.1	Copper (mg)
trace	trace	trace	trace	Zinc (mg)
trace	trace	nil	trace	Selenium (µg)
trace	unknown	unknown	nil	Vitamin A (µg)
nil	nil	nil	nil	Vitamin D (µg)
trace	unknown	unknown	nil	Vitamin E (mg)
0.02	trace	nil	nil	Vitamin B_1 (mg)
0.02	trace	nil	nil	Vitamin B_2 (mg)
0.16	3.0	2.6	nil	Niacin (mg)
0.03	0.39	0.34	nil	Vitamin B_6 (mg)
nil	nil	nil	nil	Vitamin B_{12} (µg)
6	nil	nil	nil	Folate (µg)
0.06	nil	nil	nil	Pantothenate (mg)
1.3	nil	nil	nil	Biotin (µg)
22	30.	26	nil	Vitamin C (mg)

BEVERAGE	Cream soda	Fruit juice drink carbonated	Fruit juice drink ready to drink	Ginger ale dry
PORTION SIZE	one standard can	one standard can	one carton	one mixer bottle
NUTRIENTS				
Energy (kcals)	168	129	74	17
Protein (g)	nil	trace	0.2	nil
Total fat (g)	nil	trace	trace	nil
Saturated fat (g)	nil	trace	trace	nil
Mono-unsat. fat (g)	nil	trace	trace	nil
Poly-unsat. fat (g)	nil	trace	trace	nil
Carbohydrate (g)	43.9	34.0	19.6	4.3
Sugar (g)	unknown	34.0	19.6	4.3
Fibre (g)	nil	nil	trace	nil
Sodium (mg)	40	26	10	unknown
Potassium (mg)	3	89	88	unknown
Calcium (mg)	17	23	12	unknown
Magnesium (mg)	3	23	6	unknown
Phosphorous (mg)	nil	7	4	unknown
Iron (mg)	0.33	trace	trace	unknown
Copper (mg)	trace	trace	trace	unknown
Zinc (mg)	trace	trace	trace	unknown
Selenium (µg)	trace	trace	trace	trace
Vitamin A (µg)	nil	51	unknown	nil
Vitamin D (µg)	nil	nil	nil	nil
Vitamin E (mg)	nil	trace	unknown	nil
Vitamin B_1 (mg)	nil	trace	trace	nil
Vitamin B_2 (mg)	nil	trace	trace	nil
Niacin (mg)	nil	trace	0.2	nil
Vitamin B_6 (mg)	nil	trace	0.02	nil
Vitamin B_{12} (µg)	nil	nil	nil	nil
Folate (µg)	nil	3	4	nil
Pantothenate (mg)	nil	trace	trace	nil
Biotin (µg)	nil	trace	trace	nil
Vitamin C (mg)	nil	3	46	nil

Grapefruit juice unsweetened	**Lemonade**	**Lime juice cordial** concentrate	**Lucozade**	**BEVERAGE**
one small glass	one standard can	one tumbler	one small can	**PORTION SIZE**
				NUTRIENTS
53	73	56	150	Energy (kcals)
0.6	trace	0.1	trace	Protein (g)
0.2	nil	nil	nil	Total fat (g)
trace	nil	nil	nil	Saturated fat (g)
trace	nil	nil	nil	Mono-unsat. fat (g)
trace	nil	nil	nil	Poly-unsat. fat (g)
13.3	19.1	14.9	40.0	Carbohydrate (g)
13.3	19.1	14.9	35.8	Sugar (g)
trace	nil	nil	nil	Fibre (g)
11	23	4	20	Sodium (mg)
160	50	25	68	Potassium (mg)
22	17	5	18	Calcium (mg)
13	3	2	18	Magnesium (mg)
18	trace	3	5	Phosphorus (mg)
0.32	trace	0.15	trace	Iron (mg)
0.02	trace	0.04	trace	Copper (mg)
trace	trace	unknown	trace	Zinc (mg)
2	trace	trace	trace	Selenium (µg)
0.3	trace	trace	348	Vitamin A (µg)
nil	nil	nil	nil	Vitamin D (µg)
0.3	trace	trace	nil	Vitamin E (mg)
0.06	trace	trace	trace	Vitamin B_1 (mg)
0.02	trace	trace	trace	Vitamin B_2 (mg)
0.32	trace	trace	trace	Niacin (mg)
0.03	trace	trace	trace	Vitamin B_6 (mg)
nil	nil	nil	nil	Vitamin B_{12} (µg)
10	trace	trace	trace	Folate (µg)
0.13	trace	trace	trace	Pantothenate (mg)
1.6	trace	trace	trace	Biotin (µg)
50	nil	trace	20	Vitamin C (mg)

BEVERAGE	**Mango juice** canned	**Orange squash** concentrate	**Orange juice** unsweetened	**Pineapple juice** unsweetened
PORTION SIZE	one small glass	one tumbler	one small glass	one small glass
NUTRIENTS				
Energy (kcals)	62	93	58	66
Protein (g)	0.2	1.5	0.8	0.5
Total fat (g)	0.4	0.3	0.2	0.2
Saturated fat (g)	trace	0.1	trace	trace
Mono-unsat. fat (g)	0.2	0.1	trace	trace
Poly-unsat. fat (g)	0.2	0.1	trace	trace
Carbohydrate (g)	15.7	22.5	14.1	16.8
Sugar (g)	15.4	22.5	14.1	16.8
Fibre (g)	trace	trace	0.2	trace
Sodium (mg)	14	5	16	13
Potassium (mg)	29	440	240	85
Calcium (mg)	3	18	16	13
Magnesium (mg)	unknown	23	13	10
Phosphorus (mg)	35	42	21	2
Iron (mg)	2.4	0.2	0.32	0.32
Copper (mg)	unknown	0.05	trace	0.03
Zinc (mg)	unknown	0.1	trace	0.16
Selenium (µg)	unknown	3	2	trace
Vitamin A (µg)	56	14	4.5	2
Vitamin D (µg)	nil	nil	nil	nil
Vitamin E (mg)	1.68	0.34	0.27	0.05
Vitamin B_1 (mg)	0.02	0.16	0.13	0.1
Vitamin B_2 (mg)	0.02	0.06	0.03	0.02
Niacin (mg)	0.8	0.65	0.32	0.16
Vitamin B_6 (mg)	unknown	0.13	0.11	0.08
Vitamin B_{12} (µg)	nil	nil	nil	nil
Folate (µg)	unknown	45	32	13
Pantothenate (mg)	unknown	0.37	0.21	0.11
Biotin (µg)	unknown	2.7	1.6	trace
Vitamin C (mg)	40	105	62	18

Root beer	Tomato juice	Tonic water	BEVERAGE
one standard can	one small glass	one mixer bottle	**PORTION SIZE**
			NUTRIENTS
135	22	36	Energy (kcals)
nil	1.3	nil	Protein (g)
nil	trace	nil	Total fat (g)
nil	trace	nil	Saturated fat (g)
nil	trace	nil	Mono-unsat. fat (g)
nil	trace	nil	Poly-unsat. fat (g)
35	4.8	9.7	Carbohydrate (g)
35	4.8	unknown	Sugar (g)
nil	1.0	nil	Fibre (g)
13	368	4	Sodium (mg)
3	368	nil	Potassium (mg)
17	16	1	Calcium (mg)
3	16	nil	Magnesium (mg)
nil	30	nil	Phosphorus (mg)
0.33	0.64	trace	Iron (mg)
0.03	0.1	trace	Copper (mg)
0.33	0.16	trace	Zinc (mg)
trace	trace	trace	Selenium (µg)
nil	53	nil	Vitamin A (µg)
nil	nil	nil	Vitamin D (µg)
nil	1.62	nil	Vitamin E (mg)
nil	0.03	nil	Vitamin B_1 (mg)
nil	0.03	nil	Vitamin B_2 (mg)
nil	1.12	nil	Niacin (mg)
nil	0.1	nil	Vitamin B_6 (mg)
nil	nil	nil	Vitamin B_{12} (µg)
nil	16	nil	Folate (µg)
nil	0.32	nil	Pantothenate (mg)
nil	2.4	nil	Biotin (µg)
nil	13	nil	Vitamin C (mg)

BEVERAGE	**Cocoa** made with whole milk (no sugar)	**Coffee** infusion with added full-cream milk (no sugar)	**Drinking chocolate** with milk (full cream) (no sugar)	**Horlicks** made only with milk (full cream) (no sugar)
PORTION SIZE	one mug	one mug	one mug	one mug
NUTRIENTS				
Energy (kcals)	198	18	234	257
Protein (g)	8.8	1.3	8.8	10.9
Total fat (g)	10.9	1.0	10.7	10.1
Saturated fat (g)	6.8	0.8	6.5	unknown
Mono-unsat. fat (g)	3.1	0.3	3.1	unknown
Poly-unsat. fat (g)	0.3	trace	0.3	unknown
Carbohydrate (g)	17.7	1.3	27.6	33
Sugar (g)	17.2	1.3	26.8	26
Fibre (g)	unknown	nil	unknown	unknown
Sodium (mg)	182	16	182	255
Potassium (mg)	416	252	416	520
Calcium (mg)	286	39	286	390
Magnesium (mg)	52	21	57	39
Phosphorus (mg)	260	42	257	286
Iron (mg)	0.52	0.26	0.52	0.52
Copper (mg)	0.18	trace	0.23	0.08
Zinc (mg)	1.3	0.26	1.3	1.3
Selenium (µg)	unknown	trace	unknown	unknown
Vitamin A (µg)	138	17	122	306
Vitamin D (µg)	0.08	trace	0.08	0.65
Vitamin E (mg)	0.21	0.03	0.21	unknown
Vitamin B_1 (mg)	0.1	trace	0.1	0.36
Vitamin B_2 (mg)	0.39	0.08	0.36	0.73
Niacin (mg)	0.26	1.56	0.26	4.42
Vitamin B_6 (mg)	0.13	0.03	0.13	unknown
Vitamin B_{12} (µg)	1.0	trace	0.8	unknown
Folate (µg)	13	3	13	unknown
Pantothenate (mg)	0.78	0.1	unknown	unknown
Biotin (µg)	4.7	7.8	unknown	unknown
Vitamin C (mg)	trace	nil	trace	trace

Horlicks low fat instant one sachet made with water	Milkshake made with milk shake powder and full cream milk	Milkshake made with milk shake syrup and full cream milk	Milkshake flavoured milk	BEVERAGE
one mug	one tumbler	one tumbler	plastic bottle	**PORTION SIZE**
				NUTRIENTS
86	174	150	340	Energy (kcals)
4.0	6.2	5.6	18.0	Protein (g)
0.8	7.4	6.8	7.5	Total fat (g)
unknown	unknown	4.2	4.5	Saturated fat (g)
unknown	unknown	1.8	2.0	Mono-unsat. fat (g)
unknown	unknown	0.2	trace	Poly-unsat. fat (g)
16.8	22.2	18	53.0	Carbohydrate (g)
unknown	22.2	18	47.0	Sugar (g)
unknown	trace	nil	nil	Fibre (g)
136	104	110	305	Sodium (mg)
198	280	240	750	Potassium (mg)
133	220	200	550	Calcium (mg)
unknown	24	20	65	Magnesium (mg)
unknown	178	160	445	Phosphorus (mg)
unknown	0.4	0.2	1.15	Iron (mg)
unknown	0.02	nil	trace	Copper (mg)
unknown	0.8	0.6	2.5	Zinc (mg)
unknown	unknown	2	unknown	Selenium (μg)
108	102	96	106	Vitamin A (μg)
0.37	0.06	nil	0.05	Vitamin D (μg)
unknown	0.18	0.16	0.15	Vitamin E (mg)
0.17	0.08	0.06	0.15	Vitamin B_1 (mg)
0.23	0.32	0.3	0.85	Vitamin B_2 (mg)
2.6	0.2	0.2	0.55	Niacin (mg)
unknown	0.12	0.1	0.15	Vitamin B_6 (mg)
0.3	0.8	nil	0.5	Vitamin B_{12} (μg)
44	10	10	10	Folate (μg)
unknown	unknown	0.62	1.5	Pantothenate (mg)
unknown	unknown	4	11.0	Biotin (μg)
4	2	2	trace	Vitamin C (mg)

BEVERAGE	Ovaltine made with full cream milk (no sugar)	Tea infusion with added full cream milk (no sugar)	Tea lemon instant powder made up with water (no milk or sugar)
PORTION SIZE	one mug	one mug	one mug
NUTRIENTS			
Energy (kcals)	252	21	18
Protein (g)	9.9	1.0	trace
Total fat (g)	9.9	1.0	trace
Saturated fat (g)	unknown	0.8	nil
Mono-unsat. fat (g)	unknown	0.5	nil
Poly-unsat. fat (g)	unknown	trace	nil
Carbohydrate (g)	33.5	1.3	4.9
Sugar (g)	unknown	1.3	4.9
Fibre (g)	unknown	nil	unknown
Sodium (mg)	172	16	12
Potassium (mg)	494	104	10
Calcium (mg)	286	34	trace
Magnesium (mg)	52	8	trace
Phosphorous (mg)	338	31	1
Iron (mg)	0.78	nil	0.01
Copper (mg)	0.29	0.03	trace
Zinc (mg)	1.3	0.26	trace
Selenium (μg)	unknown	trace	trace
Vitamin A (μg)	304	17	trace
Vitamin D (μg)	0.65	nil	nil
Vitamin E (mg)	unknown	0.03	unknown
Vitamin B_1 (mg)	0.36	nil	trace
Vitamin B_2 (mg)	0.73	0.08	trace
Niacin (mg)	4.42	nil	0.02
Vitamin B_6 (mg)	unknown	0.03	trace
Vitamin B_{12} (μg)	1.3	trace	nil
Folate (μg)	unknown	8	trace
Pantothenate (mg)	unknown	0.18	0.01
Biotin (μg)	unknown	2.6	0.1
Vitamin C (mg)	trace	nil	11

SECTION 4

Ready-made Meals and Eating Out

This section is devoted to the analysis of food as we eat it. It is split up into breakfast, lunch and evening meal, and gives the nutrient value for the whole meal rather than of the individual items. Since we are eating more meals and snacks away from home, this section also includes data from restaurants and composite meals made up from known portion sizes. However, there is little on the type of meals and portion sizes you would get in small restaurants, or even in those restaurants that are part of a pub or motorway service station chain. This is because there is a lack of information about this type of food, both its portion size or nutritional analysis.

The important thing about ready-made meals and meals eaten out is that more and more of our nutrients are coming from these sources. Fast food is not necessarily unhealthy; it is a question of making sure you get the balance right. If you eat a lot of chilled ready-made meals, have some vegetables with them, fresh or frozen, and make sure you eat one or two pieces of fruit daily. If you eat a lot of take-away food, then try some ready-prepared meals instead.

Breakfast

Breakfast is an important meal, but today few of us have time for anything more than a quick bowl of muesli, and many people do not eat it at all. Breakfast can be a good way of getting some high-quality starchy carbohydrate and fibre into your daily diet, and it only takes a few minutes! Breakfast cereals are usually fortified with vitamins and iron, and although some are also fortified too heavily with sugar, most provide an excellent and healthy start to the day, especially if you use semi-skimmed or skimmed milk. Toast is also nutritious, but if you are eating it every day, use a sunflower or olive-oil spread, and save butter for a weekend treat.

Cooked breakfasts used to be a very necessary start to the day when we all went to work on our bikes, but today few people really need all that protein and fat. A boiled egg or some poached smoked haddock is a better, lighter meal than bacon and egg, if you do fancy something hot. However, no holiday or weekend away would be complete without the full works; just make sure you do enough exercise during the day to deserve it!

This section ranges from simple cereals and toast, through to the full cooked breakfast. All milk referred to is full-cream milk, and butter has been used in all calculations rather than margarine or low-fat spread. For the cooked breakfasts, any fried food has been fried in blended vegetable oil. The cereals have been chosen to reflect the main types: sugar-coated, muesli, cornflake-type, biscuit-type and porridge. This section commences with cereals and moves on through toast and other breads to cooked breakfast items. It finishes with some data from McDonald's restaurants.

FOOD	Cornflakes and milk	Muesli and milk	Porridge made with milk	Sugar Puffs and milk
PORTION SIZE	average bowl	average bowl	average bowl	average bowl
NUTRIENTS				
Energy (kcals)	174	248	186	163
Protein (g)	5.6	8.5	7.7	5.0
Total fat (g)	4.1	6.9	8.2	4.1
Saturated fat (g)	2.4	2.4	unknown	2.4
Mono-unsat. fat (g)	1.1	1.1	unknown	1.1
Poly-unsat. fat (g)	0.2	0.1	unknown	0.1
Carbohydrate (g)	30.6	40.3	21.9	30.1
Sugar (g)	7.3	16.7	7.5	21.8
Fibre (g)	0.3	3.0	1.3	1.0
Sodium (mg)	388	245	992	58
Potassium (mg)	170	360	304	188
Calcium (mg)	120	175	192	119
Magnesium (mg)	15	54	46	28
Phosphorus (mg)	107	232	224	134
Iron (mg)	2.07	2.86	0.96	0.69
Copper (mg)	0.01	0.05	0.05	0.07
Zinc (mg)	0.46	1.65	1.28	0.85
Selenium (μg)	2	1	trace	1
Vitamin A (μg)	55	55	unknown	55
Vitamin D (μg)	0.66	0.03	0.05	0.03
Vitamin E (mg)	0.21	1.69	0.46	0.19
Vitamin B_1 (mg)	0.33	0.28	0.16	0.03
Vitamin B_2 (mg)	0.56	0.52	0.27	0.18
Niacin (mg)	4.6	3.35	0.32	0.85
Vitamin B_6 (mg)	0.6	0.86	0.1	0.07
Vitamin B_{12} (μg)	0.9	0.4	nil	0.4
Folate (μg)	81	76	11	10
Pantothenate (mg)	0.44	0.95	0.64	0.35
Biotin (μg)	2.5	9.4	4.8	1.9
Vitamin C (mg)	1	1	2	1

Weetabix and milk	Half a grapefruit	Danish pastry	Croissant with butter and jam	FOOD
two	average	one	one	**PORTION SIZE**
				NUTRIENTS
203	24	411	342	Energy (kcals)
7.5	0.6	6.4	5.2	Protein (g)
4.7	0.1	19.4	20.3	Total fat (g)
2.4	trace	6.2	5.4	Saturated fat (g)
1.1	trace	8.5	2.0	Mono-unsa. fat (g)
0.1	trace	3.5	0.3	Poly-unsat. fat (g)
34.8	5.4	56.4	36.8	Carbohydrate (g)
7.4	5.4	31.4	14.4	Sugar (g)
3.9	1	1.8	1.0	Fibre (g)
203	2	209	315	Sodium (mg)
288	160	187	94	Potassium (mg)
129	18	101	52	Calcium (mg)
59	7	26	17	Magnesium (mg)
208	16	108	82	Phosphorus (mg)
2.46	0.08	1.43	1.26	Iron (mg)
0.22	0.02	0.07	0.16	Copper (mg)
1.2	trace	0.55	0.57	Zinc (mg)
1	1	unknown	unknown	Selenium (µg)
55	2.3	unknown	89	Vitamin A (µg)
0.03	nil	unknown	0.15	Vitamin D (µg)
0.5	0.15	trace	0.2	Vitamin E (mg)
0.31	0.04	0.14	0.11	Vitamin B_1 (mg)
0.57	0.02	0.08	0.1	Vitamin B_2 (mg)
4.1	0.24	0.99	1.2	Niacin (mg)
0.15	0.02	0.08	0.07	Vitamin B_6 (mg)
0.4	nil	trace	trace	Vitamin B_{12} (µg)
26	21	22	44	Folate (µg)
0.63	0.22	0.55	0.3	Pantothenate (mg)
5.1	0.8	7.7	5.4	Biotin (µg)
1	29	nil	2	Vitamin C (mg)

FOOD	**Toast** with butter and marmalade	**Cornflakes** and toast with butter and marmalade	**Bacon and egg**	**Boiled egg and toast**
PORTION SIZE	two slices brown bread	average bowl and two slices brown bread	one egg and two rashers of bacon	one egg and two slices
NUTRIENTS				
Energy (kcals)	394	568	340	390
Protein (g)	6.6	12.1	20.6	12.8
Total fat (g)	17.6	21.8	28.6	23.0
Saturated fat (g)	11.0	13.5	10.4	12.5
Mono-unsat. fat (g)	4.2	5.3	12.8	6.3
Poly-unsat. fat (g)	0.9	1.1	3.1	1.1
Carbohydrate (g)	55.9	86.4	trace	35.0
Sugar (g)	23.6	30.9	trace	2.8
Fibre (g)	3.0	3.2	nil	2.8
Sodium (mg)	583	971	1051	648
Potassium (mg)	146	316	240	198
Calcium (mg)	100	220	46	118
Magnesium (mg)	40	55	18	45
Phosphorus (mg)	120	227	223	216
Iron (mg)	1.89	3.96	1.97	2.66
Copper (mg)	0.14	0.14	0.11	0.14
Zinc (mg)	0.89	1.35	2.2	1.48
Selenium (µg)	trace	2	9	6
Vitamin A (µg)	179	235	129	272
Vitamin D (µg)	0.15	0.81	1.19	1.03
Vitamin E (mg)	0.4	0.61	0.09	0.96
Vitamin B_1 (mg)	0.16	0.49	0.25	0.2
Vitamin B2 (mg)	0.08	0.64	0.29	0.25
Niacin (mg)	1.92	6.52	2.66	1.97
Vitamin B_6 (mg)	0.09	0.69	0.23	0.15
Vitamin B_{12} (µg)	trace	0.9	1.0	0.6
Folate (µg)	29	110	25	47
Pantothenate (mg)	0.26	0.7	0.93	0.91
Biotin (µg)	2.5	5.0	12.3	10.5
Vitamin C (mg)	3	4	nil	nil

Kedgeree homemade	**Full English cooked breakfast** with cornflakes and toast	**Scrambled egg on toast**	**Smoked haddock and poached egg**	**FOOD**
average		two eggs and two slices		**PORTION SIZE**
				NUTRIENTS
513	1317	612	275	Energy (kcals)
47.7	46.7	19.4	34.3	Protein (g)
26.1	72.3	44.8	14.5	Total fat (g)
7.5	27.6	24.9	7.1	Saturated fat (g)
9.9	28.3	12.6	4.6	Mono-unsat. fat (g)
5.4	10.2	2.2	1.2	Poly-unsat. fat (g)
23.4	127.9	35.8	1.7	Carbohydrate (g)
0.3	40.1	3.5	1.7	Sugar (g)
0.3	8.0	2.8	nil	Fibre (g)
1890	3176	1814	1225	Sodium (mg)
810	1135	289	590	Potassium (mg)
93	378	165	102	Calcium (mg)
66	118	59	42	Magnesium (mg)
540	666	332	385	Phosphorus (mg)
1.8	8.75	3.63	1.1	Iron (mg)
0.18	0.48	0.18	0.08	Copper (mg)
2.1	5.1	2.15	1.25	Zinc (mg)
69	26	11	46	Selenium (µg)
324	464	545	195	Vitamin A (µg)
3	2.22	2.02	1.02	Vitamin D (µg)
unknown	2.09	1.88	0.76	Vitamin E (mg)
0.15	0.97	0.25	0.09	Vitamin B_1 (mg)
0.63	1.1	0.47	0.41	Vitamin B_2 (mg)
6.3	12.61	2.04	4.68	Niacin (mg)
0.84	1.18	0.19	0.57	Vitamin B_6 (mg)
6	2.4	2.5	3.5	Vitamin B_{12} (µg)
unknown	172	61	36	Folate (µg)
1.56	2.41	1.8	1.04	Pantothenate (mg)
18	21.7	22.3	9.0	Biotin (µg)
trace	18	trace	trace	Vitamin C (mg)

FOOD	McDonald's Bacon and egg McMuffin	McDonald's Big Breakfast	McDonald's Hotcakes and sausage with butter and syrup	McDonald's Sausage and egg McMuffin
PORTION SIZE				
NUTRIENTS				
Energy (kcals)	333	631	576	427
Protein (g)	19.9	28.8	15.3	23.5
Total fat (g)	16.1	39.0	20.7	26.1
Saturated fat (g)	12.1	19.1	15.0	17.2
Mono-unsat. fat (g)	unknown	unknown	unknown	unknown
Poly-unsat. fat (g)	unknown	unknown	unknown	unknown
Carbohydrate (g)	26.9	41.2	81.9	24.6
Sugar (g)	2.1	2.6	30.8	2.7
Fibre (g)	1.8	0.9	4.5	6.7
Sodium (mg)	800	1100	1300	900
Potassium (mg)	unknown	unknown	unknown	unknown
Calcium (mg)	unknown	unknown	unknown	unknown
Magnesium (mg)	unknown	unknown	unknown	unknown
Phosphorus (mg)	unknown	unknown	unknown	unknown
Iron (mg)	unknown	unknown	unknown	unknown
Copper (mg)	unknown	unknown	unknown	unknown
Zinc (mg)	unknown	unknown	unknown	unknown
Selenium (µg)	unknown	unknown	unknown	unknown
Vitamin A (µg)	unknown	unknown	unknown	unknown
Vitamin D (µg)	unknown	unknown	unknown	unknown
Vitamin E (mg)	unknown	unknown	unknown	unknown
Vitamin B_1 (mg)	unknown	unknown	unknown	unknown
Vitamin B_2 (mg)	unknown	unknown	unknown	unknown
Niacin (mg)	unknown	unknown	unknown	unknown
Vitamin B_6 (mg)	unknown	unknown	unknown	unknown
Vitamin B_{12} (µg)	unknown	unknown	unknown	unknown
Folate (µg)	unknown	unknown	unknown	unknown
Pantothenate (mg)	unknown	unknown	unknown	unknown
Biotin (µg)	unknown	unknown	unknown	unknown
Vitamin C (mg)	unknown	unknown	unknown	unknown

Lunch

It can be difficult to know the real value of a sandwich as compared to a meal. It is easy to assume that, because we eat a meal with a knife and fork, it is not only going to be higher in energy but also more wholesome. Mothers often bemoan the fact that their children do not eat 'proper' meals, because they do not have meat and two veg but live on sandwiches. Sandwiches and snacks can be surprisingly high in energy and fat, but they can also be much healthier than so-called proper meals.

Most supermarkets and delis offer a superb selection of sandwiches with many different types of bread and exotic fillings. There are usually low-fat and low-calorie alternatives on offer, which do not contain the ubiquitous mayonnaise. When choosing your sandwich, remember 'mayo' adds plenty of unhealthy fat to an otherwise healthy meal or snack. Try to buy sandwiches without mayonnaise, but with salad or other vegetables. If your sandwich tastes too dry without it, make your own with mayonnaise but do not also add butter or margarine.

If you are dining out, the humble spud is the healthiest choice; a jacket potato with beans or chilli is an excellent high-fibre, low-fat choice, providing it is not smothered in butter. Other healthy-sounding snack meals are not quite what they seem; salads are often loaded with fat in their dressings, but the most deceptive of all is the ploughman's lunch which can contain twice as much fat and energy as a pork pie. This is due almost entirely to the large chunk of cheddar and the two butter pats you put on your French bread, but a generous helping of sweet pickle will also add lots of extra calories and sugar.

SANDWICHES – made with brown bread and butter	**Beef**	**Cheese and pickle**	**Egg mayonnaise**	**Ham**
PORTION SIZE	one round	one round	one round	one round
NUTRIENTS				
Energy (kcals)	381	474	371	320
Protein (g)	27.9	17.8	11.4	15.4
Total fat (g)	16.7	28.4	21.8	15.4
Saturated fat (g)	9.1	17.3	9.4	8.5
Mono-unsat. fat (g)	4.5	7.0	5.6	3.8
Poly-unsat. fat (g)	0.5	1.0	3.8	0.7
Carbohydrate (g)	31.9	39.1	34.4	31.9
Sugar (g)	2.2	9.0	4.7	2.2
Fibre (g)	2.5	2.8	2.5	2.5
Sodium (mg)	531	1117	706	1119
Potassium (mg)	371	178	183	265
Calcium (mg)	79	401	100	79
Magnesium (mg)	55	51	45	47
Phosphorus (mg)	249	334	199	251
Iron (mg)	3.35	1.87	2.45	2.21
Copper (mg)	0.14	0.13	0.15	0.23
Zinc (mg)	4.71	1.86	1.37	1.96
Selenium (µg)	7	5	4	4
Vitamin A (µg)	124	295	201	124
Vitamin D (µg)	0.59	0.22	0.84	0.11
Vitamin E (mg)	0.33	0.52	2.31	0.32
Vitamin B_1 (mg)	0.25	0.21	0.22	0.45
Vitamin B_2 (mg)	0.24	0.25	0.21	0.19
Niacin (mg)	5.28	1.85	1.84	3.75
Vitamin B_6 (mg)	0.43	0.14	0.15	0.2
Vitamin B_{12} (µg)	1.8	0.5	0.6	trace
Folate (µg)	41	44	45	29
Pantothenate (mg)	0.58	0.38	0.74	0.52
Biotin (µg)	3.4	3.5	6.1	2.7
Vitamin C (mg)	trace	trace	unknown	trace

Tuna and mayonnaise	Smoked salmon	Cheese and salad baguette	Ham and salad baguette	**SANDWICHES AND BAGUETTES**
one round	one round	one round	one round	**PORTION SIZE**
				NUTRIENTS
397	347	726	526	Energy (kcals)
18.6	13.8	27.3	19.3	Protein (g)
21.6	19.1	40.3	21.7	Total fat (g)
8.8	11.5	24.7	12.5	Saturated fat (g)
4.7	4.8	10.3	5.5	Mono-unsat. fat (g)
5.3	1.4	2.3	1.7	Poly-unsat. fat (g)
34.4	31.9	67.7	67.7	Carbohydrate (g)
4.7	2.2	3.5	3.5	Sugar (g)
2.5	2.5	2.2	2.2	Fibre (g)
780	1103	1239	1337	Sodium (mg)
248	251	308	374	Potassium (mg)
82	81	597	168	Calcium (mg)
55	48	52	45	Magnesium (mg)
204	188	445	263	Phosphorus (mg)
2.41	1.8	2.96	3.26	Iron (mg)
0.21	0.15	0.22	0.29	Copper (mg)
1.35	0.93	2.29	1.83	Zinc (mg)
41	7	41	37	Selenium (µg)
125	177	431	213	Vitamin A (µg)
2.75	0.16	0.32	0.16	Vitamin D (µg)
1.87	0.4	1.12	0.83	Vitamin E (mg)
0.2	0.24	0.28	0.47	Vitamin B_1 (mg)
0.12	0.12	0.33	0.19	Vitamin B_2 (mg)
9.05	4.44	1.96	3.46	Niacin (mg)
0.33	0.18	0.2	0.23	Vitamin B_6 (mg)
2.3	0.9	0.7	trace	Vitamin B_{12} (µg)
29	29	58	38	Folate (µg)
0.37	0.49	0.7	0.73	Pantothenate (mg)
3.5	2.2	3.6	2.2	Biotin (µg)
trace	trace	6	6	Vitamin C (mg)

SANDWICHES – RETAIL (Marks & Spencer)	**Chicken tikka**	**Egg and bacon** reduced fat	**Prawn and salad**	**BLT/prawn and ham selection**
PORTION SIZE	one pack	one pack	one pack	one pack
NUTRIENTS				
Energy (kcals)	423	371	341	606
Protein (g)	20.6	26.5	14.6	24.5
Total fat (g)	23.4	18.3	19.4	37.9
Saturated fat (g)	5.8	5.9	6.0	9.1
Mono-unsat. fat (g)	unknown	unknown	unknown	unknown
Poly-unsat. fat (g)	unknown	unknown	unknown	unknown
Carbohydrate (g)	32.5	24.4	27.3	42.2
Sugar (g)	5.0	4.0	5.3	4.5
Fibre (g)	3.1	5.9	3.7	5.4
Sodium (mg)	1003	1330	1050	1810
Potassium (mg)	unknown	unknown	unknown	unknown
Calcium (mg)	unknown	unknown	unknown	unknown
Magnesium (mg)	unknown	unknown	unknown	unknown
Phosphorus (mg)	unknown	unknown	unknown	unknown
Iron (mg)	unknown	unknown	unknown	unknown
Copper (mg)	unknown	unknown	unknown	unknown
Zinc (mg)	unknown	unknown	unknown	unknown
Selenium (μg)	unknown	unknown	unknown	unknown
Vitamin A (μg)	unknown	unknown	unknown	unknown
Vitamin D (μg)	unknown	unknown	unknown	unknown
Vitamin E (mg)	unknown	unknown	unknown	unknown
Vitamin B_1 (mg)	unknown	unknown	unknown	unknown
Vitamin B_2 (mg)	unknown	unknown	unknown	unknown
Niacin (mg)	unknown	unknown	unknown	unknown
Vitamin B_6 (mg)	unknown	unknown	unknown	unknown
Vitamin B_{12} (μg)	unknown	unknown	unknown	unknown
Folate (μg)	unknown	unknown	unknown	unknown
Pantothenate (mg)	unknown	unknown	unknown	unknown
Biotin (μg)	unknown	unknown	unknown	unknown
Vitamin C (mg)	unknown	unknown	unknown	unknown

Crackers and cheese	Crispbread and cottage cheese	Pitta bread and humus	Pitta bread and taramasalata	OTHER BREAD AND CRACKERS
four crackers, two portions each of cheese and butter	four crispbread and small tub of cheese	one bread and two tablespoons humus	one bread and two tablespoons taramasalata	**PORTION SIZE**
				NUTRIENTS
435	238	311	652	Energy (kcals)
13.0	19.2	11.5	9.8	Protein (g)
34.7	5.2	8.5	48.5	Total fat (g)
19.6	2.7	unknown	3.7	Saturated fat (g)
7.8	1.2	unknown	26.4	Mono-unsat. fat (g)
1.1	0.1	unknown	15.0	Poly-unsat. fat (g)
19.2	30.6	50.4	47.1	Carbohydrate (g)
trace	3.6	2.9	1.8	Sugar (g)
0.6	4.7	3.1	1.7	Fibre (g)
589	514	792	975	Sodium (mg)
67	300	197	137	Potassium (mg)
322	100	93	87	Calcium (mg)
17	50	55	23	Magnesium (mg)
232	303	165	114	Phosphorus (mg)
0.64	1.51	2.41	1.64	Iron (mg)
0.07	0.2	0.34	0.16	Copper (mg)
1.14	1.87	1.29	0.81	Zinc (mg)
6	6	unknown	unknown	Selenium (µg)
322	51	unknown	unknown	Vitamin A (µg)
0.26	0.03	nil	unknown	Vitamin D (µg)
0.98	0.29	unknown	unknown	Vitamin E (mg)
0.08	0.15	0.28	0.25	Vitamin B_1 (mg)
0.18	0.35	0.07	0.13	Vitamin B_2 (mg)
0.52	0.59	1.71	1.32	Niacin (mg)
0.07	0.21	unknown	unknown	Vitamin B_6 (mg)
0.4	0.8	nil	2.7	Vitamin B_{12} (µg)
19	44	16	19	Folate (µg)
0.24	0.89	unknown	unknown	Pantothenate (mg)
1.8	6.2	unknown	unknown	Biotin (µg)
trace	trace	1	1	Vitamin C (mg)

PUB GRUB	Chicken pie	Cornish pasty	Hot dog	Jacket potato with baked beans
PORTION SIZE	individual	one average	one	medium
NUTRIENTS				
Energy (kcals)	374	481	248	354
Protein (g)	11.7	11.6	9.7	13.8
Total fat (g)	23.0	29.6	10.5	1.1
Saturated fat (g)	9.1	10.7	3.3	0.1
Mono-unsat. fat (g)	9.6	15.2	4.1	0.1
Poly-unsat. fat (g)	3.1	2.2	1.6	0.6
Carbohydrate (g)	32.0	45.1	30.8	77.0
Sugar (g)	2.1	1.7	1.5	9.8
Fibre (g)	1.0	1.3	1.0	9.7
Sodium (mg)	559	856	616	711
Potassium (mg)	182	276	120	1537
Calcium (mg)	78	87	86	89
Magnesium (mg)	20	26	23	98
Phosphorus (mg)	117	160	156	252
Iron (mg)	1.04	2.17	1.75	3.08
Copper (mg)	0.08	0.51	0.11	0.29
Zinc (mg)	0.78	1.45	0.83	1.55
Selenium (µg)	unknown	unknown	20	6
Vitamin A (µg)	trace	trace	trace	16
Vitamin D (µg)	unknown	trace	unknown	nil
Vitamin E (mg)	unknown	1.88	0.18	0.68
Vitamin B_1 (mg)	0.53	0.14	0.24	0.78
Vitamin B_2 (mg)	0.12	0.09	0.11	0.11
Niacin (mg)	1.95	2.32	1.75	2.63
Vitamin B_6 (mg)	0.16	0.17	0.07	1.15
Vitamin B_{12} (µg)	trace	1.5	trace	nil
Folate (µg)	10	4	31	108
Pantothenate (mg)	0.83	0.87	0.4	1.06
Biotin (µg)	5.2	1.5	0.9	4.2
Vitamin C (mg)	unknown	nil	unknown	25

Jacket potato with cheese	Ploughman's, with cheddar cheese	Pork pie	Jumbo sausage in French bread	FOOD
medium	average	individual	one sausage	PORTION SIZE
				NUTRIENTS
410	1037	526	563	Energy (kcals)
17.2	43.2	13.7	21.5	Protein (g)
14.1	61.2	37.8	21.7	Total fat (g)
8.7	37.8	14.3	7.1	Saturated fat (g)
3.8	15.9	17.5	8.3	Mono-unsat. fat (g)
0.7	3.2	3.8	2.0	Poly-unsat. fat (g)
57.1	8305	34.9	75.1	Carbohydrate (g)
2.2	18.5	0.7	3.6	Sugar (g)
4.9	3.2	1.3	2.3	Fibre (g)
290	2289	1008	1434	Sodium (mg)
1165	507	210	306	Potassium (mg)
308	1041	66	196	Calcium (mg)
68	73	22	45	Magnesium (mg)
318	760	168	297	Phosphorus (mg)
1.38	3.63	1.96	3.64	Iron (mg)
0.26	0.24	0.45	0.45	Copper (mg)
1.82	3.77	1.4	2.04	Zinc (mg)
8	48	unknown	34	Selenium (µg)
145	706	trace	unknown	Vitamin A (µg)
0.1	0.47	trace	trace	Vitamin D (µg)
0.41	1.9	0.6	0.16	Vitamin E (mg)
0.68	0.35	0.22	0.24	Vitamin B_1 (mg)
0.2	0.58	0.13	0.2	Vitamin B_2 (mg)
2.02	2.46	2.52	4.56	Niacin (mg)
1.01	0.32	0.08	0.14	Vitamin B_6 (mg)
0.4	1.3	1.4	0.8	Vitamin B_{12} (µg)
92	87	4	31	Folate (µg)
0.97	1.05	0.84	0.81	Pantothenate (mg)
2.1	6.1	1.4	3.5	Biotin (µg)
25	12	nil	unknown	Vitamin C (mg)

PUB GRUB	Scotch eggs	Salad – game pie	Salad – smoked mackerel	Soup with a roll and butter
		with a tablespoon each of potato, rice, carrot, tomato and green salads and coleslaw		
PORTION SIZE	one	average	average	one bowl
NUTRIENTS				
Energy (kcals)	301	1121	985	398
Protein (g)	14.4	25.5	32.5	10.1
Total fat (g)	20.5	77.3	84.3	19.6
Saturated fat (g)	5.2	18.9	14.5	11.0
Mono-unsat. fat (g)	7.9	27.7	34.6	4.0
Poly-unsat. fat (g)	4.0	26.0	28.5	0.5
Carbohydrate (g)	15.7	86.6	25.9	48.9
Sugar (g)	trace	18.4	12.4	8.6
Fibre (g)	unknown	5.4	3.1	5.3
Sodium (mg)	804	1072	1445	1970
Potassium (mg)	156	805	972	488
Calcium (mg)	60	166	84	124
Magnesium (mg)	18	63	73	47
Phosphorus (mg)	204	311	416	146
Iron (mg)	2.16	5.14	3.27	2.89
Copper (mg)	0.28	0.47	0.35	0.28
Zinc (mg)	1.44	2.85	2.4	1.37
Selenium (µg)	unknown	9	52	14
Vitamin A (µg)	36	1624	580	186
Vitamin D (µg)	0.88	1.66	12.09	0.16
Vitamin E (mg)	unknown	10.11	8.81	0.4
Vitamin B_1 (mg)	0.1	0.59	0.61	0.22
Vitamin B_2 (mg)	0.25	0.48	0.84	0.09
Niacin (mg)	1.2	6.48	15.48	2.25
Vitamin B_6 (mg)	0.16	0.74	1.13	0.17
Vitamin B_{12} (µg)	0.6	5.4	9.2	trace
Folate (µg)	50	180	49	46
Pantothenate (mg)	1.32	1.44	1.9	0.16
Biotin (µg)	10.4	25.9	9.4	0.5
Vitamin C (mg)	unknown	36	35	trace

Evening meal

Although some people still enjoy a traditional evening meal of meat, potatoes and vegetables, for many of us this is a thing of the past, except perhaps on Sunday. Pasta and rice are convenient to store and easy to use in quick and simple-to-prepare dishes. Potatoes still have that 'fattening' label, so unjustly bestowed in the 1960s, but the truth is that all starchy foods, including potatoes, are good for us. However, we should take note that the Italians have a very small amount of sauce with their pasta and the Chinese a very large amount of rice with their main course. It is always the other things we add to these staple grains which increase the fat and energy content of the dish.

Many people still feel guilty about taking a ready-cooked meal off the supermarket shelf or a packet of fish fingers out of the freezer. These foods may have been prepared elsewhere, but their nutritional value can be as good as homemade. If you eat a lot of ready-made meals, the important thing to remember is you still need to eat a balanced diet. Variety is king, so make sure you are eating plenty of fresh or frozen vegetables, and tinned or fresh fruit, as well as your ready-made and convenience foods.

If you eat out or have a take-away meal only once a month, it will not make that much difference to your overall food intake, but if you eat take-away meals regularly, use this section to compare the fat contents. Restaurant food is also variable; starters and main courses such as pâté and anything containing mayonnaise, cream or pastry can be surprisingly high in fat. A good dessert will not usually be very low in fat or sugar, nor should it be, but some are actually healthier than a starter, or cheese and crackers, and if you can forego the cream you can even feel a little virtuous.

EATING AT HOME – home-prepared meals	**Beef stew** with jacket potato and leeks	**Chicken curry and rice**	**Roast chicken** with roast potatoes, mixed vegtables and stuffing	**Chilli con carne** with rice
PORTION SIZE	medium	medium	average	medium
NUTRIENTS				
Energy (kcals)	554	838	561	581
Protein (g)	39.4	31.8	37.5	28.9
Total fat (g)	14.1	54.4	17.7	21.0
Saturated fat (g)	4.0	unknown	3.3	6.6
Mono-unsat. fat (g)	5.2	unknown	8.1	8.4
Poly-unsat. fat (g)	2.8	unknown	4.7	2.4
Carbohydrate (g)	72	59	67.4	73.9
Sugar (g)	9.1	unknown	5.1	6.2
Fibre (g)	8.0	0.4	4.3	5.2
Sodium (mg)	1040	1207	394	552
Potassium (mg)	1871	640	1622	1065
Calcium (mg)	79	69	199	96
Magnesium (mg)	93	62	96	92
Phosphorus (mg)	432	61	400	383
Iron (mg)	5.16	5.04	3.57	5.2
Copper (mg)	0.37	0.47	0.36	0.65
Zinc (mg)	8.33	2.72	2.76	6.1
Selenium (μg)	15	7	18	14
Vitamin A (μg)	611	586	389	53
Vitamin D (μg)	1.04	trace	0.2	trace
Vitamin E (mg)	1.3	unknown	0.23	2.62
Vitamin B_1 (mg)	0.84	0.1	0.79	0.26
Vitamin B_2 (mg)	0.34	0.25	0.39	0.31
Niacin (mg)	6.96	10.94	11.57	5.8
Vitamin B_6 (mg)	1.58	0.09	1.08	0.59
Vitamin B_{12} (μg)	2.6	2.1	trace	1.8
Folate (μg)	120	65	129	38
Pantothenate (mg)	1.74	0.36	1.89	0.99
Biotin (μg)	4.3	1.8	3.6	4.0
Vitamin C (mg)	33	3	28	20

Cod in parsley sauce (frozen) with mashed potato and mixed vegetables	**Grilled fish fingers** with green beans and two potato waffles	**Lasagne** with mixed salad	**Omelette – plain** with chips and peas	**EATING AT HOME –** home-prepared meals
medium	4	medium	medium	**PORTION SIZE**
				NUTRIENTS
363	424	687	878	Energy (kcals)
26.5	20.5	36.6	24.7	Protein (g)
12.7	17.8	45.7	55.5	Total fat (g)
4.9	4.1	19.8	12.0	Saturated fat (g)
1.8	5.6	16.4	24.5	Mono-unsat. fat (g)
0.3	7.1	5.7	14.8	Poly-unsat. fat (g)
37.8	48.5	34.1	74.8	Carbohydrate (g)
5.0	2.4	13.5	2.9	Sugar (g)
2.1	5.0	3.2	7.5	Fibre (g)
604	883	1478	1397	Sodium (mg)
1031	919	1077	1425	Potassium (mg)
141	162	427	117	Calcium (mg)
69	58	68	90	Magnesium (mg)
402	392	546	554	Phosphorus (mg)
1.59	2.34	3.58	4.81	Iron (mg)
0.19	0.04	0.27	0.47	Copper (mg)
1.57	0.9	5.62	2.8	Zinc (mg)
2	26	17	16	Selenium (µg)
452	49	557	336	Vitamin A (µg)
trace	trace	1.26	1.9	Vitamin D (µg)
0.26	0.18	3.43	1.48	Vitamin E (mg)
0.49	0.19	0.36	0.56	Vitamin B_1 (mg)
0.29	0.13	0.44	0.61	Vitamin B_2 (mg)
3.46	2.44	6.72	5.2	Niacin (mg)
0.84	0.24	0.62	1.03	Vitamin B_6 (mg)
unknown	1.1	4.2	2.6	Vitamin B_{12} (µg)
118	69	60	125	Folate (µg)
1.43	0.45	1.63	1.69	Pantothenate (mg)
4.1	1.8	9.9	21.0	Biotin (µg)
20	42	17	28	Vitamin C (mg)

EATING AT HOME – home-prepared meals	**Sausages – pork** grilled with chips and baked beans	**Quiche – mushroom and cheese** with new potatoes and green salad	**Steak and kidney pie** with new potatoes and peas	**Sunday lunch** roast pork, roast potatoes, carrots; fruit crumble and custard
PORTION SIZE	3	medium	medium	medium
NUTRIENTS				
Energy (kcals)	1103	531	585	1053
Protein (g)	32.3	18.0	23.3	42.7
Total fat (g)	64.6	27.1	27.6	41.8
Saturated fat (g)	12.9	11.0	10.0	9.2
Mono-unsat. fat (g)	30.2	8.3	10.9	11.9
Poly-unsat. fat (g)	17.7	5.9	4.8	5.7
Carbohydrate (g)	104.5	57.9	65.3	134.9
Sugar (g)	10.8	5.7	4.4	54.8
Fibre (g)	10.0	3.5	6.6	9.3
Sodium (mg)	2181	788	761	566
Potassium (mg)	1907	724	795	2145
Calcium (mg)	237	308	88	299
Magnesium (mg)	119	48	56	112
Phosphorus (mg)	697	339	298	545
Iron (mg)	4.96	2.04	4.41	4.26
Copper (mg)	0.56	0.29	0.34	0.47
Zinc (mg)	3.4	1.6	3.66	4.39
Selenium (µg)	15	12	38	22
Vitamin A (µg)	16	327	162	993
Vitamin D (µg)	1.32	1.82	1.44	2.06
Vitamin E (mg)	1.6	0.87	2.4	2.71
Vitamin B_1 (mg)	0.44	0.37	0.58	1.3
Vitamin B_2 (mg)	0.39	0.4	0.6	0.54
Niacin (mg)	8.6	1.88	5.18	8.9
Vitamin B_6 (mg)	1.24	0.72	0.93	1.2
Vitamin B_{12} (µg)	1.2	1.3	3.6	1.5
Folate (µg)	94	59	72	124
Pantothenate (mg)	1.36	1.65	1.81	2.96
Biotin (µg)	9.4	10.6	9.2	8.0
Vitamin C (mg)	27	27	25	44

Chicken casserole	Chilli con carne	Pasta with ham and mushrooms	Salmon en croute	EATING AT HOME – ready-made meals (Marks & Spencer)
one ready meal	one ready meal	one ready meal	one ready meal	PORTION SIZE
				NUTRIENTS
320	277	268	292	Energy (kcals)
30.9	24.6	13.0	11.2	Protein (g)
12.9	10.5	14.8	20.8	Total fat (g)
4.4	4.2	8.0	7.4	Saturated fat (g)
unknown	unknown	unknown	unknown	Mono-unsat. fat (g)
unknown	unknown	unknown	unknown	Poly-unsat. fat (g)
20.1	20.9	23.8	16.4	Carbohydrate (g)
3.01	11.9	2.2	1.0	Sugar (g)
3.1	5.7	1.6	0.1	Fibre (g)
1002	1113	600	400	Sodium (mg)
unknown	unknown	unknown	unknown	Potassium (mg)
unknown	unknown	unknown	unknown	Calcium (mg)
unknown	unknown	unknown	unknown	Magnesium (mg)
unknown	unknown	unknown	unknown	Phosphorus (mg)
unknown	unknown	unknown	unknown	Iron (mg)
unknown	unknown	unknown	unknown	Copper (mg)
unknown	unknown	unknown	unknown	Zinc (mg)
unknown	unknown	unknown	unknown	Selenium (μg)
unknown	unknown	unknown	unknown	Vitamin A (μg)
unknown	unknown	unknown	unknown	Vitamin D (μg)
unknown	unknown	unknown	unknown	Vitamin E (mg)
unknown	unknown	unknown	unknown	Vitamin B_1 (mg)
unknown	unknown	unknown	unknown	Vitamin B_2 (mg)
unknown	unknown	unknown	unknown	Niacin (mg)
unknown	unknown	unknown	unknown	Vitamin B_6 (mg)
unknown	unknown	unknown	unknown	Vitamin B_{12} (μg)
unknown	unknown	unknown	unknown	Folate (μg)
unknown	unknown	unknown	unknown	Pantothenate (mg)
unknown	unknown	unknown	unknown	Biotin (μg)
unknown	unknown	unknown	unknown	Vitamin C (mg)

TAKEAWAY FOOD – Chinese and Indian	**Chicken in black bean sauce, sweet and sour pork and egg fried rice**	**Chicken and cashew nuts, beef and green peppers and boiled rice**	**Chicken tandoori, lamb rogan josh and naan bread**	**Chicken korma, lamb vindaloo, pilau rice and two poppadams**
PORTION SIZE	half portion of each meat dish	half portion of each meat dish	half portion of each meat dish	half portion of each meat dish
NUTRIENTS				
Energy (kcals)	1106	940	1189	1342
Protein (g)	66.7	67.2	87.4	73.9
Total fat (g)	52.0	29.2	55.5	72.7
Saturated fat (g)	8.5	7.3	12.3	12.1
Mono-unsat. fat (g)	19.6	12.3	15.1	12.6
Poly-unsat. fat (g)	19.6	7.2	5.8	6.5
Carbohydrate (g)	99.7	108	90.7	99.9
Sugar (g)	18.8	10.5	15.8	23.4
Fibre (g)	3.7	3.4	4.4	3.0
Sodium (mg)	1416	1092	1938	1642
Potassium (mg)	1321	1420	1776	1800
Calcium (mg)	96	52	428	287
Magnesium (mg)	101	140	150	206
Phosphorus (mg)	751	758	908	783
Iron (mg)	5.05	5.5	8.56	11.31
Copper (mg)	0.54	0.77	0.59	0.83
Zinc (mg)	5.25	6.92	7.41	8.57
Selenium (µg)	31	36	70	16
Vitamin A (µg)	257	319	119	61
Vitamin D (µg)	1.73	0.56	1.21	0.88
Vitamin E (mg)	1.57	1.06	5.8	9.48
Vitamin B_1 (mg)	1.14	0.38	0.69	0.7
Vitamin B_2 (mg)	0.62	0.47	0.67	0.52
Niacin (mg)	18.0	18.84	23.97	17.21
Vitamin B_6 (mg)	1.35	1.63	1.55	1.09
Vitamin B_{12} (µg)	2.7	1.8	3.5	1.8
Folate (µg)	53	56	61	43
Pantothenate (mg)	3.69	1.16	4.93	2.3
Biotin (µg)	16.5	3.0	13.7	6.5
Vitamin C (mg)	53	79	11	4

Cod and chips	Cod, chips and mushy peas	Chicken and chips	Saveloy and chips	**TAKE-AWAY FOOD –** fish and chip shop
medium	medium	medium	medium	**PORTION SIZE**
				NUTRIENTS
922	1023	842	672	Energy (kcals)
34.1	41.3	42.1	13.2	Protein (g)
52.2	53.1	48.1	39.4	Total fat (g)
14.5	14.7	13.6	7.6	Saturated fat (g)
22.9	23.0	21.6	11.1	Mono-unsat. fat (g)
12.8	13.2	10.3	6.5	Poly-unsat. fat (g)
83.9	101.2	64.1	70.6	Carbohydrate (g)
3.6	5.7	3.6	3.6	Sugar (g)
5.5	7.7	4.6	4.6	Fibre (g)
346	771	283	652	Sodium (mg)
1879	2092	1785	1490	Potassium (mg)
137	155	42	38	Calcium (mg)
108	135	97	71	Magnesium (mg)
470	595	415	267	Phosphorus (mg)
2.74	4.36	3.22	2.87	Iron (mg)
0.36	0.5	0.43	0.47	Copper (mg)
2.11	2.98	3.73	2.17	Zinc (mg)
4	4	29	4	Selenium (μg)
unknown	unknown	36	trace	Vitamin A (μg)
trace	trace	0.38	trace	Vitamin D (μg)
0.82	1.19	1.24	0.87	Vitamin E (mg)
0.32	0.32	0.24	0.26	Vitamin B_1 (mg)
0.14	0.14	0.31	0.08	Vitamin B_2 (mg)
4.36	4.36	11.16	2.7	Niacin (mg)
0.89	0.89	1.11	0.71	Vitamin B_6 (mg)
3.4	3.4	trace	trace	Vitamin B_{12} (μg)
97	97	19	1	Folate (μg)
1.03	1.03	2.27	0.78	Pantothenate (mg)
5.9	5.9	4.6	0.8	Biotin (μg)
19	19	19	19	Vitamin C (mg)

FAST FOOD – burgers	**McDonald's Hamburger**	**Burger King Double Whopper**	**Burger King Double cheeseburger with bacon**	**Composite meal** McDonald's Big Mac with medium fries
PORTION SIZE	medium	medium	medium	medium
NUTRIENTS				
Energy (kcals)	244	906	684	865
Protein (g)	13.9	49.5	43.7	33.3
Total fat (g)	8.6	56.7	43	46.5
Saturated fat (g)	4.0	unknown	unknown	17
Mono-unsat. fat (g)	unknown	unknown	unknown	unknown
Poly-unsat. fat (g)	unknown	unknown	unknown	unknown
Carbohydrate (g)	27.7	50.8	33.8	81
Sugar (g)	5.7	unknown	unknown	8.0
Fibre (g)	2.7	3.1	1.2	11.9
Sodium (mg)	400	795	1179	1100
Potassium (mg)	unknown	unknown	unknown	unknown
Calcium (mg)	unknown	unknown	unknown	unknown
Magnesium (mg)	unknown	unknown	unknown	unknown
Phosphorus (mg)	unknown	unknown	unknown	unknown
Iron (mg)	unknown	unknown	unknown	unknown
Copper (mg)	unknown	unknown	unknown	unknown
Zinc (mg)	unknown	unknown	unknown	unknown
Selenium (μg)	unknown	unknown	unknown	unknown
Vitamin A (μg)	unknown	unknown	unknown	unknown
Vitamin D (μg)	unknown	unknown	unknown	unknown
Vitamin E (mg)	unknown	unknown	unknown	unknown
Vitamin B_1 (mg)	unknown	unknown	unknown	unknown
Vitamin B_2 (mg)	unknown	unknown	unknown	unknown
Niacin (mg)	unknown	unknown	unknown	unknown
Vitamin B_6 (mg)	unknown	unknown	unknown	unknown
Vitamin B_{12} (μg)	unknown	unknown	unknown	unknown
Folate (μg)	unknown	unknown	unknown	unknown
Pantothenate (mg)	unknown	unknown	unknown	unknown
Biotin (μg)	unknown	unknown	unknown	unknown
Vitamin C (mg)	unknown	unknown	unknown	unknown

Kentucky Fried Chicken	Hot Wings	Kentucky Dippers	Composite meal chicken, fries and coleslaw	FAST FOOD – chicken (Kentucky Fried Chicken)
medium	medium	medium	medium	**PORTION SIZE**
				NUTRIENTS
220	408	322	579	Energy (kcals)
18.5	14.5	18.7	24.3	Protein (g)
14.3	17.2	20.6	32.8	Total fat (g)
unknown	unknown	unknown	unknown	Saturated fat (g)
unknown	unknown	unknown	unknown	Mono-unsat. fat (g)
unknown	unknown	unknown	unknown	Poly-unsat. fat (g)
4.8	2.0	15.1	50	Carbohydrate (g)
unknown	unknown	unknown	unknown	Sugar (g)
unknown	unknown	unknown	unknown	Fibre (g)
unknown	unknown	unknown	unknown	Sodium (mg)
unknown	unknown	unknown	unknown	Potassium (mg)
unknown	unknown	unknown	unknown	Calcium (mg)
unknown	unknown	unknown	unknown	Magnesium (mg)
unknown	unknown	unknown	unknown	Phosphorus (mg)
unknown	unknown	unknown	unknown	Iron (mg)
unknown	unknown	unknown	unknown	Copper (mg)
unknown	unknown	unknown	unknown	Zinc (mg)
unknown	unknown	unknown	unknown	Selenium (µg)
unknown	unknown	unknown	unknown	Vitamin A (µg)
unknown	unknown	unknown	unknown	Vitamin D (µg)
unknown	unknown	unknown	unknown	Vitamin E (mg)
unknown	unknown	unknown	unknown	Vitamin B_1 (mg)
unknown	unknown	unknown	unknown	Vitamin B_2 (mg)
unknown	unknown	unknown	unknown	Niacin (mg)
unknown	unknown	unknown	unknown	Vitamin B_6 (mg)
unknown	unknown	unknown	unknown	Vitamin B_{12} (µg)
unknown	unknown	unknown	unknown	Folate (µg)
unknown	unknown	unknown	unknown	Pantothenate (mg)
unknown	unknown	unknown	unknown	Biotin (µg)
unknown	unknown	unknown	unknown	Vitamin C (mg)

FAST FOOD – pizza (Pizza Hut) US data only – none available for UK	Cheese deep pan	Ham thin 'n' crispy	Pepperoni personal pan pizza	Supreme personal pan pizza
PORTION SIZE	one slice	one slice	whole pizza	whole pizza
NUTRIENTS				
Energy (kcals)	300	190	670	710
Protein (g)	15	10	28	32
Total fat (g)	14	6.0	29	31
Saturated fat (g)	unknown	unknown	unknown	unknown
Mono-unsat. fat (g)	unknown	unknown	unknown	unknown
Poly-unsat. fat (g)	unknown	unknown	unknown	unknown
Carbohydrate (g)	30	23	79	78
Sugar (g)	2.0	1.0	8	7
Fibre (g)	2.0	unknown	1	5
Sodium (mg)	510	560	1260	1380
Potassium (mg)	unknown	unknown	unknown	unknown
Calcium (mg)	unknown	unknown	unknown	unknown
Magnesium (mg)	unknown	unknown	unknown	unknown
Phosphorus (mg)	unknown	unknown	unknown	unknown
Iron (mg)	unknown	unknown	unknown	unknown
Copper (mg)	unknown	unknown	unknown	unknown
Zinc (mg)	unknown	unknown	unknown	unknown
Selenium (μg)	unknown	unknown	unknown	unknown
Vitamin A (μg)	unknown	unknown	unknown	unknown
Vitamin D (μg)	unknown	unknown	unknown	unknown
Vitamin E (mg)	unknown	unknown	unknown	unknown
Vitamin B_1 (mg)	unknown	unknown	unknown	unknown
Vitamin B_2 (mg)	unknown	unknown	unknown	unknown
Niacin (mg)	unknown	unknown	unknown	unknown
Vitamin B_6 (mg)	unknown	unknown	unknown	unknown
Vitamin B_{12} (μg)	unknown	unknown	unknown	unknown
Folate (μg)	unknown	unknown	unknown	unknown
Pantothenate (mg)	unknown	unknown	unknown	unknown
Biotin (μg)	unknown	unknown	unknown	unknown
Vitamin C (mg)	unknown	unknown	unknown	unknown

Meal out: bread roll and butter, prawn cocktail, sirloin steak, chips and salad, cheesecake, white wine - two glasses, coffee and mints	**Party food:** mini pork pie, mini sausage roll, slice quiche, small slice French bread and Danish Blue cheese, celery, cucumber and carrot crudités, 4 tbsp sour cream dip, olives, crisps and nuts	**EATING OUT –** other
		NUTRIENTS
2301	1426	Energy (kcals)
97.7	39.7	Protein (g)
138.2	110.7	Total fat (g)
54.3	25.1	Saturated fat (g)
46.6	23.4	Mono-unsat. fat (g)
27.9	10.4	Poly-unsat. fat (g)
127.1	72.2	Carbohydrate (g)
49.9	9.2	Sugar (g)
6.0	6.1	Fibre (g)
2099	2513	Sodium (mg)
2939	1069	Potassium (mg)
255	566	Calcium (mg)
181	124	Magnesium (mg)
1145	643	Phosphorus (mg)
12.31	4.22	Iron (mg)
0.62	1.74	Copper (mg)
15.52	5.05	Zinc (mg)
38	19	Selenium (µg)
714	622	Vitamin A (µg)
2.86	0.44	Vitamin D (µg)
11.28	4.67	Vitamin E (mg)
0.71	0.62	Vitamin B_1 (mg)
1.02	0.38	Vitamin B_2 (mg)
21.41	7.3	Niacin (mg)
2.38	0.51	Vitamin B_6 (mg)
9.2	1.0	Vitamin B_{12} (µg)
112	83	Folate (µg)
2.81	1.78	Pantothenate (mg)
3.0	23.6	Biotin (µg)
30	14	Vitamin C (mg)

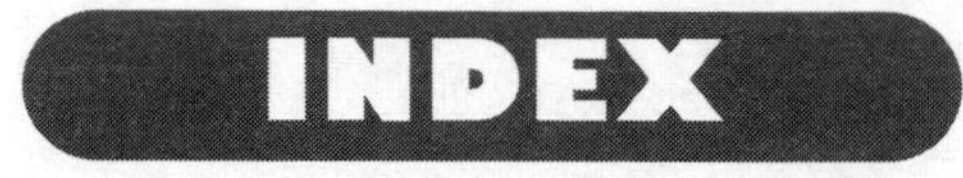

INDEX